Prevention and Management of Acute and Late Toxicities in Radiation Oncology

Gokhan Ozyigit • Ugur Selek

Editors

Prevention and Management of Acute and Late Toxicities in Radiation Oncology

Management of Toxicities in Radiation Oncology

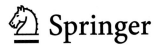 Springer

Editors
Gokhan Ozyigit
Chair and Professor
Department of Radiation Oncology
Hacettepe University, Faculty of Medicine
Ankara
Turkey

Ugur Selek
Chair and Professor
Department of Radiation Oncology
Koc University, Faculty of Medicine
Istanbul
Turkey

ISBN 978-3-030-37797-7   ISBN 978-3-030-37798-4   (eBook)
https://doi.org/10.1007/978-3-030-37798-4

This Springer imprint is published by the registered company Springer Nature Switzerland AG
The registered company address is: Gewerbestrasse 11, 6330 Cham, Switzerland

To our patients from whom we have learned to excel.

Preface

The role of radiation oncologists in multidisciplinary care is gradually becoming essential and more involved in patient care in the current era of improving technology and individualized management. As the patients' awareness and their participation in treatment decisions increase, the clinicians have been discussing more and more about the quality of life issues in addition to outcome matters. Therefore, acute and late toxicity management is more crucial than ever in our clinical practice in comparison to a decade ago. We have planned to provide a structured and comprehensive book to deliver a current evidence-based and/or practice-proven management tool to feel confident in prescribing the innovative treatments with a goal of functionally unimpaired patient during and after radiotherapy.

In this context, our book covers prevention and current management of acute and late toxicities of radiation therapy in a wide range of malignancies, while each chapter focuses on a particular anatomic site with information on normal sectional anatomy, contouring of target volumes and organs at risk, dose constraints, the pathophysiology of radiation toxicity, and treatment approaches for each potential toxicity; given under the variability of planning and delivery of intensity-modulated radiation therapy, volumetric modulated arc therapy, stereotactic radiosurgery, and stereotactic body radiotherapy.

Overall, this book will enable the selection of appropriate, evidence-based management options in individual patients who experience radiation toxicities, taking into account the organ-specific pathophysiology of radiation injury, for practicing clinical and radiation oncologists, radiotherapists, fellows, residents, and nurses.

We hope to encourage the clinicians through practical and theoretical aspects of acute and late toxicity management in modern radiation oncology, and we extend our most sincere gratitude to our patients, who stand side by side with us to fight with their cancer, and who teach us invaluable lessons to brace our faith to succeed.

Ankara, Turkey   Gokhan Ozyigit
Istanbul, Turkey   Ugur Selek

Acknowledgments

The editors are indebted to Gesa Frese and Wilma McHugh from Springer DE and Niveka Somasundaram and Mariesha Justin from SPi Global/Springer Nature for their assistance in preparing *Prevention and Management of Acute and Late Toxicities in Radiation Oncology*. We extend our most sincere gratitude to our colleagues and friends at Hacettepe University, Koç University, and Baskent University as well as our families.

Contents

Toxicity Management for Central Nervous System Tumors in Radiation Oncology

1

Guler Yavas and Gozde Yazici

1.1   Anatomy

The central nervous system (CNS) consists of the brain and the spinal cord (SC). The spinal cord is a single structure, whereas the adult brain can be defined by four major regions: the cerebrum, the diencephalon, the brain stem, and the cerebellum. The main functions of the CNS include receiving, processing, and responding to sensory information.

1.1.1   Brain

Embryologically, the brain is composed of the prosencephalon (forebrain), the mesencephalon (midbrain), and the rhombencephalon (hind brain). The prosencephalon forms the two hemispheres (telencephalon) and the diencephalon (interbrain) during the later stages of embryogenic life [1]. The weight of the brain changes from birth through adulthood. At birth the brain weighs less than 400 g, but by the beginning of the second year of life it weighs around 900 g, and the adult brain weighs between 1250 and 1450 g [2]. The cerebrum is the largest region of the human brain and the two hemispheres together account for 85% of the brain mass. The interbrain (diencephalon) is the part that links the two hemispheres of the brain. The diencephalon has four regions: the epithalamus, thalamus,

G. Yavas
Faculty of Medicine, Department of Radiation Oncology, Selcuk Meram University, Konya, Turkey

G. Yazici (✉)
Hacettepe University, Faculty of Medicine, Department of Radiation Oncology, Ankara, Turkey
e-mail: yazicig@hacettepe.edu.tr

© Springer Nature Switzerland AG 2020
G. Ozyigit, U. Selek (eds.), *Prevention and Management of Acute and Late Toxicities in Radiation Oncology*, https://doi.org/10.1007/978-3-030-37798-4_1

hypothalamus, and subthalamus. Each cerebral hemisphere is divided into five lobes entitled as: the frontal, parietal, temporal and occipital lobes, and the insula. The surfaces of the cerebral hemispheres are formed by highly folded collection of gray matter, few millimeters in width, named as the cerebral cortex. Although it is only 2–4 mm in thickness, the gray matter accounts for 40% of total brain mass. The inner region of the cortex is a central core of white matter that consists solely of neuronal pathways. Deep within the cerebral white matter is an important region of the cerebrum, a group of sub-cortical gray matter known as "basal nuclei." The basal nuclei are composed of the caudate nucleus, putamen, and globus pallidus which are important regulators of skeletal muscle movements [3].

The cavities within the cerebral hemispheres are called as the right and the left lateral ventricles, which communicate with the third ventricle via interventricular foramen (foramen of Monro). The first and the second ventricles lie within the hemispheres of the brain, and the third ventricle is located in the interbrain. The space between the pons, bulbus, and the cerebellum is called as the fourth ventricle. These ventricles are continuous with one another and with the central canal of the spinal cord. The inner surface of the ventricles is lined by ependymal cells, and protruding into each ventricle is a choroid plexus which functions in the production of cerebrospinal fluid (CSF). About 300–400 mL of CSF is produced daily. The CSF forms a liquid cushion for the brain, and helps to nourish the brain.

The brain and spinal cord is covered by three membranes which are called the meninges. The dura mater is the outermost layer of the meninges, lying directly underneath the bones of the skull and vertebral column. Inside the dura mater there is the arachnoid mater. Arachnoid mater consists of layers of connective tissue. It is avascular, and does not receive any innervation. Underneath the arachnoid mater is the sub-arachnoid space which contains CSF. The pia mater is located underneath the sub-arachnoid space. It is very thin, and is tightly adhered to the surface of the brain and spinal cord. It follows the contours of the brain. Like the dura mater, pia mater is highly vascularized with blood vessels perforating through the membrane to supply the underlying neural tissue. Therefore the dura mater and pia mater are very sensitive to pain.

1.1.2 Brain Stem

The brain stem (BS) is composed of the mesencephalon, the pons, and the medulla oblongata. The BS begins inferior to the thalamus and is positioned between the cerebrum and the spinal cord. The mesencephalon is a relatively narrow band of the BS surrounding the cerebral aqueduct (of Sylvius), extending from the diencephalon to pons. The pons is thicker portion of the brainstem, and is about 25–30 mm in length. The pons bulges from the midbrain and medulla and is separated from them by the superior and inferior pontine sulci. Posteriorly it is surrounded by the cerebellum, and they unite through the middle cerebellar peduncles. The medulla oblongata is the caudal portion of the BS [2].

1.1.3 Spinal Cord

The spinal cord runs through the spinal canal from the cranial top portion of the atlas down to the L1–2 intervertebral disc in adults. It may extend below to L3 vertebral body in children. The spinal cord ends at the level of the L1 vertebral body, and the roots extend caudally in the cauda equina to exit in the appropriate intervertebral foramina. It is 45 cm long, 30 g in weight, and approximately 1 cm in diameter [2, 4]. The spinal cord in the spinal canal is surrounded by meninges. Dorsal and ventral roots course through the intervertebral foramina.

1.1.4 Orbita (Eye, Retina, Lens)

The orbits are conical structures surrounding the organs of vision. The shape of the orbit resembles a four-sided pyramid. Orbit supports the eye and it protects this vital structure. The volume of the orbital cavity in an adult is roughly about 30 cc.

The globe of the eye, or bulbus oculi, is a bulb-like structure consisting of a wall enclosing a fluid-filled cavity. The adult eyeball is spherical in shape, and is 24 mm in length antero-posteriorly. The anterior segment of the eyeball consists of the structures ventral to the vitreous humor, including the cornea, iris, ciliary body, and lens (crystalline lens). The pupil serves as an aperture which is adjusted by the surrounding iris, acting as a diaphragm that regulates the amount of light entering the eye. Both the iris and the pupil are covered by the convex transparent cornea. The cornea is the major refractive component of the eye due to the huge difference in refractive index across the air-cornea interface. The lens is a transparent, biconvex structure. Lens and the cornea refract light to focus on the retina. The lens is made of transparent proteins called "crystallins." It is approximately 5 mm thick and has a diameter of about 9 mm for an adult [5].

The posterior segment of the eyeball is located posteriorly to the lens, and it includes the anterior hyaloid membrane, the vitreous humor, the retina, and the choroid. The retina is the light-sensitive tissue that lines thinner surface of the eye. In embryogenesis both the retina and the optic nerves originate from the diencephalon and should therefore be considered as part of the CNS.

1.1.5 Optic Pathway

The optic pathway consists of the series of cells and synapses that carry visual information from the environment to the brain for processing. It includes the retina, optic nerve, optic chiasm, optic tract, lateral geniculate nucleus, optic radiations, and striate cortex.

The optic nerve is the second cranial nerve, responsible for transmitting the sensory information for vision. The optic nerves are surrounded by the cranial meninges. The optic nerves progress from the posterior aspect of the globe, angle up through the optic canals, and unite to form the optic chiasm. At the chiasm, fibers from the nasal (medial) half of each retina cross over to the contralateral optic tract, while fibers from the temporal (lateral) halves remain ipsilateral. Each optic tract travels to its corresponding cerebral hemisphere to reach the lateral geniculate nucleus. From the lateral geniculate nucleus, the signals continue to the primary visual cortex, where further visual processing takes place [6].

1.1.6 Hippocampus

The hippocampus has a distinctive, curved shape that has been likened to the sea-horse monster of Greek mythology and the ram's horns of Amun in Egyptian mythology. The literature describes considerable age and disease-specific variability in hippocampal size (range 2.8–4.0 cm^3) and location. The hippocampus is located in the medial temporal lobe of the brain. It is a paired structure, with mirror-image halves in the left and right sides of the brain. It consists of ventral and dorsal portions, both of which share similar composition but are parts of different neural circuits. It belongs to the limbic system (Latin limbus = border) which includes the hippocampus, cingulate cortex, olfactory cortex, and amygdala. It plays important roles in long-term memory and spatial navigation [7].

1.1.7 Pituitary Gland

The pituitary gland (hypophysis cerebri) is a small organ situated in a depression of the sphenoid bone at the base of the skull called the "sella turcica." Anatomically, the pituitary gland is related superiorly to the optic chiasm, inferiorly to the sphenoid sinus, and laterally, on either side, to the cavernous sinus and the structures contained within. The pituitary gland measures approximately $10 \times 13 \times 6$ mm, weighs about 500 mg, and occupies most of the volume of the sella turcica. The gland consists of two anatomically and functionally distinct regions, the anterior lobe (adenohypophysis) and the posterior lobe (neurohypophysis). Between these lobes lies a small sliver of tissue called the intermediate lobe. The adenohypophysis is originated from the Rathke's pouch, an ectodermal diverticulum from the roof of the stomodeum, whereas the neurohypophysis is derived from the diencephalon. The adenohypophysis is divided into the pars anterior (anterior lobe) and the pars intermedia (intermediate lobe). The neurohypophysis consists mainly of the "pars posterior" (posterior lobe), part of the infundibular stem and the median eminence. The adenohypophysis secretes several hormones (somatotropin, gonadotropins, thyrotropin, adrenocorticotropin, prolactin, lipotropic hormones, and endorphins), whereas the posterior pituitary essentially stores vasopressin and oxytocin, secreted by the supraoptic and paraventricular nuclei of the hypothalamus [8].

1.2   Contouring

Over the past decades a great deal of progress has been made in the field of radiation oncology as the profession has switched from 2-dimensional to 3-dimensional to intensity modulated and stereotactic techniques. Radiation-related side effects can be improved by avoiding critical structures called organs at risk (OARs) with the help of these technical developments. The comprehensive identification and delineation of OARs are vital to the quality of radiation therapy treatment planning and the safety of treatment delivery. The delineation of intracranial OARs is one of the most crucial points in the planning of brain tumors since RT to the brain may cause serious side effects. Moreover, accurate delineation of OARs is essential for the inverse-planning process of intensity modulate radiotherapy (IMRT).

In some situations changes in anatomy because of the possible tumor extension necessitates a basic understanding of normal anatomy. During the delineation of intracranial OAR using contrast-enhanced computed tomography (CT) scans together with magnetic resonance imaging (MRI) allows better visualization and definition when compared to using CT alone. For example, in order to delineate spinal cord accurately, especially for stereotactic planning, a high-resolution T2-weighted MRI is recommended. Moreover during the delineation of optic chiasm and optic nerves using a high-resolution T1- or T2-weighted MRI rather than planning CT helps better and easier delineation. It is very important to contour on appropriate density windows for each tissue. The structures should be reviewed in the coronal and sagittal planes when contouring on axial slices to verify completeness of coverage in all dimensions [9].

1.2.1   Brain

The delineation of the brain consists of the small brain vessels, cerebellum, CSF and excludes the brainstem and large cerebellar vessels, including the sigmoid sinus, transverse sinus, and superior sagittal sinus (Figs. 1.1 and 1.2). CT bone settings in addition to brain soft tissue 350/40 WW/WL-settings are recommended. The carotid canal and cavernous sinus which are located in the middle cranial fossa are not recommended to be included [9–11].

1.2.2   Brain Stem

The cranial boarder of the brainstem (BS) is defined as bottom of optic tract or the disappearance of posterior cerebral artery which is the bottom of the lateral ventricles, and the caudal border is defined as the tip of the dens of C2 (cranial border of the spinal cord). For delineation of BS, MRI is recommended; however, the bottom section of the lateral ventricles is easily visible on both MRI and CT (Fig. 1.3). Visualization of sagittal plane may be helpful when defining the BS. From cranial to caudal, BS may be divided into three parts during contouring: the midbrain, pons,

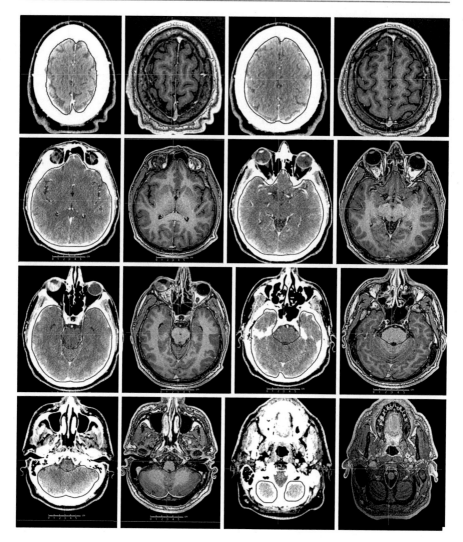

Fig. 1.1 Delineation of the brain as normal structure

and medulla oblongata [10–12]. Cochlea should also be delineated in pontocerebellar region (Fig. 1.4).

1.2.3 Spinal Cord

For delineation of the spinal cord accurately, especially for stereotactic planning, a high-resolution T2-weighted MRI or CT myelogram is recommended. The spinal cord should be delineated instead of whole spinal canal. For CNS tumors, the cranial border of the spinal cord is defined at the tip of the dens of C2, which is the caudal border of the BS, and the caudal border at the upper edge of T3 [11].

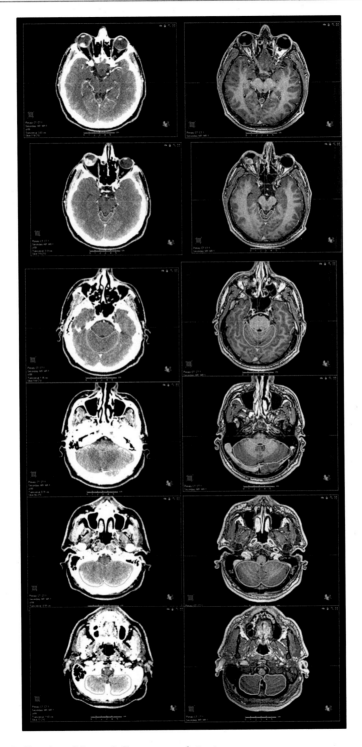

Fig. 1.2 Delineation of the cerebellum as normal structure

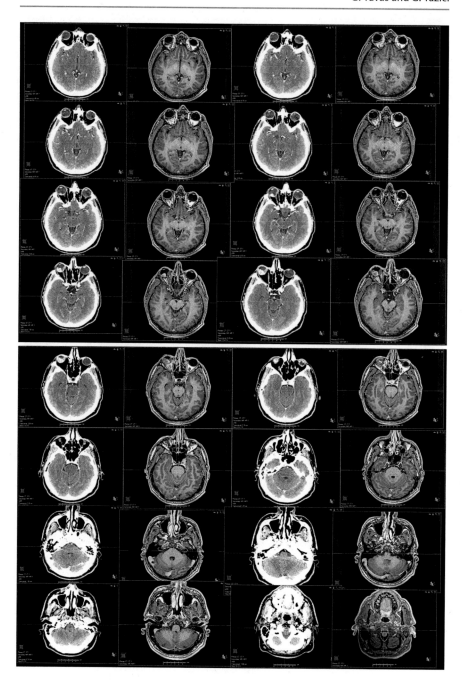

Fig. 1.3 Delineation of the brain stem as normal structure

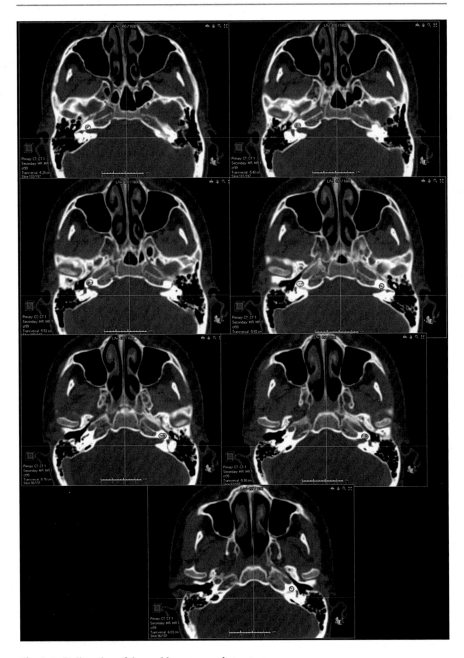

Fig. 1.4 Delineation of the cochlea as normal structure

1.2.4 Orbita (Eye, Retina, Lens)

Cornea can be easily delineated using 2–3 mm brush on both MRI and CT scans (Fig. 1.5). Lens, which is up to 10 mm in diameter, is a biconvex, avascular, non-innervated, encapsulated body composed entirely of epithelial cells and fibers. The lens can be easily delineated on CT [10, 11].

The posterior segment of the eyeball includes the anterior hyaloid membrane, vitreous humor, retina, and choroid [10, 11]. The retina is approximately 0.25 mm thick, and covers the posterior 5/6 of the globe, extending nearly as far as the ciliary body. The retina can be delineated on both MRI and CT using a 3 mm brush. The anterior border of the retina is between the insertion of the medial rectus muscle and the lateral rectus muscle, posterior to the ciliary body. The optic nerve is excluded from this contour. On axial images the anterior limit of the retina is between the insertion of the medial rectus muscle and the insertion of the lateral rectus muscle, posteriorly to the ciliary body [10, 11, 13]. Lacrimal glands should also be delineated (Fig. 1.6).

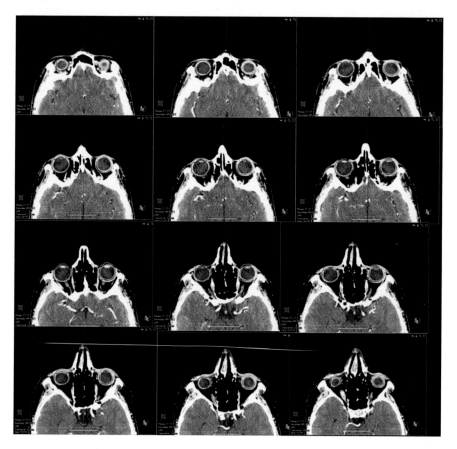

Fig. 1.5 Delineation of the orbita

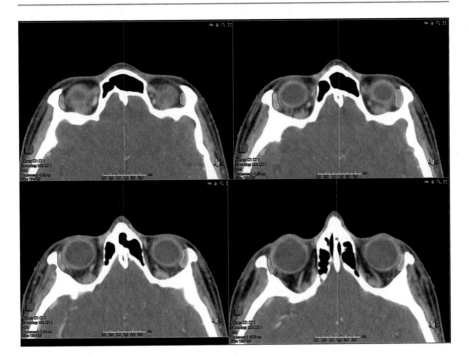

Fig. 1.6 Delineation of the lacrimal glands

1.2.5 Optic Pathway

The optic nerve is thin, usually 2–5 mm thick, and is clearly identifiable on CT. Using both CT and T1- and T2-weighted imaging/fast fluid-attenuated inversion recovery imaging of MRI is recommended for the accurate delineation of the optic nerve. Depending on the orientation of the scan plane relative to the brain, the optic nerve and chiasm can appear on multiple images (Fig. 1.7). The optic nerves should be delineated all the way from the posterior edge of the eyeball, through the bony optic canal to the optic chiasm. It is crucial to delineate the optic apparatus in continuity, since gaps in the structures will result in omission of the dose from the missing volume for that structure's dose–volume histogram.

The optic chiasm is usually 2–5 mm thick, and is located in the sub-arachnoid space of the supracellar cistern 1 cm superior to pituitary gland. Internal carotid artery forms the lateral boarder of the optic chiasm. It is demarcated inferiorly by the third ventricle. The pituitary stalk is the most important landmark since it is located just behind the crossing of the fibers. Pituitary gland is easily visible in T1-weighted MRI images because it shows hyperintense signals. Although it can be visible on both CT and MRI scans, a T1-weighted MRI with axial, sagittal, and coronal sections is recommended for better delineation [10, 11, 13].

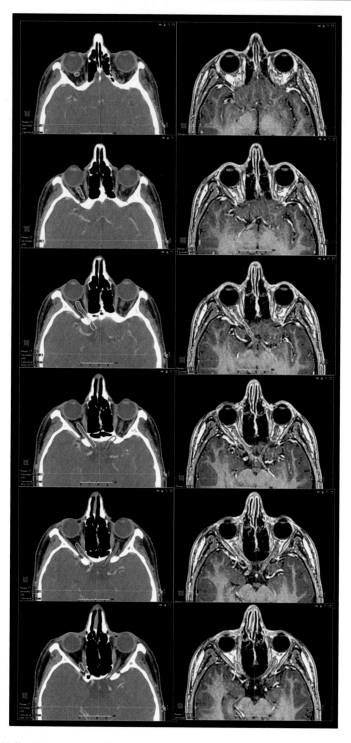

Fig. 1.7 Delineation of optic pathway

1.2.6   Hippocampus

During the recent years, the accurate delineation of the hippocampus (dentate gyrus) has been increasingly important since both the clinical and preclinical evidence suggest that irradiation to hippocampal dentate gyrus can cause neurocognitive impairment. The hippocampus is delineated as the gray matter medial to the medial boundary of the temporal horn of the lateral ventricle bordered medially by the quadrigeminal cistern as described by Gondi et al. [14] (Fig. 1.8). At the level of the curve of the temporal horn which is also called as uncal recess, the hippocampus is easily visible because it is the gray matter included in the curve and is bounded anteriorly, laterally, and medially by the CSF in the temporal horn. Amygdala, which is a gray matter located medially to the temporal horn of the lateral ventricle is easily distinguished from the hippocampus at this level. The amygdala should be excluded from the contour of the hippocampus [13]. The boundary between the hippocampus and the amygdala is not clearly visible in the more caudal slices. The hippocampus is mainly composed of gray matter therefore for the delineation of

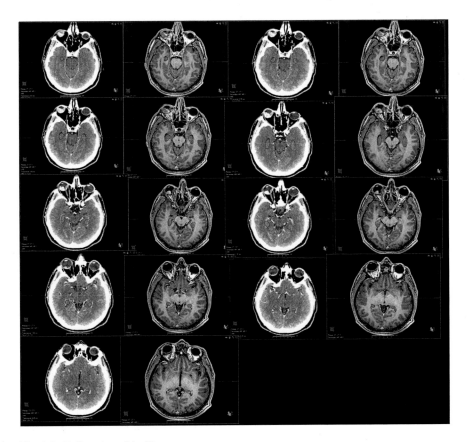

Fig. 1.8 Delineation of the hippocampus

hippocampus T1-weighted MRI scan is recommended. Very thin slice-thickness (1–2 mm) is necessary to visualize the hippocampus. In sagittal view it is easy to visualize "banana" shape hippocampus.

1.2.7 Pituitary Gland

The pituitary gland is oval-shaped structure which is craniocaudally up to 12 mm, and is located in the sella turcica. The pituitary gland is one of the smallest OARs; therefore, it is difficult to visualize it on CT images (Fig. 1.9). The lateral border of the pituitary gland is formed by the cavernous sinuses. The inner part of the sella turcica can be used as surrogate anatomical bony structure. It is better to define the pituitary gland in the sagittal images [11, 13].

1.3 Pathophysiology

Despite the significant advances in limiting overt neurotoxicity, cognitive dysfunction is still a major problem particularly for childhood CNS tumors. During the last decades the researchers focused on identifying the primary cause of tissue damage. However, the data indicates that the response of the CNS to RT is a continuous and interacting process. Although the exact mechanism is not clear, the clinical and scientific evidence helps us to understand the pathophysiology of radiation-induced brain injury. The CNS is particularly more vulnerable to ionizing irradiation when compared to other tissue types. The ionizing irradiation may cause direct or indirect DNA damage, but it may also cause a metabolic stress, which is very harmful for the CNS [15]. Understanding the mechanisms of radiation-induced CNS toxicity may help to develop strategies to either increase the radiation tolerance or treat CNS alterations caused by ionizing radiation.

The etiology of radiation-induced CNS toxicity is a multifactorial process that is influenced by patient-related factors including age, medical comorbidities, psychological and genetic predispositions, characteristics of the underlying malignancy, and any additional injuries caused by other treatment modalities such as surgery and chemotherapy [16]. The radiation-induced CNS injury is described in three phases from the radiobiological perspective: acute (within days to weeks after irradiation), early delayed (within 1–6 months post-irradiation), and late or late delayed (>6 months post-irradiation). The Radiation Therapy Oncology Group (RTOG) describes acute injury based on the clinical time expression as the injury occurring during or within 90 days of RT. Acute injury includes seizure, coma, and paralysis which are considered to be secondary to edema and disruption of the blood–brain barrier (BBB). The corticosteroid treatment improves the acute neurologic changes. Late toxicities include headache, lethargy, and severe CNS dysfunctions such as partial loss of power and dyskinesia, and coma, and occur after

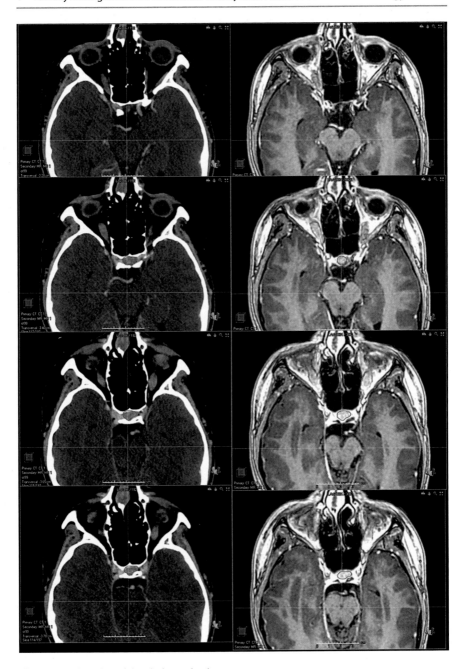

Fig. 1.9 Delineation of the pituitary gland

90 days of RT. Radiation-induced late toxicities are probably associated with increased intracranial pressure caused by the persistent vasogenic edema resulting from BBB damage [17].

Larger fraction sizes and compressed fractionation schedules are known to contribute negatively to the CNS toxicity. RTOG prospectively compared different whole brain RT fractionation schedules in patients with symptomatic brain metastases with respect to the impact on overall survival [18]. Multiple fractionation schedules ranging from 10 Gy in a single fraction to up to 40 Gy delivered over 20 fractions were delivered. Most fractionation schedules were not significantly different in terms of overall survival times, except the delivery of 10 Gy in a single fraction. 10 Gy to the entire brain in single fraction was determined to be significantly detrimental. It can be interpreted from these data that, above a certain threshold, larger fractionation sizes has detrimental impact on radiation-induced brain injury when the treatment volumes are equivalent.

Among the varieties of radiation-induced CNS toxicities, it is the late delayed effects that cause severe and irreversible neurological consequences. After the exposure of ionizing radiation, late delayed effects within the CNS have been attributable to both the parenchymal and vascular injury involving the oligodendroglial cells, neuronal progenitors, and vascular endothelial cells [19]. Late delayed toxicity of CNS irradiation may be presented with different scenarios including demyelination, proliferative and degenerative glial reactions, endothelial cell loss, and capillary occlusion. Therefore a single mechanism cannot explain these complex alterations. At least four factors contribute to the development of CNS toxicity: (1) damage to vessel structures; (2) deletion of oligodendrocyte-2 astrocyte progenitors (O-2A) and mature oligodendrocytes; (3) deletion of neural stem cell populations in the hippocampus, cerebellum, and cortex; (4) generalized alterations of cytokine expression [20]. These four contributing factors can be explained with (1) the vascular hypothesis, (2) parenchymal hypothesis, (3) the dynamic interactions between multiple cell type's hypothesis, and (4) molecular mechanisms.

1.3.1 Vascular Hypothesis

The vascular hypothesis argues that vascular damage leads to ischemia with secondary white matter necrosis. Death of endothelial cells is an early event in small vessels which may be responsible for the initial edema [21, 22]. After the early changes of the vascular wall there is progressive loss of endothelia. Thrombocytes adhere to exposed matrix which leads to the formation of thrombi. Thrombi occur within weeks and months after RT. After this, abnormal endothelial proliferation is observed. In the acute and subacute phases of vascular damage the most prominent findings are altered permeability of the vascular wall and BBB breakdown, and in the late phase the important findings are telangiectasia, hyalinosis, and fibrinoid deposits in the vessel wall.

1.3.2 Parenchymal Hypothesis

1.3.2.1 Oligodendrocytes

Since the white matter necrosis after RT is associated with demyelination, the parenchymal hypothesis initially focused on the oligodendrocytes as they are required for the formation of myelin sheaths. The progenitor cells of oligodendrocytes, known as O-2A cells, give rise to mature oligodendrocytes. It has been proposed that the radiation-induced loss of O-2A progenitor cells leads to failure to replace oligodendrocytes that eventually results in demyelination and white matter necrosis. It has been shown that the oligodendrocytes are the most radiosensitive type of glial cells, with cell death occurring rather early after relatively low doses of irradiation. Therefore, the data seemed to be consistent with the white matter selectivity of radiation-induced brain injury. However, the time course of oligodendrocyte depletion after irradiation was not consistent with that of white matter necrosis during the development of late delayed effects [19, 20].

1.3.2.2 Astrocytes

Astrocytes have many functions besides their supportive role, including modulation of synaptic transmission and secretion of neurotrophic factors such as basic fibroblast growth factor to promote neurogenesis. Astrocytes are vital for the protection of endothelial cells oligodendrocytes, and neurons from oxidative stress. It has been suggested that hippocampal astrocytes are capable of regulating neurogenesis by instructing the stem cells to adopt a neuronal fate [23]. In response to injury, astrocytes exhibit two common reactions: in acute phase cellular swelling (radiation-induced edema), and in chronic phase hyperplasia and hypertrophy. In chronic phase astrocytes undergo proliferation, exhibit hypertrophic nuclei/cell bodies, and show increased expression of glial fibrillary acidic protein (GFAP) [24–26]. These reactive astrocytes secrete a host of pro-inflammatory mediators such as cyclooxygenase (Cox)-2 and the intercellular adhesion molecule (ICAM)-1, which lead to the infiltration of leukocytes into the brain via BBB breakdown [25–27].

1.3.2.3 Microglia

Microglia are the immune cells of the brain. After injury, microglia become activated. Activated microglia can proliferate, phagocytose, and exacerbate the injury by the production of reactive oxygen species (ROS), lipid metabolites, and hydrolytic enzymes. Although microglial activation plays an important role in phagocytosis of dead cells, sustained activation is believed to contribute to a chronic inflammatory state. In-vitro studies suggested that activated microglia leads to a remarkable increase in expression of pro-inflammatory genes TNFα, IL-1β, IL-6 and Cox-2, and the chemokines. In particular, excessive generation of ROS from the injured and/or pro-inflammatory cells has been implicated in the development of late delayed effects of the ionizing radiation [27–29].

1.3.2.4 Neurons

The neurons, which are located in the gray matter, were initially thought to be a radioresistant. Therefore the neurons were believed to play no role in radiation-induced CNS injury. However, studies have demonstrated radiation-induced changes in hippocampal cellular activity, synaptic efficiency/spike generation, and neuronal gene expression [30–32]. In addition, the chronic and progressive cognitive dysfunction following cranial irradiation was shown in both children and adult patients in clinical studies; therefore, the neurons should be sensitive to radiation.

1.3.3 Neuronal Stem Cells/Neurogenesis

The hippocampus plays important roles in the consolidation of information from short-term memory to long-term memory, and in spatial memory. The dentate gyrus, which is a part of hippocampus is a highly dynamic structure and a major site of postnatal/adult neurogenesis. Residents in the hippocampus are neuronal stem cells, self-renewing cells capable of generating neurons, astrocytes, and oligodendroglio-cytes. High doses of radiation produce overt histopathological changes such as demyelination and vasculopathies within the brain parenchyma, but lower doses produce cognitive dysfunction without inducing obvious morphological changes. Although the pathogenesis of radiation-induced cognitive dysfunction is unknown, recent studies suggest that it may involve impaired neurogenesis within the sub-granular zone (SGZ) of the dentate gyrus [19, 33, 34].

1.3.4 Dynamic Interactions Between Multiple Cell Types Hypothesis

The radiation-induced late CNS injury is a dynamic process between the multiple cell types of the CNS. Oligodendrocytes, astrocytes, microglia, neurons, and vascular endothelial cells are not only passive bystanders that merely die from radiation damage but rather act as participants in an orchestrated response to radiation injury [28, 35].

1.3.5 Molecular Mechanisms

There are many suggested molecular mechanisms involved in the radiation-induced CNS toxicity including: (a) apoptosis and neurogenesis inhibition, (b) excessive production of cytokines and chemokines, (c) VEGF, hypoxia and blood–brain barrier disruption, (d) radiation-induced ROS generation.

1.3.5.1 Apoptosis and Neurogenesis Inhibition

Radiation-induced apoptosis is primarily related to mitochondrial damage followed by caspase activation. In addition, ATM gene is required for the regulation of apoptosis in some part of the brain including hippocampal dentate gyrus, external granular layer of the cerebellum and retina. In preclinical studies it has been demonstrated that apoptosis occurs in the young adult rat brain after ionizing radiation, and leads to damage in hippocampal neurons which eventually is associated with cognitive decline [20, 36, 37].

1.3.5.2 Excessive Production of Cytokines and Chemokines

Among the numerous pro-inflammatory cytokines and chemokines IL-1, IL-6, TNF-α, and TGF-β are the ones that are excessively produced immediately after radiation exposure to brain tissue [20]. Although there are many studies providing the evidence that the expression of TNF- α is directly activated by ionizing radiation, limited evidence is available with respect to the pathways describing the TNF-α gene induction in response to radiation [38]. All of these cytokines and chemokines in the irradiated tissue perpetuate and augment the inflammatory response for long periods of time, causing to possible chronic inflammation and radiation-induced CNS injury.

1.3.5.3 VEGF, Hypoxia, and Blood–Brain Barrier Disruption

The endothelial cell density after RT is reduced which gradually diminishes the integrity of BBB. This causes vasogenic edema, inflammation, and tissue hypoxia. Hypoxia causes induction of HIF-1α and VEGF. VEGF augments the vascular permeability which eventually causes disruption of BBB, worsening vasogenic edema, inflammation, and tissue hypoxia. All of these cascades further increase the VEGF concentrations. Eventually VEGF concentrations become sufficient to increase endothelial proliferation and angiogenesis which leads to a dramatic increase in endothelial cells. This situation is referred as "conditional renewal." All of these cascades end with white matter necrosis. Reports suggesting that anti-VEGF therapy can normalize BBB function in microvessels damaged during radiosurgery in the human brain and suggest that manipulating the VEGF signaling cascade may be a useful strategy for mitigating late delayed injuries resulting from brain radiation as well [19, 39].

1.3.5.4 Radiation-Induced ROS Generation

Reactive oxygen species (ROS) include free radicals, oxygen ions, and both inorganic and organic peroxides. ROS are highly reactive since they have unpaired electrons in their shells. In normal situation, the antioxidant systems protect cells against oxidative damage. However, under stress, ROS levels can increase dramatically, overwhelming antioxidant systems and resulting in significant injury to tissues. This condition is called as "oxidative stress." Increased levels of ROS might arise from macrophages, infiltrating activated leukocytes, and neurons. Tissue hypoxia resulting from vascular damage is another source of ROS generation. Moreover pro-inflammatory cytokines and growth factors increase intracellular ROS generation [19].

The brain is very vulnerable to oxidative stress. When compared to other cells, neurons and glial cells contain relatively low levels of antioxidant enzymes including catalase, glutathione peroxidase, and superoxide dismutase (SOD). Additionally, myelin membranes contain relatively high levels of peroxidizable fatty acids which make them highly susceptible to ROS. Strategies to block effector molecules or to reduce oxidative stress are attractive approaches for mitigating radiation-induced toxicity [19, 39].

1.3.5.5 Brain

Radiation-induced brain toxicity has been classified into three phases: acute, early delayed (subacute), and late delayed injury. These phases were first described by Sheline [40]. Acute brain injury occurs during and/or in days to weeks after irradiation. Early delayed brain injury is seen 1–6 months post-irradiation; however, some other researchers consider this time course as 6–12 weeks. Late delayed injury, which is the most severe, often irreversible and progressive form of the injury usually develops >6 months after irradiation.

The most common acute reactions associated with brain irradiation include headache, nausea, drowsiness, and sometimes worsening of neurologic symptoms, fatigue, hair loss (alopecia), skin erythema (radiation dermatitis). Acute side effects are usually transient and self-limiting [41–43]. The initial vascular injury causes platelet aggregation and thrombus formation in microvessels within weeks to months. Furthermore early vascular injury causes degenerative structural changes in white matter.

General neurologic deterioration during early delayed period (2–6 months after RT) is probably due to transient, diffuse demyelination. Many focal neurologic signs following irradiation of intracranial tumor have been attributed to intralesional reactions, probably indicative of tumor response or perilesional reactions including edema and demyelination. Periventricular white matter lesions start to appear on conventional MR imaging or CT during this interval, even with standard fractionated partial brain RT [41]. Similar to acute toxicities, early delayed side effects are usually reversible and resolve spontaneously.

Late delayed side effects are of the most concern when discussing radiation-induced brain toxicity. Unlike acute and early delayed side effects, late delayed toxicity is largely progressive and irreversible. Due to the limited lifespan of many adult brain tumor patients receiving irradiation to the brain, it is largely unknown what the long-term consequences of most treatments would be after many years. The classical late effect following brain irradiation is either localized or multifocal necrosis, often associated with high-dose and large brain-volume treatment. Complications include worsening neurologic signs and symptoms, seizures, and increased intracranial pressure [41]. Both conventional and more precise treatments including stereotactic radiotherapy (SRT) and stereotactic radiosurgery (SRS) have the potential to produce late delayed side effects such as cognitive alterations in short-term memory and concentration, and in rare cases dementia. Radiation-induced neuropsychological function and cognition deficits evolve in a biphasic pattern with a subacute transient decline corresponding to more common symptoms, followed by a late delayed irreversible impairment several months or years later in a much smaller proportion of surviving patients [44].

1.3.5.6 Brain Stem

Brainstem injury patients may exhibit III-XII cranial nerve palsy as well as long-beam (cone and sensory system) and cerebellar injury symptoms. The pathophysiology of the brain stem injury is similar to brain injury [45].

Patients have no clinical symptoms in mild cases; serious complaints vary and include limb weakness, hemiplegia, gait instability, temperature sensory disturbance, diplopia, dysarthria, tongue, and facial paralysis. One severe clinical manifestation of brain stem injury is syncope. Damage to descending sympathetic nerve fibers, which anatomically run along the brain stem, may result in syncope or Horner syndrome. Some patients may recover from the disease after their brainstem suffers mild radiation injury, while others may need earlier medical intervention to alleviate their symptoms. However, patients who develop severe radiation brainstem injuries have a poor prognosis due to the lack of effective medical therapies [46].

1.3.5.7 Spinal Cord

The most common early delayed side effect of the spinal cord is transient myelopathy, particularly in the cervical and thoracic spine. The most common pathophysiology of the transient myelopathy is believed to be demyelination on the posterior columns. Lhermitte's sign, or "transient radiation myelopathy," which is characterized by an electric shock sensation that radiates down the spine and extremities on flexion of the neck, is a relatively infrequent sequela of irradiation of the cervical spinal cord. It is a self-limiting condition and most patients improve during the course of several months to a year. Although Lhermitte's sign is rarely a precursor of myelitis, there have been some reports of patients who developed radiation myelopathy after experiencing Lhermitte's sign. In general, the Lhermitte's sign that predated true radiation myelitis is later in onset than the usual latency period of 2–4 months [46].

Late effects to spinal cord are less common and highly severe. A progressive myelopathy syndrome can be seen, initially presenting with a partial cord involvement and progressing to a total transverse myelopathy. Irreversible radiation myelopathy usually is not seen earlier than 6–12 months after the completion of treatment. Typically, half of the patients who develop radiation-induced myelopathy in the cervical or thoracic cord region will do so within 20 months of treatment and 75% of cases will occur within 30 months. The signs and symptoms are typically progressive over several months, but acute onset of plegia over several hours or a few days is also possible. The diagnosis of radiation myelopathy is one of exclusion; a history of radiation therapy in doses sufficient to result in injury must be present. The region of the irradiated cord must lie slightly above the dermatome level of expression of the lesion; the latent period from the completion of treatment to the onset of injury must be consistent with that observed in radiation myelopathy; and local tumor progression must be ruled out. Radiation myelopathy is a diagnosis of exclusion, and patients must be evaluated for tumor progression and paraneoplastic syndromes with MRI of the cord [47, 48].

1.3.5.8 Orbita (Eye, Retina, Lens)

Radiation-induced orbital injury is composed of a wide variety of clinical conditions from transient eyelid erythema and a mild conjunctivitis to corneal perforation and complete loss of vision, with or without loss of the globe (Fig. 1.10).

Long-term radiation effects of the human ocular adnexa are manifest by a spectrum of changes. Among these alterations are loss of meibomian glands and ducts, loss of distal glands with persistent remnants of ducts and acini, squamous metaplasia of the meibomian glands and dilated ducts filled with keratin. Late conjunctival alterations include chronic conjunctivitis, focal loss of epithelial cells, and squamous metaplasia [49].

Radiation-induced retinopathy histologically resembles diabetic retinopathy. Histologic examination reveals several consistent findings including thickening of arteriolar capillary walls, accumulation of fine fibrillar material within the walls of the vessels, myointimal proliferation, swelling of the endothelium, an enlarged elastic lamina, narrowing and occlusion of the vessel lumen, degeneration of the media and adventitia, and swelling and loss of muscular, elastic, and collagenous components. In clinic, radiation retinopathy can manifest by many disorders including cotton wool spots, macular edema, exudates, microaneurysms, telangiectasia, retinal hemorrhages, proliferative neovascularization, vitreous hemorrhage, and pigmentary changes [49].

Cataract is a well-known radiation complication. According to the anatomic location cataracts are classified into three types including, nuclear, cortical, and posterior subcapsular types. Nuclear and cortical cataracts develop from pathologic changes within the lens fiber cells; on the other hand, posterior subcapsular cataracts are associated with abnormalities at the germinative zone of the lens. Among the three different cataract types, the posterior subcapsular cataract is the one that is

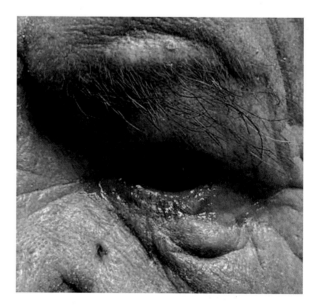

Fig. 1.10 A patient with eyelid erythema and a mild conjunctivitis after radiotherapy

most commonly associated with ionizing irradiation [50]. Radiation damage to the germinative zone of lens epithelial cell DNA is probably responsible for most post treatment cataracts. In addition to DNA damage, direct cytoplasmic effects, such as disruption of membrane channels, protein cross-linking, and ion pump abnormalities are also important in radiation-induced cataract progression [49, 51].

1.3.5.9 Optic Pathway

The most frequent clinical symptoms of radiation-induced optic neuropathy are sudden, painless, and irreversible loss of vision in one or both eyes 3 months to 9 years after RT.

The changes are similar to those associated with brain radionecrosis. Pathological specimens have revealed thickened blood vessels, endothelial cell proliferation occluding vessel lumens, and demyelinization [49, 51].

1.3.5.10 Hippocampus

The hippocampus is central to short-term declarative memory and spatial information processing. Hippocampus consists of the dentate gyrus, CA3, and CA1 regions. The dentate gyrus is a highly dynamic structure and it is an important site of postnatal/adult neurogenesis. The hippocampus is consisted of neuronal stem cells that are self-renewing cells capable of generating neurons, astrocytes, and oligodendrocytes. Neurogenesis depends on the presence of a specific neurogenic microenvironment. Both astrocytes and endothelial cells can regulate neurogenesis [23, 52].

Hippocampus is particularly vulnerable to ionizing radiation. Hippocampal dysfunction is characterized by a progressive decline in the learning, memory, and spatial information processing abilities. Although the pathophysiology of radiation-induced cognitive dysfunction has still been unknown, recent evidences suggest that it may involve impaired neurogenesis within the subgranular zone of the dentate gyrus. Whole brain radiotherapy doses as low as 2 Gy are sufficient to reduce the rate of proliferation among neuronal progenitors within the subgranular zone [53]. The cellular mechanisms underlying the vulnerability of hippocampus remain to be elucidated [53–55]. Although the neuronal progenitors within the subgranular zone of the dentate gyrus are highly radiosensitive, direct effects of radiation on synaptic plasticity in the hippocampus or in other limbic or paralimbic structures may also be involved [19].

1.3.5.11 Pituitary Gland

The pituitary gland is an endocrine gland essential for the regulation of many physiological processes including growth, thyroid gland function, reproduction, and lactation. The pituitary gland is controlled in large part by the hypothalamus, a region of the brain that lies just above the pituitary. The pituitary gland is linked to the hypothalamus through the pituitary stalk.

The hypothalamic–pituitary unit is a particularly radiosensitive region in the CNS. The clinical scenarios include panhypopituitarism, hypothalamic hypopituitarism, and hypothalamic hypogonadism. Pediatric patients are more vulnerable to pituitary dysfunction than the adult patients. The most common clinical condition for the pediatric patients is growth hormone deficiency revealing short stature and retarded growth [56].

Growth hormone deficiency is usually the first and frequently is the only manifestation of neuro-endocrine injury following cranial irradiation. GH axis is followed by the gonadotrophin, adrenocorticotrophic hormone (ACTH), and thyroid-stimulating hormone (TSH) axes; these observations in humans have been reproduced in animal models [57, 58].

1.4 Dose Constraints

Despite the increasing number of patients treated with RT for CNS tumors, limited evidence is available about the relationship between dose and toxicity. In addition, technological advances in the field of radiation therapy have emerged new treatment strategies, including stereotactic radiosurgery (SRS) and stereotactic cranial radiotherapy (SCRT), and these treatment methods require new dose restrictions for organs at risk (OAR) (Table 1.1).

Seminal papers by Rubin [59] and Emami [60] provided rational guidelines for the dose tolerance limits of normal tissues under conventional fractionation. In 2006, leaders in the American Association of Physics in Medicine (AAPM) and American Society of Therapeutic Radiology and Oncology (ASTRO) recognized that an increasing amount of dose/volume/outcome data for normal tissues had been generated. The joint efforts of the radiation oncologists and physicist (ASTRO-AAPM), called as "Quantitative Analysis of Normal Tissue Effects in the Clinic" (QUANTEC), updated the recommendations of Emami et al. using models for normal tissue complications for most sites [61, 62]. The QUANTEC papers essentially present a critical review of the literature on radiation dose/volume/outcome for normal tissue, and attempt to quantitatively analyze these data and present recommendations on dose-volume limits for normal tissue toxicity. Nonetheless QUANTEC provides limited evidence with respect to dose constraints for SRS and SCRT. Later when the clinical data emerged, new proposals defining dose/volume/toxicity for SRS and SCRT are developed.

The radiation tolerance to CNS may be affected from a number of parameters, including total dose, dose per fraction, total treatment time, fractionation schedule, volume, host-related factors (age, comorbid diseases such as diabetes mellitus), radiation quality (linear energy transfer = LET), and adjunctive therapies.

RTOG/EORTC acute and late radiation morbidity scoring criteria are summarized in Table 1.2.

1.4.1 Brain

Although the brain is composed of different anatomical regions including the gray matter, white matter, and nuclei, dose constraints to brain is uniformly applied to

Table 1.1 Dose constraints for organs at risk for central nervous system

Organ	Emami dose limits (Gy)			QUANTEC dose limits	EPTN dose limits	SRS dose limits	SRC dose limits
	1/3	2/3	3/3				
Brain	TD5/5 = 60 TD50/5 = 75	TD5/5 = 50 TD50/5 = 65	TD5/5 = 45 TD50/5 = 60	Symptomatic necrosis risk: D_{max} < 60 Gy: <3% D_{max} = 72 Gy: 5% D_{max} = 90 Gy: 10%	α/β = 2 $V_{60Gy} \leq 3$ cc	5–10 cc < 12 Gy	
Brain stem	TD5/5 = 60 TD50/5 = 75	TD5/5 = 53 TD50/5=	TD5/5 = 50 TD50/5 = 65	Permanent cranial neuropathy or necrosis risk: D_{max} < 54 Gy: <5% D1–10 cc <59 Gy: <5%	α/β = 2 Surface $D_{0.03cc}$ 60 Gy Interior $D_{0.03cc}$ 54 Gy	V0.5 cc < 10 Gy D_{max} for ≤0.035 cc: 15 Gy D_{max} <12.5 Gy	V0.5 cc < 18 Gy in 3 fractions, 6 Gy/fraction D_{max}: 23.1 Gy in 3 fractions, 7.7 Gy/fraction V0.5 cc < 23 Gy in 5 fractions, 4.6 Gy/fraction D_{max}: 31 Gy/5 fractions, 6.2 Gy/fraction
Spinal cord	5 cm TD5/5: 50 Gy TD50/5: 70 Gy	10 cm TD5/5: 50 Gy TD50/5: 70 Gy	20 cm TD5/5: 47 Gy Cauda equina: TD5/5: 60 Gy TD50/5: 75 Gy	Myelopathy risk: D_{max} = 50 Gy: 0.2% D_{max} = 60 Gy: 6% D_{max} = 69 Gy: 50%	–	13 Gy: <1% injury risk Cauda equina: D < 5 cc: 14 Gy D_{max} for ≤0.035 cc: 16 Gy Sacral plexus: D < 5 cc: 14.4 Gy D_{max} for ≤0.035 cc: 16 Gy	20 Gy/in 3 fractions: <1% injury risk Cauda equina: D < 5 cc: 21.9 Gy (7.3 Gy/fr, in 3 fractions) D_{max}: 24 Gy (8 Gy/fr, in 3 fractions) Sacral plexus: D < 5 cc: 22.5 Gy (7.5 Gy/fr, in 3 fractions) D_{max}: 24 Gy (8 Gy/fr, in 3 fractions)
Lacrimal gland			TD5/5: 35 Gy TD50/5: 50 Gy		Dmean < 25 Gy		

(continued)

Table 1.1 (continued)

Organ	Emami dose limits (Gy)			QUANTEC dose limits	EPTN dose limits	SRS dose limits	SRC dose limits
	1/3	2/3	3/3				
Cornea			TD50/5: 50 Gy		$\alpha/\beta = 3$ $D_{0.03cc} \leq 50$ Gy		
Retina			TD5/5: 45 Gy TD50/5: 65 Gy		$\alpha/\beta = 3$ $D_{0.03cc} \leq 45$ Gy		
Lens	–	–	TD5/5: 10 Gy TD50/5: 18 Gy		$\alpha/\beta = 1$ $D_{0.03cc} \leq 10$ Gy		
Optic nerve	–	–	TD5/5: 50 Gy TD50/5: 65 Gy	Optic neuropathy risk: $D_{max} < 55$ Gy: <3% D_{max} 55–60 Gy:3–7% $D_{max} > 60$ Gy: >7–20%	$\alpha/\beta = 2$ $D_{0.03cc} \leq 55$ Gy	$D_{max} <12$ Gy $D < 0.2$ cc: 8 Gy D_{max} for ≤0.035 cc: 10 Gy	$D < 0.2$ cc: 15.3 Gy (5.1 Gy/fr, in 3 fractions) D_{max}: 23.1 Gy (5.8 Gy/fr, in 3 fractions) D0.2 cc: 23 Gy (4.6 Gy/fr, in 5 fractions) D_{max}: 25 Gy (5 Gy/fr, in 5 fractions)
Optic chiasm			TD5/5: 50 Gy TD50/5: 65 Gy	$D_{max} < 55$ Gy: <3% D_{max} 55–60 Gy:3–7% $D_{max} > 60$ Gy: >7–20%	$\alpha/\beta = 2$ $D_{0.03cc} \leq 55$ Gy	$D_{max}<12$ Gy $D < 0.2$ cc: 8Gy D_{max} for ≤0.035 cc: 10 Gy	$D < 0.2$ cc: 15.3 Gy (5.1 Gy/fr, in 3 fractions) D_{max}: 23.1 Gy (5.8 Gy/fr, in 3 fractions) D0.2 cc: 23 Gy (4.6 Gy/fr, in 5 fractions) D_{max}: 25 Gy (5 Gy/fr, in 5 fractions)
Hippocampus					$\alpha/\beta = 2$ D40% <7.3 Gy		
Pituitary gland					$\alpha/\beta = 2$ Dmean ≤ 45 Gy	Dmean <15 Gy	

QUANTEC quantitative analysis of normal tissue effects in the clinic, *EPTN* The European Particle Therapy Network, *SRS* stereotactic radiosurgery, *SCRT* stereotactic cranial radiotherapy

Table 1.2 The RTOG/EORTC acute and late radiation morbidity scoring criteria [17]

Organ	Acute toxicity				Chronic toxicity			
	Grade 1	Grade 2	Grade 3	Grade 4	Grade 1	Grade 2	Grade 3	Grade 4
Brain	Fully functional status with minor neurological findings, no medication needed	Neurological findings present sufficient to require home care/nursing assistance may be required/ medications including steroids/ antiseizure agents may be required	Neurological findings requiring hospitalization for initial management	Serious neurological impairment that includes paralysis, coma, or seizures >3 per week despite medication/ hospitalization required	Mild headache Slight lethargy	Moderate headache Great lethargy	Severe headaches Severe CNS dysfunction (partial loss of power or dyskinesia)	Seizures or paralysis Coma
Spinal cord	Fully functional status with minor neurological findings, no medication needed	Neurological findings present sufficient to require home care/nursing assistance may be required/ medications including steroids/ antiseizure agents may be required	Neurological findings requiring hospitalization for initial management	Serious neurological impairment that includes paralysis, coma, or seizures >3 per week despite medication/ hospitalization required	Mild Lhermitte's syndrome	Severe Lhermitte's syndrome	Objective neurological findings at or below cord level treated	Monoplegia, paraplegia, or quadriplegia

(continued)

Table 1.2 (continued)

Organ	Acute toxicity				Chronic toxicity			
	Grade 1	Grade 2	Grade 3	Grade 4	Grade 1	Grade 2	Grade 3	Grade 4
Eye	Mild conjunctivitis w/ or w/o scleral injection/increased tearing	Moderate conjunctivitis w/ or w/o keratitis requiring steroids and/or antibiotics/dry eye requiring artificial tears/iritis with photophobia	Severe keratitis with corneal ulceration/objective decrease in visual acuity or in visual fields/acute glaucoma/panophthalmitis	Loss of vision (uni or bilateral)	Asymptomatic cataract Minor corneal ulceration or keratitis	Symptomatic cataract Moderate corneal ulceration Minor retinopathy or glaucoma	Severe keratitis Severe retinopathy or detachment Severe glaucoma	Panophthalmitis/blindness

entire cerebral parenchyma. The brain is particularly sensitive to fraction sizes >2 Gy and, twice-daily fractionation schedules. The total dose, fraction size, and volume are the major variables that influence the radiation necrosis. The radiation necrosis is more likely to be symptomatic in some parts of the brain including corpus callosum and brain stem; however, location alone does not influence the susceptibility for the radiation necrosis [63].

Emami et al. reported the dose constraints for the brain as $TD_{5/5}$ of 60 Gy, 50 Gy and 45 Gy and a $TD_{50/5}$ of 75 Gy, 65 Gy and 60 Gy if 1/3, 2/3 or the entire brain is treated with RT, respectively [60]. Later QUANTEC conducted an extensive review of the modern literature and suggested new dose constraints for the brain in 3-dimensional era. QUANTEC's recommendations were based on a heterogeneous group of studies with varied dose and fractionation schedules. Studies were compared using the biologically effective dose (BED) with an α/β ratio of 3. A dose response relationship was found for radiation necrosis. The incidence of radiation necrosis increases from 3% with a $D_{max} < 60 Gy$ to 5% at $D_{max} = 72$ Gy and to 10% when $D_{max} = 90$ Gy. For twice-daily fractionation, a steep increase in toxicity appears to occur when the BED is >80 Gy. For large fraction sizes (>2.5 Gy), the incidence and severity of toxicity is unpredictable according to QUANTEC [63]. The European Particle Therapy Network (EPTN) proposes $V_{60\,Gy} \leq 3$ cc in EQD_2 based on the relevant literature. The α/β ratio is proposed as 2 Gy for radionecrosis [64].

The cognitive deterioration is another serious delayed late toxicity of brain irradiation. Children are more susceptible to radiation-induced cognitive decline than adults. The neurocognitive decline caused by cranial RT has been studied in several settings for children. Cognitive changes occur after ≥ 18 Gy to the entire brain in children. There is some evidence that different regions of the brain, particularly the supratentorial area, are more vulnerable to radiation-induced cognitive deterioration [63]. The effect of irradiation on the cognitive performance of adults is less well defined. There is very limited evidence with respect to the cognitive decline in adult patients with using 2 Gy per fractions.

For radiosurgery, the incidence of necrosis depends on the dose, volume, and region irradiated. The Radiation Therapy Oncology Group (RTOG) conducted a dose-escalation study that sought to define the maximal dose for targets of different sizes; all subjects had previously undergone whole brain irradiation. The maximum tolerated doses were found as 24 Gy, 18 Gy, and 15 Gy for tumors ≤20 mm, 21–30 mm, and 31–40 mm in maximum diameter, respectively [65]. The rates of acute and late unacceptable toxicities in patients treated with these doses were 0 and 10% and 0 and 20%, respectively. The volume of brain receiving ≥12 Gy has been shown to correlate with both the incidence of radiation necrosis and asymptomatic radiologic changes.

1.4.2 Brain Stem

The brain stem has many basic functions, including regulation of heart rate, breathing, sleeping, and eating. Therefore brainstem damage is a severe and potentially lethal complication and can present as a wide spectrum of clinical features depending on the location and the extent of the damage.

Emami et al. defined TD5/5 for the brainstem necrosis as 50 Gy, 53 Gy, and 60 Gy when the entire, 2/3 and 1/3 of the brainstem are treated, respectively [60]. The $TD_{50/5}$ of the entire brainstem was estimated as 65 Gy. Based on the available clinical evidence it seems to be reasonable to treat entire brainstem up to 54 Gy using conventional fractionation [66, 67]. Smaller volumes of the brainstem (1–10 mL) may be irradiated to maximum doses of 59 Gy with 2 Gy/daily fraction doses; however, the risk appears to increase markedly for $D_{max} > 64$ Gy [66, 68]. According to EPTN guideline, $D_{0.03cc}$ is suggested as $\leq$54 Gy in $EQD2_2$, in particular to the interior of the brainstem. Whenever institutions opt to use higher doses, they recommend that $D_{0.03cc}$ of the brainstem surface should be kept at 60 Gy $EQD2_2$. According to AAPM report 101, in SRS, three fractions of SCRT and five fractions of SCRT $V_{0.5cc}$ of the brainstem should be <10 Gy, 18 Gy, and 23 Gy, respectively. The maximum point doses of the brainstem is recommended as 15 Gy, 23 Gy, and 31 Gy for SRS, three fractions of SCRT and five fractions of SCRT, respectively [64]. There is no evidence that the tolerance of the children differ from the adult.

1.4.3 Spinal Cord

Radiation-induced spinal cord injury can result in paralysis, sensory deficits, pain, and bowel/bladder incontinence. Radiation myelopathy may present as a transient early delayed or late delayed reaction. The incidence of radiation myelopathy correlates with the total radiation dose, dose per fraction, and the length of spinal cord irradiated [69].

Emami et al. defined the tolerance dose for the spinal cord in conventionally fractionated radiation therapy, to be 50 Gy for cord lengths of 5 and 10 cm, and 47 Gy for 20 cm, given a probability of myelopathy of less than 5% within 5 years. TD50/5 was defined as 70 Gy for both 5 and 10 cm. The end point is myelitis and necrosis [60]. Radiation myelopathy is rare at doses below 50 Gy, and the dose required to produce a 5% risk of causing this dreaded complication is probably near 60 cGy with conventional fractionation. If other-than-conventional fraction sizes are used, the dose levels required to produce this risk are different, and in practice there are well-defined methods to adjust prescribed doses accordingly to maintain a low risk.

Schultheiss published an article with respect to the de novo irradiation to the spinal cord [70]. In this article it is reported that the probabilities of myelopathy were 0.03%, 0.2%, and 5% at 45 Gy, 50 Gy, and 59.3 Gy, respectively. According to QUANTEC using conventional fractionation of 1.8–2 Gy/fraction to the full-thickness cord, the estimated risk of myelopathy is <1% and <10% at 54 Gy and 61 Gy, respectively, with strong dependence on dose/fraction (alpha/beta = 0.87 Gy) [69]. The risk of reported myelopathy involving full cord cross-section is 0.2, 6, and 50% for D_{max} doses of 55 Gy, 60 Gy, and 69 Gy, respectively. Reports of myelopathy from SRS to spinal lesions appear rare (<1%) when the maximum spinal cord dose is limited to 13 Gy in a single fraction or 20 Gy in three fractions. For single fraction

SBRT, Ryu et al. reported a partial volume tolerance of the human spinal cord of at least 10 Gy to 10% of the spinal cord volume when spinal cord volume was defined from 6 mm above and to 6 mm below the treatment target [71]. Sahgal et al. suggested 10 Gy as the maximum safe threshold for single fraction SBRT to the thecal sac [72]. In RTOG 0631 study, the spinal cord dose constraints were D10 and D0.35cc of 10 Gy and D_{max} of 14 Gy for the involved spine [73].

1.4.4 Orbita (Eye, Retina, Lens)

Partial or total orbital irradiation may lead various clinical scenarios from transient erythema of peri-orbital skin to permanent blindness, with or without loss of the globe. When establishing dose-effects data, it is very crucial to distinguish between single and a few large radiation fractions versus multiple small fractions. Larger fractions are generally more damaging than the same dose delivered with conventional irradiation. The overall treatment time and the relative biological effectiveness (RBE) of the radiation are also important. Keratitis, edema, and small ulcers can occur after 30 Gy when large fractions, for example, 10 Gy are used but are avoided when conventional fractionation is used up to 50 Gy [49].

Loss of eye lashes is usually encountered with doses >20 Gy in conventional fractionation; however, it can occur with 10 Gy delivered over 3 days. Higher RT doses such as >50 Gy with conventional fractionation may lead to moist desquamation, secondary infection, and consequential long-term scarring as a result of non-healing ulceration [74]. Symptoms and signs of RT-induced conjunctivitis include conjunctival injection, watering, and discomfort. Acute conjunctivitis is common with doses ≥30 Gy and was observed in 46% of patients treated for orbital lymphoma to a median dose of 27 Gy. Furthermore total doses ≥35 Gy resulted in a significant incidence in late complications [75]. Chronic conjunctivitis, conjunctival keratinization, and squamous metaplasia may be seen after doses exceeding 50 Gy and in doses >60 Gy permanent scarring of the conjunctiva may cause symblepharon [74].

Radiation-induced lacrimal gland injury may cause impairment of tear production, which eventually lead to dry eye syndrome. The dry eye syndrome can progress to visual loss secondary to corneal opacification, ulceration, and vascularization. The risk of atrophy and fibrosis of the lacrimal gland increases sharply with doses ≥50 Gy in conventional fractionation. RT doses of >60 Gy, can cause permanent loss of secretion of tears and lead to profound keratoconjunctivitis sicca [74]. Emami et al. suggested the TD 5/5 and TD50/5 of the gland to be 35 Gy and, 50 Gy, respectively [60]. It is estimated that the risk of radiation-induced lacrimal gland atrophy and fibrosis is negligible with $D_{max} < 30$ Gy, with a steeply increasing risk >40 Gy, and a 100% rate of severe dry eye with $D_{max} > 57$–60 Gy [74, 76]. The EPTN consensus group stated that the mean dose of the lacrimal gland (Dmean) should not exceed 25 Gy. There are no data with respect to the α/β value of the lacrimal gland; however, it is suggested as 3 Gy for late toxicity similar to that of parotid gland [64].

Corneal edema has been reported after 40–50 Gy, resulting from loss of the intact epithelial barrier or endothelial dysfunction. Corneal ulceration has been reported with radiation doses of >60 Gy with conventional fractionation and with 20 Gy delivered in a single fraction [77, 78]. It has been estimated that the corneal TD of 50/5 is 50 Gy with conventional fractionation, and with hypofractionated treatments, the TD 5/5 may be 30 Gy or less depending on the schedule used. EPTN proposes that the $D_{0.03cc}$ to the cornea should not exceed 50 Gy, and α/β value of the cornea is estimated as three for late toxicity [64].

The retina is a part of the CNS, and expresses RT toxicity as a late-reacting tissue. Clinically radiation retinopathy mimics diabetic retinopathy, hypertensive retinopathy, and leukemic retinopathy since all have microaneurysms, cotton wool pots, capillary dilatation, telangiectasia, and capillary closure histolopathologically. Occasionally 35 Gy of total doses may result in clinically detectable vascular damage. The risk of retinopathy increases when D_{max} is >45–50 Gy with conventional fractionation. Emami et al. suggest that the TD 5/5 and TD50/5 of retina as 45 Gy and 65 Gy, respectively [60]. The EPTN consensus group proposes the $D_{0.03cc}$ of the retina should be kept below 45 Gy. They estimate an α/β value of 3 Gy for late toxicity of the retina [64].

According to Emami et al. the end point chosen for complication of the lens is formation of cataract which requires surgical intervention. Emami et al. suggest that the $TD_{5/5}$ and $TD_{50/5}$ of lens is 10 Gy and 18 Gy, respectively [60]. An increased risk of cataract is associated with increasing fraction size and shorter overall treatment time. Recently, the International Commission on Radiological Protection (ICRP) defined 0.5 Gy as the new threshold dose for lens opacities, which is based on the data from population based studies in diagnostic imaging and occupational exposure [78]. The EPTN consensus group proposes the $D_{0.03cc}$ to the lens to be kept below 10 Gy. They estimate α/β value of 1 Gy for late toxicity of the lens in the absence of solid data [64]. Recommended maximum dose constraints for adult patients range between 5–10 Gy.

1.4.5   Optic Pathway

Radiation-induced optic neuropathy was first described in 1956 by Forrest et al. [79]. Emami et al. suggested a TD5/5 of 50 Gy and a TD50/5 of 65 Gy [60]. The QUANTEC proposed that that the incidence of radiation-induced optic neuropathy was unusual for a D_{max} <55 Gy using conventional fractionation and the risk of toxicity markedly increases at doses >60 Gy. In the region between 55 and 60 Gy with conventional fractionation, the optic neuropathy risk is approximately 3–7% [80]. The only exception of the QUANTEC data is for patients with pituitary tumors, where the toxicity has been reported at doses as low as 45 Gy in 1.8 Gy/fraction. There is strong evidence that the radiation tolerance to optic nerve is increased with a reduction in fraction dose. The estimated dose limit for SRS is 12 Gy. For SRS, in the dose range of 8–12 Gy, radiation-induced optic neuropathy is rare; however, the risk becomes >10% when the dose is increased to 12–15 Gy. For particle therapy the accepted D_{max} value for the radiation-induced optic neuropathy is <54 Gy (RBE). The EPTN group supports the use of $D_{0.03}$ as 55 Gy for the optic nerve and suggests using an α/β ratio of 2 Gy for late toxicity [74].

The clinical outcome of the optic chiasm toxicity is bitemporal hemianopsia or total blindness instead of unilateral visual loss. The constraints for chiasm are as following: maximum dose less than 54 Gy, as primary criteria since the radiation-induced optic neuropathy is unusual for does <55 Gy, less than 60 Gy as secondary criteria, since the optic neuropathy risk is <7% for doses ≤60 Gy [13]. The EPTN group supports the use of $D_{0.03}$ as 55 Gy for the optic chiasm and suggests using an α/β ratio of 2 Gy for late toxicity [74].

1.4.6 Hippocampus

In the QUANTEC there was insufficient evidence with respect to the hippocampal dose constraints, due to the lack of detailed brain dose-volume data. Gondi et al. found that doses greater than 7.3 Gy to 40% of the bilateral hippocampus were associated with impaired memory function in a small retrospective series of 18 patients affected by low-grade adult brain tumors [81]. In another study by Gondi et al. (RTOG 0933) the hippocampal sparing whole brain RT yielded preservation of quality of life and memory [82]. In this study, dose to 100% of the hippocampus could not exceed 9 Gy, and maximal hippocampal dose could not exceed 16 Gy in ten fractions. Many studies are currently underway, investigating hippocampal avoidance in several clinical settings; however, we are still awaiting results. Imaging studies have revealed that doses exceeding 40 Gy resulted in significant atrophy of the hippocampus. The EPTN consensus for hippocampal dose constraint is that D40% of both hippocampi combined should be kept below 7.3 Gy, and accepted α/β ratio is 2 Gy [74].

1.4.7 Pituitary Gland

The somatotroph axis is the most vulnerable and isolated GH deficiency may occur with doses as low as 18 Gy. The impairment of GH production occurs in 30% of patients who receive 30 Gy, and in 50% of patients who receive doses between 30 and 50 Gy. Gonadotrophin deficiency is usually a long-term complication following a radiation dose of 30–40 Gy with a cumulative incidence of 20–50% after long-term follow-up. In contrast, irradiation may cause premature activation of the hypothalamus–pituitary–gonadal axis resulting in precocious puberty after doses of 30 Gy. TSH and ACTH deficiency occur after doses >30 Gy with a long-term cumulative frequency of 3–9% but the frequency may significantly increase in the long-term follow-up if the doses are higher than 50 Gy. Hyperprolactinemia, due to a radiation-induced reduction in the inhibitory neurotransmitter dopamine, has been described in female adults treated with radiation doses >40 Gy [13, 58]. The EPTN consensus panel proposes a Dmean of 45 Gy to the pituitary gland for the prevention of panhypopituitarism and accepted α/β ratio is 2 Gy for late toxicity [64]. There is no currently available dose limits for the hypothalamus.

Data referring to the development of hypopituitarism related to gamma knife radiosurgery shows that keeping the mean radiation dose to the pituitary under 15 Gy and the dose to the distal infundibulum under 17 Gy may prevent the development of radiation-induced hypopituitarism [83].

1.5 Treatment

As discussed above, the progressive damage to the CNS after irradiation is increasingly thought to be caused by radiation-induced and long-lived free radicals, ROS, and pro-inflammatory cytokines, resulting in a deterioration of neurological function. Strategies aimed at blocking effector molecules or otherwise reducing oxidative stress are attractive for preventing or mitigating radiation-induced CNS toxicity. One approach to impeding the actions of reactive oxidants is to administer drugs that induce endogenous antioxidant biochemical processes. Several drugs which block pro-inflammatory cytokines and ROS are currently available and in wide clinical use including angiotensin-converting enzyme (ACE) inhibitors, statins, superoxide dismutase (SOD) mimetics, VEGF inhibitors, COX-2 inhibitors, inhibitors of pro-inflammatory cytokines (e.g., halofuginone), and stem cell mobilizers (e.g., granulocyte colony stimulating factor, G-CSF) [19].

Another way for decreasing radiation-induced CNS toxicity in the clinic is the organ sparing approach. Attempts at sparing brain sub-compartments from injury are extrapolated from whole brain RT studies. RTOG 0933 used IMRT to spare the neural stem cell population in the adult hippocampus in patients receiving whole brain RT for brain metastases. At 4 months after the treatment, a limited benefit in memory and quality of life in the short term was demonstrated [82]. However, it is unknown what other neurocognitive parameters might be affected by hippocampal sparing. Therefore, a phase III randomized trial evaluating the effects of hippocampal sparing is ongoing.

1.5.1 Brain

Acute effects are characterized by symptoms of fatigue, dizziness, and signs of increased intracranial pressure. The acute effects are considered to be secondary to edema and disruption of the blood–brain barrier (BBB). Other common acute reactions associated with brain irradiation include hair loss and skin edema. Acute side effects occurring during standard fractionated brain RT using contemporary techniques are typically mild and manageable with basic supportive care.

The onset of fatigue is generally several weeks after the first radiation treatment. Up to 90% of patients undergoing partial brain irradiation for glioblastoma experience at least grade 1 symptoms (disturbance with some tiredness, but activity not curtailed), and approximately half experience mild to moderate symptoms (decreased activity and increased tiredness, sleeping much of the day, most activities curtailed). Symptoms typically begin by 2 weeks from the start of RT, peak at the end of the treatment course or within one to 2 weeks after treatment completion, and then slowly resolve over the next several months. Typically, the fatigue persists for several months after the completion of RT; however, it may be chronic in a small percentage of patients. One characteristic feature of the radiation-associated fatigue is lack of improvement with rest. Somnolence syndrome, which is a rare condition after partial brain irradiation, is defined by a cluster of symptoms including drowsiness, clumsiness, lethargy, and slow mental processing. The syndrome has been reported to occur in 13–79% of patients [84, 85]. The symptoms typically peak in severity 6 weeks following irradiation, and can continue for another 6 weeks.

In a randomized double-blind study of prophylactic d-threo-methylphenidate HCl (d-MPH) vs. placebo in 68 patients with primary or metastatic brain tumors undergoing cranial RT there was no difference in fatigue or quality of life levels between the two groups [86, 87]. Neither progestational steroids nor paroxetine were found to be superior to placebo in the treatment of cancer-related fatigue. It has been suggested that corticosteroid use during cranial irradiation may reduce somnolence symptoms; however, the benefit of corticosteroids in preventing the occurrence or reducing the severity of somnolence syndrome remains controversial.

Although there are limited data with respect to the use of methylphenidate (Ritalin) during RT, it can be used during whole brain RT with a usual dose of 10 mg bid, escalating to 30 mg bid in 1–2 weeks if tolerated. In a double-blind trial that was terminated prematurely, 68 patients with primary or metastatic brain tumors were randomly assigned to methylphenidate or placebo during RT [88]. After 8 weeks, there was no difference in fatigue or cognition compared to placebo. Another drug that may be used in radiation-induced fatigue is modafinil; however, there are limited and conflicting data on the use of it [89].

Hair loss and radiation dermatitis are also common acute side effects of cranial irradiation. Temporary alopecia is a dose-dependent treatment effect that occurs approximately 2–3 weeks after radiation exposure and usually resolves within 2–3 months after completion of RT. The severity and permanence of alopecia is directly related to dose. Doses, as low as 2 Gy in a single fraction have been shown to cause temporary alopecia [90]. There is no any effective treatment for the prevention of the radiation-induced hair loss or acceleration of hair re-growth.

Radiation dermatitis due to cranial irradiation is usually mild and may be treated with soothing moisturizers. The treatment methods for acute radiation-induced dermatitis include steroid treatment, creams, ointments, and hydrocolloid dressings, depending on the reaction grading. Typically 1% hydrocortisone or Aquaphor is needed for patient comfort. Rarely, areas of skin receiving particularly high doses may demonstrate dry or moist desquamation that may benefit from bacteriostatic topical treatments. Moist desquamation behind the ears and external auditory canals may develop following whole brain irradiation. In addition to topical agents cortisporin otic suspension helps to improve the symptoms [89, 91].

Mild headaches during cranial irradiation may be encountered and often patients do not require medication. For headaches that are more severe, acetaminophen is typically adequate to resolve the symptom. Another reason for headache may be mass effect from tumor. The headache from mass effect is important to differentiate as the management is different. Progression of neurologic deficits and new or worsening somnolence, together with headaches, may signal increased peritumoral edema and/or tumor progression. Glucocorticoids, to reduce cerebral pressure, are the primary approach when cerebral edema and tumor mass effect are suspected, rather than pain medications. Patients with recognized significant pretreatment cerebral edema should begin oral or parenteral glucocorticoids (e.g., dexamethasone 2–4 mg daily) prior to initiating radiation. Maintaining the dose for the first 2 weeks of RT can prevent clinical deterioration due to transiently worsened peritumoral edema. An increase in glucocorticoid dose is sometimes beneficial if symptoms worsen during the course of radiation treatment due to reactive cerebral edema. Nausea and vomiting may occur occasionally as a side effect of cranial irradiation. Antiemetics or corticosteroids are used to prevent or mitigate symptoms.

Early delayed effects occur 6–12 weeks post-irradiation which include persistent fatigue and transient focal neurologic symptoms. There are no known interventions or therapies to prevent or treat the early delayed reactions of the brain.

Late radiation-induced brain toxicities occur after 90 days of irradiation and include headache, lethargy, and severe CNS dysfunction including partial loss of motor power, dyskinesia, and coma. The late delayed effects may lead to severe irreversible neurological consequences.

Radiation necrosis is a serious complication that typically develops 1–3 years after radiation, although the range is quite broad and cases have been reported more than 10 years after radiation. Radiation necrosis may be associated with focal neurological signs such as seizures, dysfunction of the cranial nerves, and increased intracranial pressure caused by the persistent vasogenic edema resulting from BBB damage. In MRI scans it manifests as diffuse non-specific changes in white matter. Tissue necrosis typically develops at or adjacent to the original site of tumor, the location that receives the highest radiation dose. The clinical course of brain necrosis is highly variable [92]. Management is primarily symptomatic. The treatment decisions require a balance between the often-competing goals of symptom control and avoidance of side effects. Patients who are symptomatic due to vasogenic edema and associated mass effect are commonly managed with a moderate dose of corticosteroids. Once symptoms are controlled, glucocorticoids can then be gradually tapered over the course of several weeks. Follow-up imaging after one to 2 months is generally recommended. Traditionally, physicians have tried to combat CNS radiation necrosis with antiplatelet agents, anticoagulants, and high-dose vitamins; however, none of these approaches has proved to be effective in controlled clinical trials. More recently, the VEGF-A monoclonal antibody bevacizumab (Avastin) has shown some promise in reversing neurological symptoms and radiographic changes in patients with radiation necrosis [92–94]. Surgical resection of the necrotic tissue is sometimes required, particularly in cases in which there is diagnostic uncertainty as to whether the radiographic changes are indicative of tumor progression or treatment-induced tissue necrosis, or in patients with severe necrosis who cannot use bevacizumab. Surgery can provide palliative benefit by reducing the mass effect and decreasing the steroid requirements postoperatively. Therapeutic anticoagulation, antiplatelet therapy, and hyperbaric oxygen therapy have been reported to provide benefit in small case series but their efficacy has not been established prospectively yet [95, 96].

Cranial irradiation, particularly whole brain RT, has been shown to result in a spectrum of neurocognitive deficits in children and in adults. Although historically considered a late side effect, cognitive deterioration resulting from whole brain RT has been shown to appear as early as 3–4 months after RT [97–100].

Cognitive dysfunction, may be encountered with total doses as low as 20 Gy in adults and 24 Gy in children given with conventional fractions of 1.8–2 Gy. Symptoms range from cognitive slowing, poor concentration, difficulty in multitasking, decreased short-term and later eventually long-term memory, word-finding problems, and decreased IQ (particularly in children), to a progressive Alzheimer's-like dementia, which is also characterized by urinary incontinence and gait disturbance [89]. Several pharmacologic interventions have been tested in randomized trials to minimize or improve cognitive function in patients treated with focal or whole brain radiation; however, the results are conflicting. Lacking better options, drugs such as methylphenidate and donepezil, are generally well tolerated and may be beneficial in a subset of patients, along with neurocognitive rehabilitation aiming compensatory strategies. There are also some preventive strategies such as hippocampus sparing RT and the use of concomitant memantine, an oral N-methyl-D-aspartate (NMDA) receptor antagonist. The cognitive dysfunction related to cranial irradiation will be discussed in hippocampus part in detail [97].

1.5.2 Brain Stem

Radiation-related brain stem toxicity can be managed as the radiation-related brain toxicity.

1.5.3 Spinal Cord

Radiation-induced spinal cord injury has been described with several syndromes, the most prominent of which are a self-limited transient myelopathy and the more serious chronic progressive myelopathy. Acute paralysis secondary to ischemia, hemorrhage within the spinal cord, and lower motor neuron syndrome, are much less common disabling manifestations of radiation injury. Factors that decrease the spinal cord tolerance to radiation include prior spinal cord pathology, combination chemotherapy, and immunocompromised status [101].

Although acute CNS injury has been reported following acute brain RT, there is no experimental or clinical evidence that radiation induces acute spinal cord toxicity.

The most common early delayed side effect of the spinal cord is transient myelopathy, particularly in the cervical and thoracic spine. Although it is difficult to estimate the incidence of Lhermitte's sign, it is reported as 4–10% in two large observational series in patients with Hodgkin lymphoma and nasopharyngeal cancer. An increased risk of developing Lhermitte's sign was demonstrated for patients who received either ≥ 2 Gy per fraction (one fraction per day) or ≥ 50 Gy total dose to the cervical spinal cord [102, 103]. The Lhermitte's sign manifests as a shock-like sensation radiating down the spine with neck flexion. It is a self-limiting condition and most patients improve during the course of several months to year, without any medication. Although Lhermitte's sign is rarely a precursor of myelitis, there have been some reports of patients who developed radiation myelopathy following Lhermitte's sign. In general, the Lhermitte's sign that predated true radiation myelitis was later in onset than the usual latency period of 2–4 months [46]. Besides ionizing radiation, demyelinating diseases including multiple sclerosis, vitamin B12 deficiency, and structural abnormalities of the spinal canal may cause Lhermitte's sign. No active intervention is required and the syndrome usually resolves spontaneously over a period of months to a year. If the discomfort is severe, carbamazepine, pregabalin or gabapentin may be beneficial. In a randomized, placebo-controlled, double-blind trial of 128 head and neck cancer survivors the benefit for pregabalin alone in the treatment of radiation -related neuropathic pain was evaluated [104]. The authors found that the patients who received pregabalin had greater pain alleviation, better mood states, and higher quality of life compared with patients in the placebo group.

Late effects to the spinal cord are less common and more severe than acute and early delayed effects. Late injury to the spinal cord typically presents as a chronic, progressive myelopathy, initially as partial cord involvement and progressing to a total transverse myelopathy. Unlike transient myelopathy, it is usually irreversible. The differential diagnosis includes epidural spinal cord compression, intramedullary metastasis, and paraneoplastic necrotic myelopathy. There is no treatment with established benefit. The most common first treatment for chronic progressive radiation myelopathy is glucocorticoid. Symptomatically, some patients will respond at least partially to a trial of glucocorticoids. The lowest effective doses should be used and in unresponsive patients steroids should be tapered. Other strategies have been extensively studied in preclinical settings but have little clinical data to support their use. The strongest supporting evidence is for anti-angiogenic agents such as bevacizumab. In a randomized trial for CNS radiation necrosis, the majority of the bevacizumab-treated patients showed improvement in clinical symptoms and signs and a reduction in the volume of necrosis on T2-weighted FLAIR and T1-weighted gadolinium-contrast MR [105].

For the prevention of radiation myelopathy several agents including hyperbaric oxygen, anticoagulation with heparin and warfarin, vitamin E, magnesium, and growth factors (e.g., platelet-derived growth factor, insulin like growth factor 1, vascular endothelial growth factor, and basic fibroblast growth factor) have been studied; however, there is no clinically-proven strategy to prevent the onset of radiation myelopathy [95, 106].

There are also some other delayed injuries of the spinal cord, which are encountered rarely; however, deserves mentioning are lower motor neuron syndrome (LMNS), as a hemorrhagic injury from a radiation-induced telangiectasia, and cavernous angioma. The LMNS is a disorder that follows radiation therapy by 3–25 years. The earliest descriptions of the LMNS date back to World War II. Patients slowly develop progressive weakness of lower extremities with little or no sensory loss and normal, or almost normal, bladder and bowel function. Radiation-related LMNS was originally thought to reflect damage to the anterior horn cells; it is in fact, a radiculopathy rather than a neuronopathy. The differential diagnosis of post-irradiation LMNS includes neural infiltration by recurrent neoplasm and nerve sheath tumors. Many patients remain ambulatory for many years although weakness continues to progress. There is no known cure for this condition [107]. Damage to spinal cord blood vessels can lead to telangiectasia and even cavernous malformations, which can result in an acute hemorrhage. There is usually sudden onset of weakness and sensory change, sometimes associated with pain. The MRI shows evidence of acute hemorrhage. Patients usually recover [108, 109].

1.5.4   Orbita (Eye, Retina, Lens)

Radiation-induced clinical syndromes of the lid and ocular adnexa encompass a wide spectrum, from transient lid erythema and a mild conjunctivitis to corneal perforation and loss of the globe [49].

The periocular skin undergoes acute and late phase reactions following radiotherapy. Radiation dermatitis and madarosis are classed as acute effects, whereas telangiectasia, skin atrophy, and depigmentation present as late effects. The initial reaction is seen within 2 weeks of fractionated RT. The aim of the treatment of the radiation- induced periocular skin changes is aimed at improving patient comfort and preserving the integrity of the globe. The optimal treatment of the radiation-induced cutaneous eyelid toxicity including atrophy, cutaneous telangiectasia, and madarosis (permanent hair loss) is uncertain; however, ensuring cleanliness, using appropriate dressings for moist desquamation, and allowing time for healing are all suggested. Corticosteroid cream may improve erythema, but aqueous or sucralfate creams are no better than washing with mild soap and water. The use of artificial tears may be partially effective in Meibomian gland dysfunction. Trichiasis and distichiasis can be effectively managed by using epilation, electrolysis, cryotherapy, argon laser ablation, or surgery. Ectropion and entropion may be surgically treated by restoring eyelid tension, reapposing the lid, and restoring appropriate direction of tear flow [74]. The ruby laser and radiofrequency ablation are also effective treatment options for trichiasis [110].

Xerophthalmia occurs due to damage of glands within the eyelid, decreased conjunctival mucous production, and reduced lacrimal gland secretion. Early effects are conjunctival inflammation, chemosis, and tear film instability with a resultant dry eye sensation. These generally subside but may, on occasion, be persistent. The evidence-based treatment options for the radiation-induced conjunctivitis are relatively unknown because of limited number of publications about the topic. Preservative-free artificial tears administered 4–8 times daily may relieve irritation. Unless there is no strong evidence of bacterial infection, topical antibiotics should be avoided since may aggravate conjunctival injection. Viral conjunctivitis may be effectively treated with artificial tears and a topical antiviral agent. Bacterial conjunctivitis may be treated with a topical broad-spectrum antibiotic selected according to local antibiotic guidelines, unless a specific organism is cultured. In case of metaplastic conjunctiva, excision with buccal mucosa graft may be suggested [74]. Topical retinoic acid ointment may reverse conjunctival keratinization due to squamous metaplasia [111].

Radiation-induced lacrimal gland damage may cause dry eye syndrome, which can progress to visual loss secondary to corneal opacification, ulceration, and vascularization. In order to prevent radiation-induced lacrimal gland injury, lacrimal shielding can be used in appropriate patients. For the patients with radiation-induced xerophthalmia topical lubricants, cautery to retain tears, moist chamber goggles, punctual occlusion with plugs, or tarsorrhaphy may be recommended. There is no proven difference in efficacy between different topical dry eye treatments, including artificial tears (saline, hypromellose, and others), ocular lubricants (polyacrylic or hyaluronic acid), and gels [74, 112]. Moist chamber goggles are effective in patients with keratoconjunctivitis sicca, as they increase humidity and prevent evaporation. However, goggles are rarely worn continually, for cosmetic reasons. In patients with dry eye syndrome contact lenses should be avoided as they can further exacerbate dry eye symptoms. Novel treatment options including autologous serum eye drops are effective for treating severe drying of the ocular surface [113].

Radiation-induced corneal injury may result in corneal edema, keratitis sicca, punctate epithelial erosions, and corneal ulceration. These side effects may be prevented with using internal eye shields in appropriate patients. There is limited evidence with respect to the management of corneal toxicities following RT. Punctate epithelial erosions may be encouraged to heal by using topical lubrication to prevent ulceration. Close ophthalmological monitoring is recommended in moderate to severe cases when topical steroids and antibiotics may be required to relieve discomfort and treat infection, respectively. Hypertonic saline ointment and topical steroids can often improve or resolve corneal edema, but long-term steroid use should be avoided as this can cause extracellular matrix breakdown. Persistent, painful corneal edema may require a bandage contact lens or penetrating keratoplasty (corneal graft) [74].

The sclera is predominantly the avascular part of the eye, and is therefore more radioresistant than other ocular tissues. However, scleral atrophy and necrosis have been reported [114]. In addition scleral atrophy may be complicated by corneoscleritis and endophthalmitis with bacterial or fungal organisms. In case of infection topical antibiotics or antifungals may be required.

Acute complications of the anterior chamber including transient early iritis and iridocyclitis are rarely encountered. Late reactions are rarely seen since iris is relatively radioresistant. However, severe persistent iritis has been observed after hypofractionated RT doses of 30–40 Gy and after doses ≥70 Gy given with conventional fractionation [74, 115]. Neovascular glaucoma is also a late severe complication of the eyes. Sparing the anterior chamber is an important strategy in appropriate patients. The patients with diabetes should be carefully followed-up with respect to iritis and neovascular glaucoma. The primary treatments for iritis and neovascular glaucoma are topical steroids and cycloplegic drops, respectively. If performed early, laser panretinal photocoagulation (PRP) or peripheral cryotherapy may regress the new iris vessel formation and prevent the progression of glaucoma. If the disease progress the changes cannot be reversed with using PRP. Intravitreal bevacizumab along with the standard ablative treatments options seems to be promising for the management of iris neovascularization associated with neovascular glaucoma. Neovascular glaucoma may rarely progress to blind and painful eye, if so the blind eye may be enucleated. The resultant secondary glaucoma is often refractory to pharmacological management and requires surgical intervention including trabeculectomy [74].

Radiation-induced acute lens toxicity is not reported. Cataract is a well-known late complication of the ionizing irradiation. Radiation cataract usually presents first as a posterior subcapsular opacification; however, in some cases an anterior subcapsular change is noted initially. Often there is a delayed onset, especially with low dose exposure. Lens opacities may remain stable for years, and later progress to a mature cataract. Cataract development is strongly correlated with the chronic use of steroids in these patients. Cataract risk may be reduced with using lens shielding in appropriate situations. IMRT may be used to reduce cataract risk. Additionally there is some evidence that administration of heparin may have a protective effect [116]. The treatment is the same as in nonradiation-induced cataracts, namely cataract removal and prosthetic lens placement. Pars plana lensectomy, vitrectomy, and simultaneous intraocular lens implantation are effective for RT induced-cataracts in children [74].

The retina is a part of the CNS, and expresses RT toxicity as a late-reacting tissue. Acute retinal toxicity during RT is not reported. Radiation retinopathy has a delayed presentation as a progressive pattern of degenerative and proliferative vascular changes. The signs include capillary occlusion, dilatation, microaneurysm formation, telangiectasia, intraretinal microvascular abnormalities, neovascularization, and retinal pigment epithelial changes. Visual symptoms depend on the anatomic site of retinopathy and its severity. The complications of the radiation-related retinopathy include vitreous hemorrhage, retinal detachment, and macular edema. The latency between RT and onset of clinically significant retinopathy can range from 1 month to 15 years, but most commonly occurs between 6 months and 3 years. The onset is more rapid where treatment regimens involve high-dose, single-fraction radiotherapy. Clinically significant retinopathy risk may be reduced by minimizing the volume of the irradiated retina, delivering fully fractionated RT to the lowest effective dose, and by excluding the macula from the high-dose region if possible. Unfortunately no proven therapy exists for radiation retinopathy. The studies evaluating the role of hyperbaric oxygen, intravitreal triamcinolone, and laser photocoagulation therapy have been studied; however, none of them had promising results.

Vitreous hemorrhage and retinal detachment can be managed by vitrectomy and retinal detachment surgery [117, 118].

1.5.5 Optic Pathway

Acute optic nerve toxicity is not reported during RT. Radiation-induced optic neuropathy, which is first described by Forest et al., presents as painless, monocular loss of vision that is sudden, but may follow transient episodes of blurring [119]. Optic neuropathy typically develops over one to several weeks and beginning around 6–24 months after radiation. The incidence of mild, transient radiation effects on the optic nerves is not well reported. There are limited studies evaluating the role of anticoagulation therapy, systemic corticosteroids or hyperbaric oxygen therapy for the treatment of radiation-induced optic neuropathy, particularly for the acute phase; however, none of them could show a benefit. At present, there is no proven effective treatment for radiation-induced optic neuropathy; however, the risk of may be minimized by using the lowest effective total dose, prescribing a low dose per fraction, and by constraining the volume of optic nerve irradiated. Newer therapies including intravitreal triamcinolone acetonide injections and bevacizumab have shown promise in preventing visual loss from anterior optic neuropathy. High-dose losartan which is an angiotensin 1 receptor blocker and ramipril alleviate radiation-induced optic neuropathy and preserve the functional integrity of the optic nerve, but these therapies remain unproven [74].

1.5.6 Hippocampus

The hippocampus is critical in memory formation and learning, and is extraordinarily sensitive to cranial RT, with even low doses of ionizing radiation demonstrating a significant reduction in neurogenesis and deficits in memory. Cranial irradiation can result in a spectrum of neurocognitive deficits in the years following treatment in children and in adults. Important data on the impact of RT on neurocognitive function have been derived from studies in adults with primary brain tumors and brain metastases, as well as in survivors of childhood malignancies [97].

Pharmacological treatment may be an appropriate intervention in order to improve cognition in patients previously treated for cancer. However, the data to support its use are limited, and no randomized clinical trials have been performed. Although formal randomized trials specifically evaluating their impact on cognitive function have not been performed, CNS stimulants, including modafinil and methylphenidate (Ritalin) have been evaluated in patients with cognitive declines. The limited data suggest they may improve cognitive function [88, 97].

More importantly, there are many strategies to reduce the risk of neurocognitive decline after whole brain RT and some of them are still under active investigation (1) hippocampal avoidance RT (2) memantine (3) donepezil (4) anti-inflammatory agents.

1.5.6.1 Hippocampal Avoidance RT

Advanced RT techniques, including IMRT, SRS, SCRT or proton beam therapy, have been suggested as a way to spare neurogenic niches, such as the hippocampus, when treating brain tumor patients. Since the hippocampus is an infrequent site for the brain metastases, in RTOG 0933 study Gondi et al., sought to answer the question whether avoidance of the hippocampus via highly conformal RT techniques resulted in preserved memory function compared with historical controls [82]. This study enrolled a total of 113 patients, and 42 were alive and analyzable at the study endpoint of 4 months. All patients received whole brain RT delivered to a dose of 30 Gy in ten fractions with hippocampal-avoidance. The mean relative decline in the Hopkins Verbal Learning Test-Revised Delayed Recall (HVLT-R DR) from baseline to 4 months was 7%, and it was superior to the prespecified historic comparison value of 30% observed in the control arm of large trial comparing whole brain RT plus motexafin gadolinium with whole brain RT alone [120]. The probability of HVLT-R total recall (HVLT-R TR) deterioration at 4 months was 19%, again it was superior to previous randomized trial of WBRT with or without SRS, in which the probability of HVLT-R TR deterioration at 4 months was 24% in those treated with SRS alone and 52% in those treated with WBRT plus SRS [98].

Although these findings are encouraging, it is a nonrandomized phase II study and the cognitive benefits of hippocampal avoidance need to be proven in a phase III trial. In particular, median overall survival in the trial was superior to prior trials, making it difficult to exclude improved survivorship as an explanation for the apparent improvement in neurocognitive performance. Currently two phase III randomized studies are being conducted investigating the role of hippocampal sparing in the setting of WBRT (NRG CC001) and prophylactic cranial irradiation for small cell lung cancer patients (NRG CC003).

1.5.6.2 Memantine

Glutamate is the principle excitatory amino acid neurotransmitter in cortical and hippocampal neurons. One of the receptors activated by glutamate is the N-methyl-D-aspartate (NMDA) receptor and is involved in learning and memory. Ischemia can induce excessive NMDA stimulation and lead to excitotoxicity, suggesting that agents that block pathologic stimulation of NMDA receptors may protect against further damage in patients with vascular dementia. Recent reports suggest that NMDA receptor antagonists, such as memantine, can protect against further damage in patients with vascular dementia by preventing this excitotoxicity [121, 122]. Memantine gained initial FDA approval in the treatment of Alzheimer's and vascular dementia after two phase III randomized, placebo-controlled trials showing improved cognitive metrics with minimal side effects [123, 124].

Due to the overlapping mechanisms of the neurotoxicity in vascular dementia and radiation-induced vasculopathy, the RTOG 0614 trial examined the role of memantine in the preservation of cognitive function in patients receiving WBRT [125]. In this study, 554 patients were randomly assigned to WBRT and memantine or to WBRT and placebo. Memantine was administered concurrently with 37.5 Gy whole brain RT (15 fractions of 2.5 Gy) at a dose of 5 mg daily and escalated to a final dose of 10 mg delivered twice daily and continued for a total of 24 weeks. The use of memantine during and after whole brain RT resulted in better cognitive function over time, specifically delaying time to cognitive decline and reducing the rates of decline in memory, executive function, and processing speed.

1.5.6.3 Donepezil

Donepezil is a reversible non-competitive acetyl cholinesterase inhibitor that is approved for Alzheimer-type dementia, vascular dementia, multiple sclerosis, and Parkinson's disease [126]. Shaw et al. reported positive results in an open-label phase II study of 34 adult patients with primary and metastatic brain tumors who had undergone a course of partial or whole brain irradiation ≥30 Gy at least 6 months before enrollment and who received donepezil (5 mg per day for 6 weeks followed by 10 mg per day for 18 weeks) for 24 weeks. They observed significant improvements in cognitive functioning (attention, concentration, memory, and verbal fluency), self-reported cognitive problems, mood, fatigue, and quality of life [127]. After this encouraging results, donepezil has been explored in a double-blinded, placebo-controlled trial in patients with a history (≥6 mo prior) of either whole brain or partial brain RT of ≥30 Gy for treatment of either primary or metastatic brain tumors [128]. In this study, both interim and final evaluation failed to demonstrate a significant difference in overall cognitive function with the addition of donepezil, although there were modest improvements in several cognitive functions, especially in patients with greater pretreatment impairments.

1.5.6.4 Anti-Inflammatory Agents

Cranial irradiation induces inflammatory response in the hippocampus which eventually causes reduced neurogenesis and cognitive decline. Non-steroidal anti-inflammatory drugs (NSAIDs) are thought to help with cognitive dysfunction after RT by modulating inflammatory response to RT. Although there are some preclinical studies, clinical trials are needed to establish the role of NSAIDs in radiation-induced cognitive decline [97].

1.5.7 Pituitary Gland

Children treated with RT doses ≥18 Gy to the hypothalamic-pituitary axis are at risk for GH deficiency. Those treated with doses >30 to 40 Gy are at risk for deficiencies of LH, FSH, TSH, and ACTH. The most common abnormality is growth hormone (GH) deficiency (50%), followed by gonadotropin deficiency (25%), hyperprolactinemia (24%), adrenocorticotrophic hormone (ACTH) deficiency (19%), and central hypothyroidism (16%) [13, 58]. Radiation-induced anterior pituitary hormone deficiencies are irreversible and progressive. Regular testing is mandatory to ensure timely diagnosis and early hormone replacement therapy.

Growth hormone deficiency is the first and is frequently the only manifestation of neuro-endocrine injury following cranial irradiation. GH has consistently shown to be the most radiosensitive pituitary axis, with series reporting a prevalence of GH deficiency between 50 and 100% after RT for sellar region irradiation. Radiation-induced GH deficiency is progressive with time, developing more frequently in the first 10 years after radiation delivery. GH replacement therapy is suggested fort the patients with radiation-induced GH deficiency. Guidelines recommend waiting for at least 1 year after completion of cancer-directed therapy before initiating GH treatment [57, 129].

Gonadotropin deficiency may be encountered approximately in 25% of the patients. Childhood cancer survivors are at risk for pubertal derangements including precocious puberty, pubertal delay, and pubertal arrest (hypogonadotropic hypogonadism). For the treatment of precocious puberty it may be beneficial to temporarily suppress the hypothalamic-pituitary-gonadal axis by employing long-acting formulations of GnRH agonists. Pubertal delay or arrest, hypogonadotropic hypogonadism, due to LH and FSH deficiency is also a major problem for childhood survivors. For these patients, treatment with estrogen therapy in females and testosterone in males may be indicated to induce pubertal development [130]. For the adult patients with gonadotropin deficiency adult-dose sex steroid replacement therapy is indicated.

Endocrine Society Guidelines recommend lifelong annual screening for thyroid-stimulating hormone and adrenocorticotropic hormone deficiency in childhood cancer survivors treated for tumors in the region of the hypothalamic–pituitary axis and those exposed to $\geq$30 Gy hypothalamic–pituitary radiation [129]. Lifelong levothyroxine is indicated for patients with TSH deficiency. Serum TSH should be monitored to assess dosing adequacy and medication compliance. Dose should be titrated to maintain normal free T4 levels. Patients with ACTH deficiency require glucocorticoid replacement therapy including hydrocortisone, prednisone, or prednisolone at physiologic doses based on a daily production rate of hydrocortisone of 7 mg/m^2 per day. Patients with diabetes insipidus (DI) due to anti diuretic hormone (ADH) deficiency require hormone replacement with desmopressin acetate [129].

Management of radiation-induced CNS toxicities is summarized in Table 1.3.

1.6   Rx: Sample Prescriptions for CNS Toxicity

1.6.1   Brain and Brain Stem

1.6.1.1 Fatigue
- Methylphenidate (Ritalin®): 10 mg bid, escalating to 30 mg bid in 1–2-week increments as tolerated.

1.6.1.2 Radiation Necrosis
- Glucocorticoid: 4–8 mg of oral dexamethasone (e.g., Kordexa®) daily.
- Bevacizumab: either 7.5 mg/kg every 3 weeks or 5 mg/kg every 2 weeks.
- Anticoagulant: Enoxaparin® 30 mg IV bolus, then 1 mg/kg/day.

Table 1.3 Management of radiation-induced CNS toxicities

Organ	Acute Reactions	Treatment	Chronic Reactions	Treatment
Brain Brain stem	Fatigue	Methylphenidate (Ritalin), Modafinil	Radiation necrosis	Corticosteroids Bevacizumab Antiplatelet agents Anticoagulants Hyperbaric oxygen Laser interstitial thermal therapy Surgical resection of the necrotic tissue
	Hair loss	–	Cognitive deterioration	Methylphenidate Memantine Donepezil Anti-inflammatories Hippocampal sparing RT
	Radiation dermatitis	Topical steroids, moisturizing creams, ointments, hydrocolloid dressings		
	Headache	Acetaminophen, glucocorticoids		
	Nausea and vomiting	Antiemetic, corticosteroids		
Spinal cord	Transient myelopathy (early delayed)	Carbamazepine Gabapentin Pregabalin	Radiation myelopathy	Glucocorticoid Bevacizumab Antiplatelet agents Anticoagulants Hyperbaric oxygen High-dose vitamins Surgery
			Lower motor neuron syndrome	Unknown
			Spinal cord hemorrhage	Unknown

Structure	Acute effects	Acute management	Late effects	Late management
Eyelid	Loss of the eyelashes Xerophthalmia	Artificial tears	Cutaneous telangiectasis atrophy Permanent hair loss, (madarosis) Depigmentation Entropion Ectropion	Corticosteroid Ensuring cleanliness Artificial tear Surgery
			Trichiasis Distichiasis	Epilation Electrolysis Cryotherapy Argon laser ablation Radiofrequency ablation Ruby laser Surgery
Conjunctiva	Conjunctival infection	Artificial tears Topical antibiotics Topical antivirals	Conjunctival telangiectasias Subconjunctival hemorrhage Chronic conjunctivitis	
Lacrimal gland	Dryness of the eye	Artificial tears Topical lubricants	Dry eye syndrome Keratoconjunctivitis sicca Blurred vision Photophobia	Topical lubricants Moist chamber goggles Punctual occlusion with plugs Cautery to retain tears Tarsorrhaphy
Cornea	Corneal edema Keratitis sicca, punctate epithelial erosions	Hypertonic saline ointment Topical steroids Topical lubricants Topical steroids Topical antibiotics	Corneal ulceration Corneal decompensation	Corneal graft
Sclera			Atrophy Necrosis	–

(continued)

Table 1.3 (continued)

Organ	Acute Reactions	Treatment	Chronic Reactions	Treatment
Iris	Iritis Iridocylitis		Persistent iritis Neovascular glaucoma Secondary glaucoma	Topical steroids Cycloplegic drops Laser panretinal photocoagulation (PRP) peripheral cryotherapy Intravitreal bevacizumab Surgical intervention (trabeculectomy)
Lens	–		Cataract	Surgery (Phacoemulsification with artificial lens implantation).
Retina	–		Radiation retinopathy Vitreous hemorrhage retinal detachment	Unknown Surgery Surgery
Optic nerve	–		Optic neuropathy	Systemic steroids Intraocular steroids Heparin Warfarin Anticoagulants Bevacizumab Losartan Ramipril
Hippocampus			Neurocognitive deficits	Hippocampal avoidance whole brain RT (prevention) Memantine (prevention) Donepezil (prevention) Methylphenidate

		Hormone replacement therapy
Pituitary gland	–	Hormonal abnormalities Growth hormone (GH) Luteinizing hormone (LH) Follicle-stimulating hormone (FSH) Thyroid-stimulating hormone (TSH) Adrenocorticotropic hormone (ACTH) Antidiuretic hormone (ADH), also known as vasopressin	

1.6.2 Spinal Cord

1.6.2.1 Radiation Myelopathy
- Glucocorticoids: dexamethasone (e.g., Kordexa®) 4–8 mg per day.
- Gabapentin: Neurontin® 100–300 mg at bedtime.
- Anticoagulant: Enoxaparin® 30 mg IV bolus, then 1 mg/kg/day.

1.6.3 Orbita

1.6.3.1 Viral Conjunctivitis
- Trifluridine, TFT-Thilo®, eye drop, five times daily, for herpes simplex infection.

1.6.3.2 Lacrimal Gland Dry Eye Syndrome
- Artificial tears (saline, hypromellose, and others): Refresh®, TheraTear®, and Systane®.
- Ocular lubricants (polyacrylic or hyaluronic acid): Polyethylene glycol 400® (PG-PEG 400 0.4–0.3% drops: as often as needed); Systane Nighttime Lubricant Eye Ointment: 1–2 times/day.
- Gels: HYLO®-GEL eye drops.

1.6.3.3 Lubricant Antibiotic Ointments
- Erythromycin 0.5% ophthalmic ointment (up to six times a day).
- Polymyxin B trimethoprim (Polytrim) ophthalmic solution (every 3 h (maximum of 6 doses per day) for a period of 7–10 days).
- Sulfacetamide 10% ophthalmic ointment (A small amount (about 1/2 in. ribbon) into the conjunctival sac(s) of the infected eye(s) every 3–4 h and at bedtime) Duration of therapy: 7–10 days.

1.6.4 Radiation-Induced Optic Neuropathy

- Prednisone: Deltacortil® 80 mg/day.

1.6.5 Hippocampus: Neurocognitive Dysfunction

- Memantine: 5 mg daily and escalated to a final dose of 10 mg delivered twice daily and continued for a total of 24 weeks.
- Donepezil: 5 mg/day was given for 6 weeks and then increased to 10 mg/day for 18 weeks (total duration: 24 weeks).

1.6.6 Pituitary Gland: Hormone Replacement Therapy

- ACTH deficiency: glucocorticoid replacement therapy (e.g., hydrocortisone, prednisone, or prednisolone) at physiologic doses based on a daily production rate of hydrocortisone of 7 mg/m²/day (e.g., Cortisone Acetate 25 mg q AM, 12.5 mg q3PM).
- TSH deficiency: Levothyroxine (Synthroid®) 1.6 mg/kg daily.
- GH deficiency: Somatotropin human recombinant growth hormone: Saizen®: 0.05 mg/kg/day.

References

1. Tillmann B. Atlas der Anatomie des Menschen. Heidelberg: Springer; 2005. p. 120–2.
2. Patestas MA, Gartner LP. A textbook of neuroanatomy. 2nd ed. Hoboken: Wiley; 2016. p. 68–83.
3. Netter FH. Atlas of human anatomy. 4th ed. Barcelona: Elsevier, Masson; 2007.
4. Felten DL, O'Banion MK, Maida MS. Spinal cord. In: Netter's atlas of neuroscience. Amsterdam: Elsevier; 2016. p. 77–83.
5. Irsch K, Guyton D. Anatomy of eyes. In: Encyclopedia of biometrics. Boston: Springer; 2009. p. 11–6.
6. Jacobson S, Marcus EM, Pugsley S. Neuroanatomy for the neuroscientist. 3rd ed. Cham: Springer; 2017. p. 3–26.
7. Duvernoy HM. Introduction. In: The human hippocampus. 3rd ed. Berlin: Springer-Verlag; 2005. p. 1.
8. Kannan CR. The anatomy of the pituitary gland. In: Essential Endocrinology. Boston: Springer; 1986.
9. Wright JL, Yom SS, Awan MJ, Dawes S, Fischer-Valuck B, Kudner R, Mailhot Vega R, Rodrigues G. Standardizing normal tissue contouring for radiation therapy treatment planning: an ASTRO consensus paper. Pract Radiat Oncol. 2019;9(2):65–72.
10. Eekers DB, In't Ven L, Roelofs E, Postma A, Alapetite C, Burnet NG, European Particle Therapy Network of ESTRO, et al. The EPTN consensus-based atlas for CT- and MR-based contouring in neuro-oncology. Radiother Oncol. 2018;128(1):37–43.
11. Brouwer CL, Steenbakkers RJ, Bourhis J, Budach W, Grau C, Grégoire V, van Herk M, et al. CT-based delineation of organs at risk in the head and neck region: DAHANCA, EORTC, GORTEC, HKNPCSG, NCIC CTG, NCRI, NRG oncology and TROG consensus guidelines. Radiother Oncol. 2015;117(1):83–90.
12. Sun Y, Yu XL, Luo W, Lee AW, Wee JT, Lee N, et al. Recommendation for a contouring method and atlas of organs at risk in nasopharyngeal carcinoma patients receiving intensity-modulated radiotherapy. Radiother Oncol. 2014;110(3):390–7.
13. Scoccianti S, Detti B, Gadda D, Greto D, Furfaro I, Meacci F, et al. Organs at risk in the brain and their dose-constraints in adults and in children: a radiation oncologist's guide for delineation in everyday practice. Radiother Oncol. 2015;114(2):230–8.
14. Gondi V, Tolakanahalli R, Mehta MP, Tewatia D, Rowley H, Kuo JS, et al. Hippocampal-sparing whole-brain radiotherapy: a "how-to" technique using helical tomotherapy and linear accelerator–based intensity-modulated radiotherapy. Int J Radiat Oncol Biol Phys. 2010;78(4):1244–52.

15. Smart D. Radiation toxicity in the central nervous system: mechanisms and strategies for injury reduction. Semin Radiat Oncol. 2017;27(4):332–9.
16. Ahles TA, Root JC, Ryan EL. Cancer- and cancer treatment-associated cognitive change: an update on the state of the science. J Clin Oncol. 2012;30:3675–86.
17. Cox JD, Stetz J, Pajak TF. Toxicity criteria of the Radiation Therapy Oncology Group (RTOG) and the European Organization for Research and Treatment of Cancer (EORTC). Int J Radiat Oncol Biol Phys. 1995;31:1341–6.
18. Kramer S, Henrickson F, Zelen M. Therapeutic trials in the management of metastatic brain tumors by different time/dose fraction schemes of radiation therapy. Natl Cancer Inst Monogr. 1977;46:213–21.
19. Kim JH, Brown SL, Jenrow KA, Ryu S. Mechanisms of radiation-induced brain toxicity and implications for future clinical trials. J Neuro-Oncol. 2008;87:279–86.
20. Belka C, Budach W, Kortmann RD, Bamberg M. Radiation induced CNS toxicity--molecular and cellular mechanisms. Br J Cancer. 2001;85(9):1233–9.
21. Phillips TL. An ultrastructural study of the development of radiation injury in the lung. Radiology. 1966;87:49–54.
22. Zollinger HU. Radiation vasculopathy. Pathol Eur. 1970;5:145–63.
23. Song H, Steven CF, Gage FH. Astroglia induce neurogenesis from adult neuronal stem cells. Nature. 2002;417:39–44.
24. Seifert G, Schilling K, Steinhauser C. Astrocyte dysfunction in neurological disorders: a molecular perspective. Nat Rev Neurosci. 2006;7:194–206.
25. Zhou H, Liu Z, Liu J, Wang J, Zhou D, Zhao Z, Xiao S, Tao E, Suo WZ. Fractionated radiation-induced acute encephalopathy in a young rat model: cognitive dysfunction and histologic findings. AJNR Am J Neuroradiol. 2011;32:1795–800.
26. Seth P, Koul N. Astrocyte, the star avatar: redefined. J Biosci. 2008;33:405–21.
27. Kyrkanides S, Olschowka JA, Williams JP, Hansen JT, O'Banion MK. TNF alpha and IL-1beta mediate intercellular adhesion molecule-1 induction via microglia-astrocyte interaction in CNS radiation injury. J Neuroimmunol. 1999;95:95–106.
28. Greene-Schloesser D, Robbins ME, Peiffer AM, Shaw EG, Wheeler KT, Chan MD. Radiation-induced brain injury: a review. Front Oncol. 2012;2:73.
29. Lee WH, Sonntag WE, Mitschelen M, Yan H, Lee YW. Irradiation induces regionally specific alterations in pro-inflammatory environments in rat brain. Int J Radiat Biol. 2010;86:132–44.
30. Gangloff H, Haley TJ. Effects of X-irradiation on spontaneous and evoked brain electrical activity in cats. Radiat Res. 1960;12:694–704.
31. Bassant MH, Court L. Effects of whole-body irradiation on the activity of rabbit hippocampal neurons. Radiat Res. 1978;75:593–606.
32. Rosi S, Andres-Mach M, Fishman KM, Levy W, Ferguson RA, Fike JR. Cranial irradiation alters the behaviorally induced immediate-early gene arc (activity-regulated cytoskeleton associated protein). Cancer Res. 2008;68:9763–70.
33. Madsen TM, Kristjansen PE, Bolwig TG, et al. Arrested neuronal proliferation and impaired hippocampal function following fractionated brain irradiation in the adult rat. Neuroscience. 2003;119:635–42.
34. Fike JR, Rola R, Limoli CL. Radiation response of neural precursor cells. Neurosurg Clin N Am. 2007;18:115–27.
35. Tofilon PJ, Fike JR. The radioresponse of the central nervous system: a dynamic process. Radiat Res. 2000;153:357–70.
36. Belka C, Rudner J, Wesselborg S, Stepczynska A, Marini P, Lepple-Wienhues A, Faltin H, Bamberg M, Budach W, Schulze-Osthoff K. Differential role of caspase-8 and BID activation during radiation-and CD95-induced apoptosis. Oncogene. 2000;19:1181–90.
37. Chong MJ, Murray MR, Gosink EC, Russell HR, Srinivasan A, Kapsetaki M, Korsmeyer SJ, McKinnon PJ. Atm and Bax cooperate in ionizing radiation-induced apoptosis in the central nervous system. Proc Natl Acad Sci U S A. 2000;97:889–94.
38. Hallahan DE, Virudachalam S. Intercellular adhesion molecule 1 knockout abrogates radiation induced pulmonary inflammation. Proc Natl Acad Sci U S A. 1997;94:6432–7.

39. Kim JH, Jenrow KA, Brown SL. Mechanisms of radiation-induced normal tissue toxicity and implications for future clinical trials. Radiat Oncol J. 2014;32(3):103–15.
40. Sheline GE. Radiation therapy of brain tumors. Cancer. 1977;39(Supp2):873–81.
41. Sundgren PC, Cao Y. Brain irradiation: effects on normal brain parenchyma and radiation injury. Neuroimaging Clin N Am. 2009;19(4):657–68.
42. Ljubimova NV, Levitman MK, Plotnikova ED, Eidus LK. Endothelial cell population dynamics in rat brain after local irradiation. Br J Radiol. 1991;64(766):934–40.
43. Reinhold HS, Calvo W, Hopewell JW, van der Berg AP. Development of blood vessel-related radiation damage in the fimbria of the central nervous system. Int J Radiat Oncol Biol Phys. 1990;18(1):37–42.
44. Tallet AV, Azria D, Barlesi F. Neurocognitive function impairment after whole brain radiotherapy for brain metastases: actual assessment. Radiat Oncol. 2012;7:77.
45. Haas-Kogan D, Indelicato D, Paganetti H, Esiashvili N, Mahajan A, Yock T, et al. National Cancer Institute workshop on proton therapy for children: considerations regarding brainstem injury. Int J Radiat Oncol Biol Phys. 2018;101(1):152–68.
46. Rong X, Tang Y, Chen M, Lu K, Peng Y. Radiation-induced cranial neuropathy in patients with nasopharyngeal carcinoma. A follow-up study. Strahlenther Oncol. 2012;188(3):282–6.
47. Fein DA, Marcus RB Jr, Parsons JT, Mendenhall WM, Million RR. Lhermitte's sign: incidence and treatment variables influencing risk after irradiation of the cervical spinal cord. Int J Radiat Oncol Biol Phys. 1999;27:1027–33.
48. Wara WM, Phillips TL, Sheline GE, Schwade JG. Radiation tolerance of the spinal cord. Cancer. 1975;35:1558–62.
49. Gordon KB, Char DH, Sagerman RH. Late effects of radiation on the eye and ocular adnexa. Int J Radiat Oncol Biol Phys. 1995;31(5):1123–39.
50. Khan DZ, Lacasse MC, Khan R, Murphy KJ. Radiation cataractogenesis: the progression of our understanding and its clinical consequences. J Vasc Interv Radiol. 2017;28(3):412–9.
51. Worgul BV, Merriam GR, Medvedovsky C. Cortical cataract development: an expression of primary damage to the lens epithelium. Lens Eye Toxicity Res. 1989;6:559–71.
52. Palmer TD, Takahashi J, gage FH. Vascular niche for adult hippocampal neurogenesis. J Comp Neurol. 2000;425:479–94.
53. Mizumastu S, Monje M, Morhardt R, et al. Extreme sensitivity of adult neurogenesis to low doses of x-irradiation. Cancer Res. 2003;63:4021–7.
54. Sun AM, Li CG, Han YQ, Liu QL, Xia Q, Yuan YW. X-ray irradiation promotes apoptosis of hippocampal neurons through up-regulation of Cdk5 and p25. Cancer Cell Int. 2013;13(1):47.
55. Peissner W, Kocher M, Treuer H, Gillardon F. Ionizing radiation-induced apoptosis of proliferating stem cells in the dentate gyrus of the adult rat hippocampus. Brain Res Mol Brain Res. 1999;71:61–8.
56. Appelman-Dijkstra NM, Kokshoorn NE, Dekkers OM, Neelis KJ, Biermasz NR, Romijn JA, Smit JW, Pereira AM. Pituitary dysfunction in adult patients after cranial radiotherapy: systematic review and meta-analysis. J Clin Endocrinol Metab. 2011;96(8):2330–40.
57. Fernandez A, Brada M, Zabuliene L, Karavitaki N, Wass JA. Radiation-induced hypopituitarism. Endocr Relat Cancer. 2009;16(3):733–72.
58. Darzy KH, Shalet SM. Hypopituitarism following radiotherapy. Pituitary. 2009;12(1):40–50.
59. Rubin P, Cooper RA, Phillips TL. Radiation biology and radiation pathology syllabus. Set RT1: radiation oncology, vol. 2. Chicago: American College of Radiology; 1975. p. 2–7.
60. Emami B, Lyman J, Brown A, Coia L, Goitein M, Munzenrider JE, Shank B, Solin LJ, Wesson M. Tolerance of normal tissue to therapeutic irradiation. Int J Radiat Oncol Biol Phys. 1991;21(1):109–22.3.
61. Bentzen SM, Constine LS, Deasy JO, Eisbruch A, Jackson A, Marks LB, Ten Haken RK, Yorke ED. Quantitative analyses of normal tissue effects in the clinic (QUANTEC): an introduction to the scientific issues. Int J Radiat Oncol Biol Phys. 2010;76(3 Suppl):S3–9.4.
62. Marks LB, Yorke ED, Jackson A, Ten Haken RK, Constine LS, Eisbruch A, Bentzen SM, Nam J, Deasy JO. Use of normal tissue complication probability models in the clinic. Int J Radiat Oncol Biol Phys. 2010;76(3 Suppl):S10–9.

63. Lawrence YR, Li XA, el Naqa I, Hahn CA, Marks LB, Merchant TE, Dicker AP. Radiation dose–volume effects in the brain. Int J Radiat Oncol Biol Phys. 2010;76(3):S20–7.
64. Lambrecht M, Eekers DBP, Alapetite C, Burnet NG, Calugaru V, Coremans IEM, European Particle Therapy Network of ESTRO, et al. Radiation dose constraints for organs at risk in neuro-oncology; the European Particle Therapy Network consensus. Radiother Oncol. 2018;128(1):26–36.
65. Shaw E, Scott C, Souhami L, Dinapoli R, Kline R, Loeffler J, Farnan N. Single dose radiosurgical treatment of recurrent previously irradiated primary brain tumors and brain metastases: final report of RTOG protocol 90-05. Int J Radiat Oncol Biol Phys. 2000;47:291–8.
66. Mayo C, Yorke E, Merchant TE. Radiation associated brainstem injury. Int J Radiat Oncol Biol Phys. 2010;76(3 Suppl):S36–41.
67. Lee TF, Fang FM, Chao PJ, Su TJ, Wang LK, Leung SW. Dosimetric comparisons of helical tomotherapy and step-and-shoot intensity-modulated radiotherapy in nasopharyngeal carcinoma. Radiother Oncol. 2008;89(1):89–96.
68. Merchant TE, Chitti RM, Li C, Xiong X, Sanford RA, Khan RB. Factors associated with neurological recovery of brainstem function following postoperative conformal radiation therapy for infratentorial ependymoma. Int J Radiat Oncol Biol Phys. 2010;76:496–503.
69. Kirkpatrick JP, van der Kogel AJ, Schultheiss TE. Radiation dose–volume effects in the spinal cord. Int J Radiat Oncol Biol Phys. 2010;76(3):S42–9.
70. Schultheiss TE, Kun LE, Ang KK, Stephens LC. Radiation response of the central nervous system. Int J Radiat Oncol Biol Phys. 1995;31(5):1093–112.
71. Ryu S, Jin JY, Jin R, Rock J, Ajlouni M, Movsas B, et al. Partial volume tolerance of the spinal cord and complications of single-dose radiosurgery. Cancer. 2007;109:628–36.
72. Sahgal A, Ma L, Gibbs I, Gerszten PC, Ryu S, Soltys S, et al. Spinal cord tolerance for stereotactic body radiotherapy. Int J Radiat Oncol Biol Phys. 2010;77:548–53.
73. Ryu S, Pugh SL, Gerszten PC, Yin FF, Timmerman RD, Hitchcock YJ, Movsas B, Kanner AA, Berk LB, Followill DS, Kachnic LA. RTOG 0631 phase II/III study of image-guided stereotactic radiosurgery for localized (1-3) spine metastases: phase II results. Int J Radiat Oncol Biol Phys. 2011;81(2):S131–2.
74. Jeganathan VSE, Wirth A, MacManus MP. Ocular risks from orbital and periorbital radiation therapy: a critical review. Int J Radiat Oncol. 2011;79:650–9.
75. Kozelsky TF, Garrity JA, Kurtin PJ, Leavitt JA, Martenson JA, Habermann TM. Orbital lymphoma: radiotherapy outcome and complications. Radiother Oncol. 2001;59:139–44.
76. Parsons JT, Bova FJ, Mendenhall WM, Million RR, Fitzgerald CR. Response of the normal eye to high dose radiotherapy. Oncology (Williston Park). 1996;10:837–47.
77. Smith GT, Deutsch GP, Cree IA, Liu CS. Permanent corneal limbal stem cell dysfunction following radiotherapy for orbital lymphoma. Eye (Lond). 2000;14:905–7.
78. Stewart FA, Akleyev AV, Hauer-Jensen M, Hendry JH, Kleiman NJ, MacVittie TJ, et al. ICRP PUBLICATION 118: ICRP statement on tissue reactions and early and late effects of radiation in normal tissues and organs—threshold doses for tissue reactions in a radiation protection context. Ann ICRP. 2012;41:1–322.
79. Forrest AP, Brown DAP, Morris SR, Illingsworth CF. Pituitary radon implant for advanced cancer. Lancet (London, England). 1956;270:399–401.
80. Mayo C, Martel MK, Marks LB, Flickinger J, Nam J, Kirkpatrick J. Radiation dose–volume effects of optic nerves and chiasm. Int J Radiat Oncol Biol Phys. 2010;76(3):S28–35.
81. Gondi V, Hermann BP, Mehta MP, Tomé WA. Hippocampal dosimetry predicts neurocognitive function impairment after fractionated stereotactic radiotherapy for benign or low-grade adult brain tumors. Int J Radiat Oncol Biol Phys. 2013;85:348–54.
82. Gondi V, Pugh SL, Tome WA, Caine C, Corn B, Kanner A, Rowley H, et al. Preservation of memory with conformal avoidance of the hippocampal neural stem-cell compartment during whole brain radiotherapy for brain metastases (RTOG 0933): a phase II multi-institutional trial. J Clin Oncol. 2014;32:3810–6.

83. Marek J, Jezková J, Hána V, Krsek M, Bandúrová L, Pecen L, Vladyka V, Liscák R. Is it possible to avoid hypopituitarism after irradiation of pituitary adenomas by the Leksell gamma knife? Eur J Endocrinol. 2011;164:169–78.
84. Powell C, Guerrero D, Sardell S, Cumins S, Wharram B, Traish D, Gonsalves A, Ashley S, Brada M. Somnolence syndrome in patients receiving radical radiotherapy for primary brain tumours: a prospective study. Radiother Oncol. 2011;100(1):131–6.
85. Faithfull S, Brada M. Somnolence syndrome in adults following cranial irradiation for primary brain tumours. Clin Oncol (R Coll Radiol). 1998;10:250–4.
86. Minton O, Richardson A, Sharpe M, Hotopf M, Stone P. A systematic review and meta-analysis of the pharmacological treatment of cancer-related fatigue. J Natl Cancer Inst. 2008;100:1155–66.
87. Butler JM Jr, Case LD, Atkins J, Frizzell B, Sanders G, Griffin P, Lesser G, et al. A phase III, double-blind, placebo-controlled prospective randomized clinical trial of d-threo-methylphenidate HCl in brain tumor patients receiving radiation therapy. Int J Radiat Oncol Biol Phys. 2007;69(5):1496–501.
88. Breitbart W, Alici Y. Psychostimulants for cancer-related fatigue. J Natl Compr Cancer Netw. 2010;8(8):933–42.
89. Shaw EG, Robbins ME. The management of radiation-induced brain injury. Cancer Treat Res. 2006;128:7–22.
90. Lawenda BD, Gagne HM, Gierga DP, Niemierko A, Wong WM, Tarbell NJ, Chen GT, Hochberg FH, Loeffler JS. Permanent alopecia after cranial irradiation: dose-response relationship. Int J Radiat Oncol Biol Phys. 2004;60(3):879.
91. Wei J, Meng L, Xue H, Chao Q, Wang B, Xin Y, Jiang X. Radiation-induced skin reactions: mechanism and treatment. Cancer Manag Res. 2019;11:167–77.
92. Winter SF, Loebel F, Loeffler J, Batchelor TT, Martinez-Lage M, Vajkoczy P, Dietrich J. Treatment-induced brain tissue necrosis: a clinical challenge in neuro-oncology. Neuro-Oncology. 2019;21:1118.
93. Lubelski D, Abdullah KG, Weil RJ, Marko NF. Bevacizumab for radiation necrosis following treatment of high grade glioma: a systematic review of the literature. J Neuro-Oncol. 2013;115(3):317–22.
94. Tye K, Engelhard HH, Slavin KV, et al. An analysis of radiation necrosis of the central nervous system treated with bevacizumab. J Neuro-Oncol. 2014;117(2):321–7.
95. Glantz MJ, Burger PC, Friedman AH, Radtke RA, Massey EW, Schold SC Jr. Treatment of radiation-induced nervous system injury with heparin and warfarin. Neurology. 1994;44(11):2020.
96. Chuba PJ, Aronin P, Bhambhani K, Eichenhorn M, Zamarano L, Cianci P, Muhlbauer M, Porter AT, Fontanesi J. Hyperbaric oxygen therapy for radiation-induced brain injury in children. Cancer. 1997;80(10):2005.
97. Wilke C, Grosshans D, Duman J, Brown P, Li J. Radiation-induced cognitive toxicity: pathophysiology and interventions to reduce toxicity in adults. Neuro-Oncology. 2018;20(5):597–607.
98. Chang EL, Wefel JS, Hess KR, Allen PK, Lang FF, Kornguth DG, Arbuckle RB, Swint JM, Shiu AS, Maor MH, Meyers CA. Neurocognition in patients with brain metastases treated with radiosurgery or radiosurgery plus whole-brain irradiation: a randomised controlled trial. Lancet Oncol. 2009;10(11):1037–44.
99. Li J, Bentzen SM, Renschler M, Mehta MP. Regression after whole-brain radiation therapy for brain metastases correlates with survival and improved neurocognitive function. J Clin Oncol. 2007;25(10):1260–6.
100. Meyers CA, Smith JA, Bezjak A, Mehta MP, Liebmann J, Illidge T, et al. Neurocognitive function and progression in patients with brain metastases treated with whole-brain radiation and motexafin gadolinium: results of a randomized phase III trial. J Clin Oncol. 2004;22(1):157–65.

101. Rock JP, Ryu S, Yin FF, Schreiber F, Abdulhak M. The evolving role of stereotactic radiosurgery and stereotactic radiation therapy for patients with spine tumors. J Neuro-Oncol. 2004;69(1–3):319–34.
102. Fein DA, Marcus RB Jr, Parsons JT, Mendenhall WM, Million RR. Lhermitte's sign: incidence and treatment variables influencing risk after irradiation of the cervical spinal cord. Int J Radiat Oncol Biol Phys. 1993;27(5):1029.
103. Leung WM, Tsang NM, Chang FT, Lo CJ. Lhermitte's sign among nasopharyngeal cancer patients after radiotherapy. Head Neck. 2007;27(3):187.
104. Jiang J, Li Y, Shen Q, Rong X, Huang X, Li H, Zhou L, Mai HQ, et al. Effect of pregabalin on radiotherapy-related neuropathic pain in patients with head and neck cancer: a randomized controlled trial. J Clin Oncol. 2019;37(2):135–43.
105. Levin VA, Bidaut L, Hou P, Kumar AJ, Wefel JS, Bekele BN, Grewal J, Prabhu S, Loghin M, Gilbert MR, Jackson EF. Randomized double-blind placebo-controlled trial of bevacizumab therapy for radiation necrosis of the central nervous system. Int J Radiat Oncol Biol Phys. 2011;79(5):1487–95.
106. Andratschke NH, Nieder C, Price RE, Rivera B, Ang KK. Potential role of growth factors in diminishing radiation therapy neural tissue injury. Semin Oncol. 2005;32(2 Suppl 3):S67.
107. Esik O, Vönöczky K, Lengyel Z, Sáfrány G, Trón L. Characteristics of radiogenic lower motor neurone disease, a possible link with a preceding viral infection. Spinal Cord. 2004;42(2):99–105.
108. Allen JC, Miller DC, Budzilovich GN, Epstein FJ. Brain and spinal cord hemorrhage in long-term survivors of malignant pediatric brain tumors: a possible late effect of therapy. Neurology. 1991;41(1):148.
109. Jabbour P, Gault J, Murk SE, Awad IA. Multiple spinal cavernous malformations with atypical phenotype after prior irradiation: case report. Neurosurgery. 2004;55(6):1431.
110. Moore J, de Silva SR, O'Hare K, Humphry RC. Ruby laser for the treatment of trichiasis. Lasers Med Sci. 2009;24:137–9.
111. Tseng SC. Topical tretinoin treatment for severe dry-eye disorders. J Am Acad Dermatol. 1986;15:860–6.
112. Doughty MJ, Glavin S. Efficacy of different dry eye treatments with artificial tears or ocular lubricants: a systematic review. Ophthalmic Physiol Opt. 2009;29:573–83.
113. Shtein RM, Shen JF, Kuo AN, Hammersmith KM, Li JY, Weikert MP. Autologous serum-based eye drops for treatment of ocular surface disease: a report by the American Academy of ophthalmology. Ophthalmology. 2019. https://doi.org/10.1016/j.ophtha.2019.08.018.
114. Durkin SR, Roos D, Higgs B, Casson RJ, Selva D. Ophthalmic and adnexal complications of radiotherapy. Acta Ophthalmol Scand. 2007;85(3):240–50.
115. Merriam GRSA, Focht EF. The effects of ionizing radiations on the eye. Radiat Ther Oncol. 1972;6:346–85.
116. Belkacemi Y, Ozsahin M, Pène F, Rio B, Laporte JP, Leblond V, Touboul E, Schlienger M, Gorin NC, Laugier A. Cataractogenesis after total body irradiation. Int J Radiat Oncol Biol Phys. 1996;35:53–60.
117. Gall N, Leiba H, Handzel R, Pe'er J. Severe radiation retinopathy and optic neuropathy after brachytherapy for choroidal melanoma, treated by hyperbaric oxygen. Eye (Lond). 2007;21:1010–2.
118. Wen JC, McCannel TA. Treatment of radiation retinopathy following plaque brachytherapy for choroidal melanoma. Curr Opin Ophthalmol. 2009;20:200–4.
119. Forrest AW. Tumors following radiation about the eye. Trans Am Acad Ophthalmol Otolaryngol. 1961;65:694–717.
120. Mehta MP, Rodrigus P, Terhaard CH, Rao A, Suh J, Roa W, Souhami L, et al. Survival and neurologic outcomes in a randomized trial of motexafin gadolinium and whole-brain radiation therapy in brain metastases. J Clin Oncol. 2003;21:2529.
121. Rooney JW, Laack NN. Pharmacological interventions to treat or prevent neurocognitive decline after brain radiation. CNS Oncol. 2013;2(6):531–41.

122. Orrego F, Villanueva S. The chemical nature of the main central excitatory transmitter: a critical appraisal based upon release studies and synaptic vesicle localization. Neuroscience. 1993;56:539–55.
123. Tariot PN, Farlow MR, Grossberg GT, Graham SM, McDonald S, Gergel I, Memantine Study Group. Memantine treatment in patients with moderate to severe Alzheimer disease already receiving donepezil: a randomized controlled trial. JAMA. 2004;291(3):317–24.
124. Wilcock G, Möbius HJ, Stöffler A, MMM 500 Group. A double-blind, placebo-controlled multicentre study of memantine in mild to moderate vascular dementia (MMM500). Int Clin Psychopharmacol. 2002;17(6):297–305.
125. Brown PD, Pugh S, Laack NN, Wefel JS, Khuntia D, Meyers C, et al. Memantine for the prevention of cognitive dysfunction in patients receiving whole-brain radiotherapy: a randomized, double-blind, placebo-controlled trial. Neuro-Oncology. 2013;15(10):1429–37.
126. Malouf R, Birks J. Donepezil for vascular cognitive impairment. Cochrane Database Syst Rev. 2004;1:CD004395.
127. Shaw EG, Rosdhal R, D'Agostino RB Jr, Rosdhal R, D'Agostino RB Jr, Lovato J, Naughton MJ, Robbins ME, Rapp SR. Phase II study of donepezil in irradiated brain tumor patients: effect on cognitive function, mood, and quality of life. J Clin Oncol. 2006;24:1415.
128. Rapp SR, Case LD, Peiffer A, Naughton MM, Chan MD, Stieber VW. Donepezil for irradiated brain tumor survivors: a phase III randomized placebo-controlled clinical trial. J Clin Oncol. 2015;33(15):1653–9.
129. Sklar CA, Antal Z, Chemaitilly W, Cohen LE, Follin C, Meacham LR, Murad MH. Hypothalamic-pituitary and growth disorders in survivors of childhood cancer: an endocrine society clinical practice guideline. J Clin Endocrinol Metab. 2018;103(8):2761.
130. Palmert MR, Dunkel L. Clinical practice. Delayed puberty. N Engl J Med. 2012;366(5):443–53.

Toxicity Management for Head and Neck Tumors in Radiation Oncology-I

2

Sezin Yuce Sari

2.1 Salivary Glands

2.1.1 Anatomy

The salivary glands are exocrine glands that produce saliva. They include three paired major glands (i.e., parotid, submandibular, and sublingual) and more than 600 minor glands located in the upper aerodigestive tract, oropharynx, oral cavity, nasal cavity, paranasal sinuses, and nasopharynx. Stimulated salivary production is predominantly derived from the parotid glands, whereas unstimulated salivary production is primarily from the submandibular, sublingual, and minor salivary glands [1].

The parotid gland is located superficially and inferiorly to the ramus of the mandible and anteriorly to the sternocleidomastoid (SCM) muscle, superficially covering the posterior part of the masseter muscle. The name of the parotid gland comes from its close vicinity to the ear; "para" meaning "near" and "otis" meaning "ear." The gland is enclosed by the parotid fascia and consists of a superficial lobe and a deep lobe which are separated by the extracranial facial nerve passing through the gland. The larger superficial lobe extends irregularly and overlaps the posterior part of the masseter muscle and the majority of the mandibular ramus. The deep lobe is located posterior and medial to the ramus of the mandible, and the tip of the deep lobe extends medially to the parapharyngeal space.

The guidelines for the delineation of salivary glands recommend the retromandibular vein, carotid artery, and extracranial facial nerve be included in parotid gland contours [2, 3]. The parotid gland is restricted with the external auditory canal and mastoid process superiorly; the posterior part of the submandibular space inferiorly; the masseter, medial, and lateral pterygoid muscles, and posterior border of

S. Yuce Sari (✉)
Faculty of Medicine, Department of Radiation Oncology, Hacettepe University, Ankara, Turkey

© Springer Nature Switzerland AG 2020
G. Ozyigit, U. Selek (eds.), *Prevention and Management of Acute and Late Toxicities in Radiation Oncology*, https://doi.org/10.1007/978-3-030-37798-4_2

the mandible anteriorly; the anterior belly of the SCM muscle, lateral side of the posterior belly of the digastric muscle, and mastoid process posteriorly; subcutaneous fat and the platysma muscle laterally; and the posterior belly of the digastric muscle, styloid process, parapharyngeal space, and SCM muscle medially.

The submandibular gland is located between the two bellies of the digastric muscle and the lower border of the mandible, extending upward the mandible. The gland is composed of a large superficial lobe and a smaller deep process. The inferior surface of the gland is adjacent to submandibular lymph nodes. The deep process is located medial to the mylohyoid and lateral to the hyoglossus muscles, and inferior to the lingual and superior to the hypoglossal nerves, respectively.

The borders for the submandibular gland contouring are the mylohyoid and medial pterygoid muscles or inferior border of the inferior pterygoids or level of C3 vertebra on the superior; the appearance of the fat of the submandibular triangle on the inferior; lateral surface of the hyoglossus and mylohyoid muscles on the anterior; the parapharyngeal space, cervical vessels, posterior belly of the digastric muscle, and SCM muscle on the posterior; the platysma muscle, medial surface of the medial pterygoid muscle, and medial surface of the mandibular bone on the lateral; and the cervical vessels, hyoid bone, hyoglossus muscle, lateral surface of the mylohyoid muscle, superior and middle of the pharyngeal constrictor muscle, and posterior belly of the digastric muscle on the medial aspects, respectively [2, 3].

Sublingual glands are not routinely contoured. However, the guidelines have proposed the mucous membrane covering the floor of the mouth (if not seen, the crossing of the lingual septum with the intrinsic tongue muscles) as the superior, the geniohyoid muscle and anterior part of the mylohyoid muscle as the inferior, the mylohyoid muscle and the anterior part of the surface of the mandible as the anterior, the hyoglossus muscle as the posterior, the mylohyoid muscle and anterior part of the medial surface of the mandible as the lateral, and the genioglossus muscle as the medial aspects, respectively [2, 3].

Minor salivary glands cannot be delineated separately. The radiation dose to the oral cavity, lips, soft palate, and cheeks affects the salivary function of these glands. The delineation of the oral cavity is detailed in later sections of the current chapter.

2.1.2 Contouring

Delineation of the salivary glands is shown in Figs. 2.1 and 2.2.

2.1.3 Dose Constraints

The mean salivary gland dose is correlated with salivary function and a number of studies have proposed mean doses ranging between 20 Gy and 30 Gy to the parotid gland [4–7]. Besides, Eisbruch et al. [4] recommended V15 < 66–67%, V30 < 43–45%, and V45 < 24–26% for the parotid. Salivary function of the parotid gland is minimally affected with a mean dose of <10–15 Gy in conventional

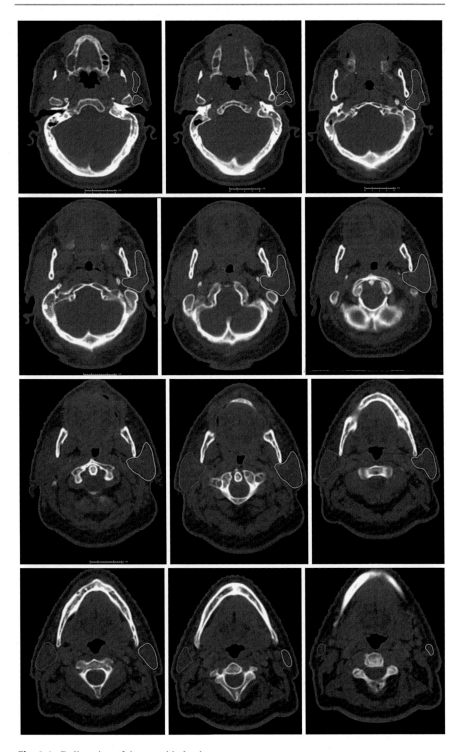

Fig. 2.1 Delineation of the parotid glands

Fig. 2.2 Delineation of
the submandibular glands

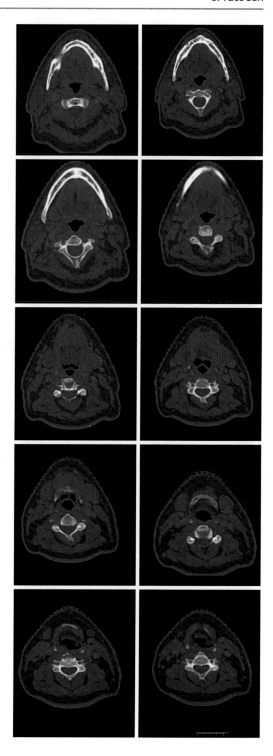

fractions. However, it gradually decreases with doses between 20 and 40 Gy, and a >75% decrease occurs over 40 Gy [5, 8]. It is important to keep in mind that although the position of the medial parotid gland changes very little during RT, the lateral edges shrink resulting in an increased mean dose to the whole gland [7]. Sparing at least one parotid or even one submandibular gland results in a decreased rate of xerostomia [9].

A dose of 7.2 Gy to the parotid was shown to reduce the salivary flow by half, and 36 Gy reduced it to the nadir level, with further reduction occurring after completion of RT without recovery during the following 2 years [10]. The largest series on the effect of RT dose on xerostomia reported a mean dose of 39 Gy resulted in a 50% risk of 1-year xerostomia without a threshold dose [11]. The authors recommended a mean dose of 20 Gy to lower the risk of xerostomia. On the other hand, improvement in salivary function was observed 2 years following RT compared to the rate at 3 months when the patients were treated with parotid-sparing IMRT with a mean parotid dose of 34 Gy [12]. This salivary function-preserving quality of IMRT was further confirmed by randomized trials comparing it to 2D-RT [13, 14]. In a small prospective series of 36 patients with parotid carcinoma, the QoL deteriorated during postoperative RT but returned to its baseline level 1 year after RT [15].

Submandibular gland sparing can also reduce the risk of xerostomia. Murdoch-Kinch et al. [16] reported that a mean dose of >40 Gy to the submandibular gland decreased the salivary function related to the particular gland. It was also shown that if the parotid gland received a mean dose of 30 Gy the risk of xerostomia increased by 20% when the mean dose to the submandibular gland was 50 Gy compared to 0 Gy [17]. Besides, surgical transfer of the submandibular gland out of the high-dose RT field resulted in 30% spare of the pretreatment stimulated salivary function [18].

Blanco et al. [5] reported poorer salivary function in patients that received mean doses >25 Gy to both parotid glands but the salivary capacity typically exceeded the 25% level with <25 Gy. Meirovitz et al. [19] recommended the volume of the contralateral parotid gland receiving >40 Gy should be <33% for complete salivary production recovery 24 months following RT. In the light of available data, the Quantitative Analysis of Normal Tissue Radiation Effects in the Clinic (QUANTEC) recommends a mean dose of <20 Gy to one parotid gland or <25 Gy to both parotid glands to avoid severe xerostomia which is defined as a long-term salivary function <25% of baseline [20]. The authors also reported that a mean dose of <35 Gy to the submandibular gland can reduce the risk of xerostomia. In general, the mean dose to each parotid is recommended <26 Gy with V15 < 65%, V30 < 45%, and V40 < 33% [20–22], and the mean dose to each submandibular gland is recommended <32–39 Gy [21, 23], if the localization of the target volume permits (Table 2.1). However, it is not practical to spare the adjacent salivary gland when an intraparotid, level Ib, or level II cervical lymph node metastasis is present as it will increase the risk of regional failure at that site [24].

Table 2.1 Dose constraints for the salivary glands

Organ at risk	Mean dose	Other
Parotid gland	<26 Gy (each)	V15 < 65% V30 < 45% V40 < 33%
Submandibular gland	<32 Gy	

2.1.4 Pathophysiology

Exceeding the tolerance dose for salivary glands results in inflammation and degeneration of the salivary gland parenchyma which leads to the reduction in salivary flow which is called xerostomia [22]. There are two hypotheses to explain the mechanism of radiation-induced damage to the salivary glands. The first one is called granulation, in which RT induces the peroxidation of lipids causing damage to the membranes of the secretory granules in acinar cells. Following, the proteolytic enzymes discharge from these granules resulting in cell lysis. According to this hypothesis, the volume of the glands is not altered; however, the secretory function is diminished. The second hypothesis mentions about the failure in cellular function due to selective damage to the membrane at the expense of the water-secretion receptor and death of stem cells which both lead to inhibition of cell renewal [25].

The decrease in the salivary flow begins within the first week of RT and persists or even progresses during the course of treatment and several months after the end of RT. The severity of xerostomia depends on the total dose of radiation to the glands and volume of the glandular tissue within the RT field. No correlation was shown with patient gender, age, or use of chemotherapy [20]. However, xerostomia risk was higher with impaired pretreatment salivary function and use of drugs that negatively affect salivary function. The recovery of the gland may occur within approximately 2 years after RT and it can even be to 100% unless there is severe damage [4–6]. However, in most cases, xerostomia is irreversible with a possible 30% increase in salivary function within 5 years [20, 26].

As saliva is required for important oral functions such as swallowing, taste, and speech, permanent impairment of the salivary function has several clinical consequences leading to a substantial decrease in the quality of life. The patient will complain about dryness of the mouth and lips, increased thirst, altered taste, difficulty in swallowing solid food, fissures at lip commissures, burning sensation of the tongue, a dorsal tongue surface atrophy. Beside the reduction of saliva production, the salivary viscosity also increases which results in impaired lubrication of oral tissues and compromised buffering capacity leading to a propensity for oral infections, increased risk of dental caries, difficulty in wearing dentures, and progressive periodontal disease.

2.1.5 Treatment

The first recommendation for patients that will undergo RT should be to carefully maintain their oral hygiene to minimize the clinical risks related to xerostomia. The patient should be lead to a dentist and offered preventive strategies such as regular tooth brushing and flossing, using remineralizing solutions, rinsing with antimicrobials such as chlorhexidine and povidone iodine, and using sialogogues such as pilocarpine and bethanechol. Mechanical stimulation can be achieved mainly by chewing gum without sugar (containing xylitol and sorbitol with antimicrobial effect) as well as electrostimulation, acupuncture, and hyperbaric chambers.

Chemical and physical radioprotectors can be used to reduce long-term xerostomia. Amifostine (WR-2721) is a pro-drug which is dephosphorylated by the plasma membrane alkaline phosphatase to its active metabolite of free thiol WR-1065. It is a free radical scavenger which can reduce radiation effects on normal tissues if administered just prior to each RT fraction. Amifostine resulted in reduced acute and chronic grade 2 or higher xerostomia when administered concurrently with RT in a randomized phase III trial [27]. Munter et al. [28] showed that amifostine significantly increased the combined parotid and submandibular gland tolerance dose by a mean dose of approximately 9 Gy. Hypotension and nausea may occur as dose limiting toxicities of amifostine. The concern of possible tumor-protective effects of amifostine was ruled out in a recent meta-analysis [29]. However, the preventive effect of amifostine was shown in the 2D RT era, and it is now questionable whether it still has any benefit when administered with IMRT which has a significant xerostomia-prevention effect per se [30–32]. Currently, there is no universal standard recommendation across treatment centers for the use of this radioprotector.

Temporarily wetting the oral mucosa by saliva substitutes, artificial saliva preparations, or mucosa lubricant is a palliative strategy to relieve discomforting symptoms due to xerostomia. Pilocarpine, cevimeline, and bethanechol are parasympathomimetic systemic drugs used in the management of RT-induced xerostomia which can also act as a radioprotector if used during RT [33, 34]. However, the efficiency of these drugs requires the presence of functional tissue. The salivary flow increases within 30 minutes after oral pilocarpine intake, and maximal benefit is achieved by long-term use. Pilocarpine may cause hyperhidrosis, nausea, dizziness, and cardiovascular and pulmonary toxicity. All therapies currently available for the treatment of xerostomia provide only temporary relief, and require multiple applications for a long period of time. Gene therapy and stem cells are currently being studied for the treatment of xerostomia [35].

2.2 Temporomandibular Joint

2.2.1 Anatomy

The temporomandibular joint (TMJ), as the name implies, is a bilateral synovial articulation between the mandible at the inferior and the temporal bone of the cranium at the superior. As the two TMJs operate simultaneously, they facilitate the lowering and lifting, forward and backward projections, and lateral movements of the mandible, thus permitting phonation, nutrition, and buccal hygiene. While delineating this structure, the head of the mandible, the articular disc, and the articular surface of the temporal bone should be included [36]. The superior border is where the articular cavity disappears, the inferior border is where the head of the mandible appears or one slice superior to the sigmoid notch of the neck of mandible, the anterior border is the articular condyle of the temporal and anterior border of the mandibular condyle, the posterior border is the surface of the glenoid, and the lateral border is the lateral border of the mandibular condyle or the surface of the glenoid fossa.

2.2.2   Contouring

Delineation of the temporomandibular joints is shown in Fig. 2.3.

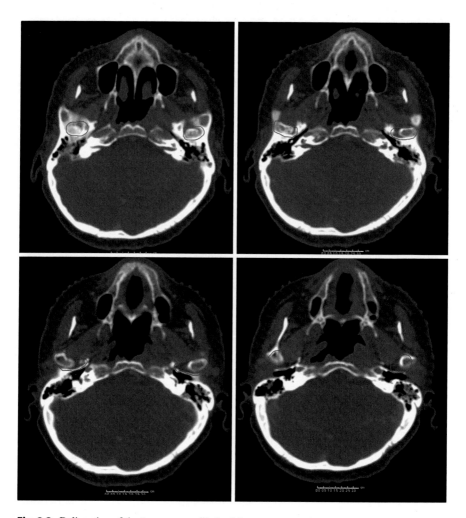

Fig. 2.3 Delineation of the temporomandibular joint

2.2.3 Dose Constraints

The risk of trismus increases with doses over 50 Gy to the TMJ [23]. Teguh et al. [37] recommended the D2% of the TMJ be restricted to <60 Gy. Other proposed doses are D33% < 65 Gy, D66% < 60 Gy, and D100% < 60 Gy [23] (Table 2.2). The rate of trismus was reported 5–38% with 70 Gy [38, 39].

2.2.4 Pathophysiology

Exceeding the tolerance dose of the TMJ results in trismus which can be defined as the difficulty or even impossibility of opening the mouth resulted from the tonic contraction of the masseter muscle (Fig. 2.4). Trismus is the consequence of

Table 2.2 Dose constraints for the temporomandibular joint

Organ at risk	Mean dose	Other
Temporomandibular joint	<50 Gy	D2% < 60 Gy D33% < 65 Gy D66% < 60 Gy Dmax <60 Gy

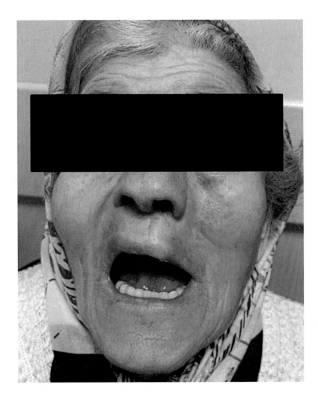

Fig. 2.4 A patient with trismus after radiotherapy

fibrosis leading to fibroatrophy, characterized by cartilaginous thinning and depletion of the synovial fluid around the masticatory muscles and the TMJ due to RT and surgery [40].

The lateral pterygoid muscle has two heads: a superior head that originates on the external face of the lateral lamina of the pterygoid process and on the tuberosity of the maxilla. The inferior head has its origin on the temporal surface of the large wing of the sphenoid. They end on the pterygoid fovea of the condylar process of the mandible and on the articular disc of the TMJ. Its duty is the closing of the mouth and the protrusion of the mandible for the superior head while the lower head opens the mouth. The medial pterygoid muscle starts from the pterygoid fossa, from the lateral lamina of the pterygoid process, and partly from the pyramidal process of the palatine bone. It ends on the medial side of the mandibular angle and pterygoid tuberosity. Its contraction allows the closure of the mouth. Finally, the masseter muscle consists of two parts. A superior part that starts from the inferior border and two-thirds of the anterior zygomatic arch and ends at the mandibular angle at the level of the masseteric tuberosity. The deep part starts from the posterior third and from the inside of the zygomatic arch and ends on the external surface of the mandibular ramus. Its contraction also allows the closure of the mouth. The temporal muscle also plays a role in closing the mouth and retropulsion of the mandible. A dose >50 Gy to the pterygoid muscles causes a 24% risk of trismus [37]. Trismus leads to complications of pain, difficulty in speaking, malnutrition, and dental hygiene. Following IMRT, there is a 5% risk of trismus [38].

2.2.5 Treatment

There is no medical treatment for trismus. Hyperbaric oxygen treatment, pentoxifylline, or botulinum toxin injections into the masticator muscles did not show convincing results [35]. Botulinum toxin can effectively reduce local pain produced by muscle spasms associated with trismus but is not a long-term solution. Forced mouth opening under general anesthesia can improve trismus, but the effect is also not long-term and there is a considerable risk of fracture and adjacent soft tissue rupture. However, stretching exercises applied by an experienced physiotherapist may be useful by strengthening musculature, improving the mobility, flexibility, and elasticity of the TMJ, and by improving blood circulation [41]. In patients that are refractory to physical therapy, surgical treatment (coronoidectomy) can be an option if there is no tumor present in the TMJ.

2.3   Oral Cavity

2.3.1   Anatomy

The oral cavity, as an organ at risk, includes the dorsal and ventral surface of the tongue (including the base), floor of the mouth, and hard and soft palates, which is named as "extended oral cavity." For simplicity and consistency of delineation, the extended oral cavity is defined as the structure posterior to the internal arch of the mandible and maxilla. The mucosa anterior and lateral to these bones is included in the contour of the lips and buccal mucosa, respectively. The oral cavity is restricted to the mucosa of the hard palate and mucosal reflections near the maxilla superiorly; the mucosa of the base of the tongue and hyoid on the posterior, and the mylohyoid muscle and anterior belly of the digastric muscle on the anterior inferiorly; the inner surface of the mandible and maxilla anteriorly and laterally; and the posterior borders of the soft palate, uvula, and base of the tongue posteriorly [3]. Any air that may be present in the oral cavity is excluded from this volume.

2.3.2 Contouring

Delineation of the oral cavity is shown in Fig. 2.5.

2.3.3 Dose Constraints

The mean dose to the oral cavity is recommended <30 Gy, V20 < 80%, and V30 < 46% [23, 42]. Other recommendations include V45 < 40% and V50 < 20% [43] (Table 2.3).

2.3.4 Pathophysiology

Radiation-induced loss of the basal cells in the epithelium of the oral mucosa results in oral mucositis (Fig. 2.6). Poor oral hygiene, periodontal caries, malnutrition, and tobacco and alcohol consumption increase the risk as well as high total and fraction doses of RT, concomitant chemotherapy use, and previous surgery. The symptoms of mucositis usually start during the third week of RT and can persist up to 1 month after RT is completed or even longer with concurrent chemotherapy. The initial sign is mucosal blanching within the RT field but it can progress to patchy or confluent mucositis. Other signs and symptoms include tenderness, pain, erythema, edema, and difficulty in swallowing. A pseudomembrane and a painful ulcerated surface resulting from membrane sloughing can occur. Oral candidiasis is a frequent infection of the oropharynx in patients receiving HNC RT. This infection may aggravate mucositis since the yeast colonizes the injured mucosa. Mucosal healing usually occurs rapidly after the completion of RT.

Atrophy and degeneration of taste buds may result as a consequence of oral cavity irradiation. Taste buds are susceptible to irradiation, and sensations of sweet, sour, salty, or bitter can be affected. Incidence of taste changes is dependent on RT dose. Though recovery may be observed within a few months following treatment in some patients, persistent changes may also occur.

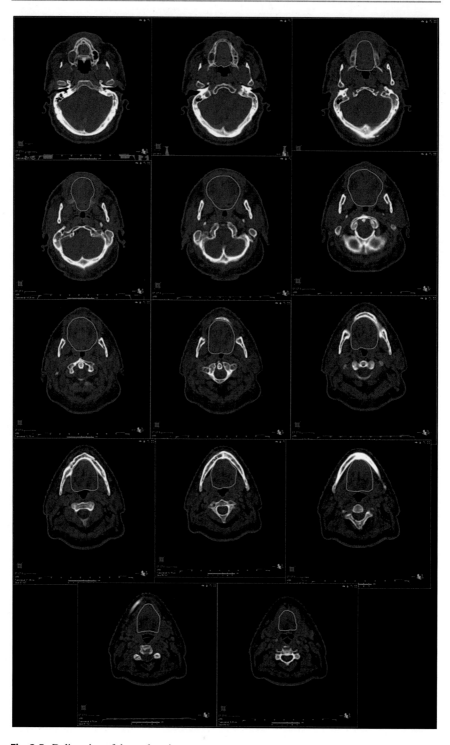

Fig. 2.5 Delineation of the oral cavity

Table 2.3 Dose constraints for the oral cavity

Organ at risk	Mean dose	Other
Oral cavity	<30 Gy	V20 < 80% V30 < 46% V45 < 40% V50 < 20%

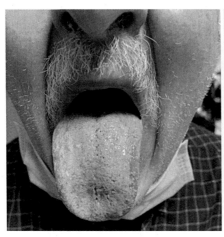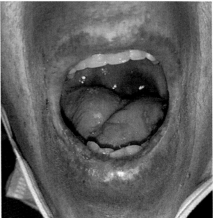

Fig. 2.6 Mucositis after radiotherapy

There are several international scoring scales for mucositis. One of the most used scales is from the Radiation Therapy Oncology Group (RTOG) which has four grades [44]. This scoring system defines grade I oral mucositis as one leading to mild pain without requiring analgesics, grade II as patchy mucositis or one that requires analgesic use, grade III as confluent mucositis or one that requires narcotic analgesic use, and grade IV as mucositis with ulcers, necrosis, or bleeding. The World Health Organization scoring scale includes four grades based on both clinician-based observations and patient-reported functional symptoms [44]. The National Cancer Institute-Common Terminology Criteria for Adverse Events (NCI-CTCAE) is often used to document the side effects caused by cancer treatment [44]. This scale defines grade 1 as mucositis with mild or no symptoms, grade 2 as mucositis with moderate pain or ulcer not interfering with oral intake, grade 3 as mucositis with severe pain interfering with oral intake, grade 4 as mucositis with life-threatening symptoms, and grade 5 as death.

2.3.5   Treatment

The patients should be warned to minimize the exposure of the affected mucosa by tobacco, alcohol, or poorly fitting dentures. Instructions for oral hygiene and mouth care should be given. The Mucositis Study Group of the Multinational Association of Supportive Care in Cancer and International Society of Oral Oncology (MASCC/ISOO) has published clinical practice guidelines for mucositis prevention secondary to cancer therapy in which a standardized oral care protocol including brushing with a soft tooth brush, flossing, and non-medicated rinse use (saline or sodium bicarbonate rinses) is recommended during treatment [45]. Reduced salivary function as a result of xerostomia may cause accumulation of food and debris, which requires more frequent hygiene. Cleaning of the oral cavity after meals is important. Frequent rinsing (4–6 times daily) of the oral cavity with 0.9% saline is a common practice in many centers. The use of drying agents such as alcohol or glycerine-based products may be beneficial. A meticulous dental assessment several weeks before RT starts is required to allow for adequate time interval for tissue healing if invasive oral procedures such as dental extraction are indicated. Along with meticulous dental hygiene, there is a number of agents used to prevent the development of oral mucositis, mostly under clinical evaluation, such as palifermin, dusquetide, GC4419, clonidine lauriad, benzydamine, low-level laser therapy, and natural agents including plant extracts, manuka honey, vitamin A, aloe vera, chamomile, and glutamine [46].

Once mucositis has been developed, saline and bicarbonate lavage can be used in the management of non-confluent mucositis. Initially, patients can be treated with an over-the counter pain reliever, but once patients develop grade II or III mucositis, they will commonly require narcotic analgesics for adequate pain control. Topical xylocaine can also be used to relieve oral discomfort. Topical antifungals such as nystatin and clotrimazole may be used in the management of oral candidiasis. Systemic antifungals such as fluconazole and ketoconazole may also be used if necessary. If taste has been affected, patients should be instructed to chew foods longer to allow for more contact of foods with taste buds. Also, smelling the foods before eating can be recommended since taste and smelling senses are interlinked. The nutritional status of the patient should also be optimized. The combination of dysphagia and mucositis can result in significant nutritional compromise necessitating intravenous hydration and parenteral nutritional supplementation.

2.4   Vestibulocochlear Nerve

2.4.1   Anatomy

The vestibulocochlear nerve is the eighth cranial nerve (CN VIII) composed of the vestibular and cochlear nerves, both purely sensory in function. The vestibulocochlear nerve carries special somatic afferent fibers from structures of the internal ear. The cochlear nerve enables the sense of hearing, while the vestibular nerve is responsible for equilibrium, spatial orientation, and motion. After the cochlear nerve originates from the sensory receptors of the organ of Corti which lies in the cochlea of the internal ear, it enters the internal acoustic meatus where it joins with the vestibular nerve to form the vestibulocochlear nerve. The cochlear nerve then travels along the vestibular nerve through the internal acoustic meatus to the posterior cranial fossa, through the pontine cistern and then enters the brainstem in the cerebellopontine angle along with the facial nerve (CN VII). The information is further transmitted to the thalamus and auditory cortex of the temporal lobe. The vestibular nerve, on the other hand, arises from the sensory receptors located within the membranous labyrinth. Most of the vestibular nerve fibers terminate in the brainstem in the vestibular nuclei, but some fibers run directly to the reticular nuclei of the brainstem without synapsing, and also to the cerebellar nuclei.

The nerve itself cannot be visualized on imaging. Therefore, the cochlea where it derives from is delineated instead [23]. It is recommended to delineate the cochlea at least in two slices in the bony window of CT [36]. The cochlea lies forward and laterally to the internal auditory canal. The internal ear is composed of two parts: the bony labyrinth, composed of a series of small bony cavities constituting the cochlea on the anterior, the vestibule in the center, and the semicircular canals on the posterior, and the membranous labyrinth, composed in the central part of the vestibule of the saccule and the utricle which is connected to the three semicircular canals. On the other side of the vestibule, the cochlea is hollowed out by three channels: the vestibular ramp that abuts the oval window, the tympanic ramp that abuts the round window, and the cochlear canal. The bony and membranous labyrinth is mainly responsible for hearing and balance, respectively.

The cochlea is delineated with the petrous apex of the temporal pyramid on the superior, the carotid canal on the inferior, the medial wall of the tympanic cavity on the lateral, the temporal pyramid on the medial, the anterior and superior surface of the petrous bone on the anterior, and the anterior aspect of the internal auditory canal on the posterior aspect, respectively. As an OAR, the cochlea can be delineated as a separate organ, or together with the internal auditory canal.

2.4.2 Contouring

Delineation of the vestibulocochlear nerve is shown in Fig. 2.7.

2.4.3 Dose Constraints

Sensorineural hearing loss has been observed with doses >60 Gy to the inner ear. Bhandare et al. [47] reported clinical hearing loss in 37% of patients receiving 60.5 Gy compared to 3% with lower doses. Chan et al. [48] reported a significantly higher rate of hearing loss at a high frequency in patients with nasopharyngeal carcinoma treated with RT and concurrent chemotherapy compared to RT alone (55% vs. 33.3%) the difference was not statistically significant at a low frequency (7.9% vs. 16.7%). Most hearing loss is seen >4000 Hz although normal frequency ranges

Fig. 2.7 Delineation of
the vestibulocochlear
nerve. Green: internal
acoustic canal, red:
cochlea, blue: inner ear

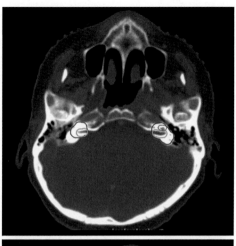

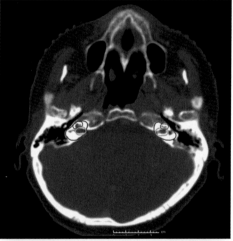

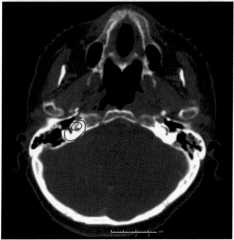

Table 2.4 Dose constraints for the cochlea

OAR	Mean dose	Other
Cochlea	<40 Gy	Dmax < 60% D2% <40 Gy

between 1000 and 3000 Hz for daily use. In a prospective study, a $\geq$ 10 dB hearing loss 2 years following RT was reported in 40% of patients for 8000 Hz, and in 50% for 3000 Hz [49]. The authors recommended a threshold dose of 45 Gy for $\geq$2000 Hz which also depends on age and baseline hearing capacity. The mean threshold dose for the cochlea and tuba of Eustachius for sensorineural hearing loss varies between 40 and 50 Gy [48–50]. After a latency around 1.5–2 years, hearing loss stabilizes. No dose–response relationship has been published for vestibular damage [51].

Other publications recommend the D2% <40 Gy, maximum dose <60 Gy and mean dose $\leq$40–45 Gy, <35 Gy, or even $\leq$10 Gy to the cochlea [52, 53]. In general, the mean dose should be as low as possible and, in all cases, should be kept <40 Gy (Table 2.4). This dose should further be decreased in the event of other risk factors for hearing loss such as older age, pre-existing hearing deficiency, or concurrent chemotherapy with platinum [54, 55]. In hypofractionated regimens, the recommended maximum dose to the cochlea is <9–10 Gy in 1 fraction, <17 Gy in 3 fractions, and <23–25 Gy in five fractions [23, 56, 57].

2.4.4 Pathophysiology

In the physiology of hearing, the external ear collects, conveys, and amplifies the sound waves which cause the auricular labyrinth to vibrate toward the middle ear. The energy of the sound waves is transformed into mechanic vibrations of the bony structure of the middle ear which leads the kinetic impulse be transmitted to the perilymph within the cochlea. Through the endolymph in the membranous labyrinth of the cochlear duct, sound waves are transmitted causing vibration of the membranes that separate the scalae of the cochlea. This stimulates hair cells of the auditory system, producing an electrical signal that is transmitted along the acoustic nerve to the auditory cortex. Radiotherapy affects both the endothelium and nerve structures negatively. The irradiation of the internal ear results in the atrophy of sensory neuronal cells and fibrosis and ossification of the fluid spaces in a few weeks or months after RT is initiated. Besides, RT also leads to the atrophy and degeneration of nerve structures and production of inflammatory mediators which manifests as degeneration and atrophy of Corti's ganglion and the cochlear nerve causing edema and compression of the cochlear nerve in the ear canal [47, 51]. The symptoms include tinnitus, labyrinthitis, vertigo with balance alteration, and sensorineural deafness which can lead to cognitive impairment, and, at the end, decrease in the quality of life. Vascular insufficiency (alteration of the endothelium) has been proposed as the etiology of sensorineural hearing loss.

Sensorineural hearing loss was detected in more than 30% of the patients assessed treated with RT for HNC, and the risk increases up to >40% with the use of cisplatin-based concurrent chemotherapy [48, 58].

2.4.5 Treatment

There is no standard treatment of sensorineural hearing loss caused by RT. Conservative measures include systemic steroids to improve inflammation and edema in the inner ear after RT-induced damage and to reduce the compression of the acoustic nerve due to inflammatory swelling [35]. Hyperbaric oxygen treatment can be used for its role on vascular damage and ischemia. In patients with RT-induced bilateral profound sensorineural hearing loss, cochlear implants are a viable rehabilitation option. No harmful effects of cochlear implant surgery and activity on vestibular function and balance have been reported [59].

2.5 Mandible

2.5.1 Anatomy

The mandible is a horse shoe-shaped, medial, symmetrical bone in which the lower teeth are located. It is divided into three parts: a body and two branches united by the two mandibular angles. The head of the mandible is joined to the articular fossa and articular tubercle of the temporal bone by the TMJ. These mismatched surfaces are separated by an articular disc [36].

When contouring, the mandible is defined as the entire mandibular bone of a single piece including the alveoli but excluding the teeth [3, 23]. The use of CT bone view settings is recommended while contouring [3].

2.5.2 Contouring

Delineation of the mandible is shown in Fig. 2.8.

2.5.3 Dose Constraints

Depending on the target localization, the D2% of the mandible should be <65 Gy [60]. Five percent risk of the development of osteoradionecrosis (ORN) in 5 years (TD 5/5) is increased if the mean dose is >60–65 Gy and >60 Gy for patients with and without teeth, respectively [23] (Table 2.5). The recommended maximum dose is 65 Gy. Cooper et al. [61] reported no ORN with doses <65 Gy but the rate of ORN was 80% with doses >75 Gy, more frequent in dentulous than edentulous patients.

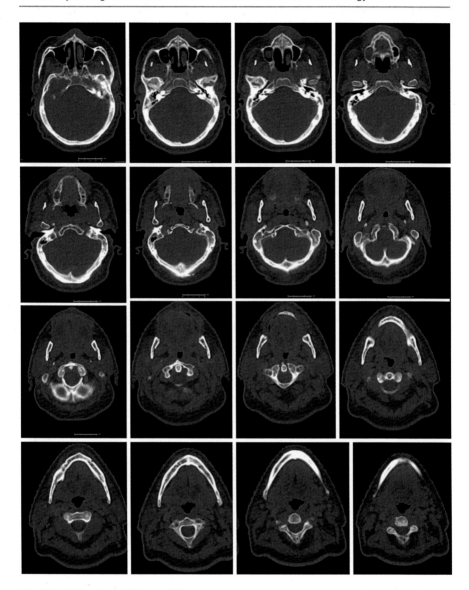

Fig. 2.8 Delineation of the mandible

Table 2.5 Dose constraints for the mandible

Organ at risk	Mean dose	Other
Mandible	<60–65 Gy	D2% < 65 Gy Dmax < 65 Gy

2.5.4 Pathophysiology

Exceeding doses of RT to the mandible leads to osteocytic damage, injury to the small vasculature of the haversian systems and the periosteum and fibrosis which negatively affects the bone's capability to resist trauma and avoid infections [62, 63]. As the compromised bone loses self-repair ability, pathologic fractures may occur along with pain, fistula, infection, and sensational loss. What makes the mandible predisposed to this risk is its terminal vascularization (radiation-induced fibrosis is not compensated for by the facial artery and occlusion of the lower alveolar artery occurs) and mineralized nature (the bone density is higher in the regions of the molar and premolar teeth which are the most commonly damaged) [63–65]. The patient presents with a painful and denuded region on the mandible, with purulent drainage and sometimes with fistula formation (to the mucosal or skin surface). The risk of ORN increases with trauma, oral infections, and intimate association of primary tumor with the bone. Osteoradionecrosis typically occurs within the first 3 years after diagnosis of HNC. There is an incidence of 1–5% of mandibular ORN following RT [66]. The risk is increased with the extraction of posterior maxillary teeth post-RT [67].

2.5.5 Treatment

One can prevent mandibular ORN by maintaining meticulous oral hygiene, eliminating trauma, avoiding removable dental prostheses when the denture bearing area is within the necrosis field, maintaining adequate nutritional intake, and discontinuing alcohol and tobacco consumption. If attempts to preserve teeth are unsuccessful, post-RT dental extractions should be performed cautiously due to the risk of initiating ORN. Dental extractions should be performed followed by primary suturing and under antibiotic prophylaxis. In case infection occurs, topical or systemic antibiotics are prescribed. Analgesics can be indicated for pain management. Local resection of the loose bony spicules can be possible.

Pentoxifylline, tocopherol, and clodronate have been used to overcome fibrosis in the TMJ [35]. Pentoxifylline is a methylxanthine derivative which inhibits fibroblast proliferation, extracellular matrix production, and collagenase activity stimulation. Tocopherol (vitamin E) is an antioxidant agent acting as a free radical scavenger by downregulating the procollagen gene expression and protecting the cell membrane against lipid peroxidation. These agents inhibit TNF-α and TGF-β for their anti-inflammatory actions. Clodronate is a bisphosphonate that directly activates osteoblasts and reduces the activity of osteoclasts, resulting in bone resorption inhibition, increase in bone synthesis, and decrease in fibroblast proliferation.

If these treatments fail and the patients suffer from progressing pain, hyperbaric oxygen treatment can be performed to increase the oxygenation of the irradiated tissue, enhance angiogenesis, increase osteoblast repopulation and fibroblast function. Surgical resection and reconstruction of the irradiated mandible can be an option in severe cases with fracture and/or fistula [35].

2.6   Rx: Sample Prescriptions

Dental and Oral Mucosa Prophylaxis
- Chlorhexidine gluconate 0.12% oral rinse (Peridex®): 15 ml (marked in cup) twice daily oral rinsing for 30 s after toothbrushing.
- Povidone-iodine oral antiseptic 1% (Betadine® mouthwash): One cup every 2–4 h daily oral rinsing for 30 s.

Xerostomia Prophylaxis
- Amifostine (Ethyol®): 200 mg/m^2 once daily as a 3-min iv infusion, starting 15–30 min prior to standard fraction RT.

Xerostomia Treatment
- Pilocarpine hydrochloride: Start with 5 mg tablets three times daily and titrate according to the therapeutic response and tolerance, up to 15–30 mg per day (not to exceed 10 mg per dose). Use at least 12 weeks uninterruptedly for maximum benefit.
- Bethanechol: 10–50 mg three or four times daily. The effect usually starts within 30 min, reaches maximum within 60–90 min, and persists for about 1 h.
- Cevimeline hydrochloride (Evoxac®): 30 mg three times a day.

Oral Mucositis Prophylaxis
Palifermin (Kepivance®): 60 mcg/kg/day iv bolus injection for three consecutive days before and three consecutive days after myelotoxic therapy for a total of six doses. The first three doses are administered prior to myelotoxic therapy with the third dose 24–48 h before myelotoxic therapy. The last three doses are administered after myelotoxic therapy is complete.

Benzydamine HCl 0.15% solution (Tantum®): ≥15 ml gargle or rinse for at least 30 s 3–4 times daily.

Glutamine (Abound®): two servings (packets) per day, after dissolved with liquid.

Antifungal Treatment
- Topical
  - Lidocaine (Xylocaine®): No more than 10 g (500 mg lidocaine base) in a single dose. The total maximum dose administered in a 24-h period should not exceed 20 g (1000 mg lidocaine base).
  - Clotrimazole: Gently massage into the affected and surrounding skin areas twice a day.
- Systemic
  - Fluconazole (Diflucan®): 200 mg on the first day, followed by 100 mg once daily, should be continued for at least 2 weeks to decrease the likelihood of relapse.
  - Ketoconazole (Nizoral®): 200 mg (one tablet) daily. In case of clinical responsiveness dose may be increased to 400 mg (two tablets) once daily.

Hearing Loss
- Glucocorticoids: dexamethasone (Kordexa®, Dekort®) 4–16 mg daily.

TMJ Treatment
- Pentoxifylline (Trental®): One tablet (400 mg) three times daily with meals. Continue for at least 8 weeks balancing efficacy with digestive and central nervous system side effects.
- Tocopherol: 15 mg oral q.i.d., should not exceed 1000 mg/day.
- Sodium clodronate (Bonefos®): Starting dose is 1600 mg daily, if clinically necessary, may be increased, but is not recommended to exceed 3200 mg daily. The duration of treatment is recommended to be life-long.

References

1. Dawes C, Wood CM. The contribution of oral minor mucous gland secretions to the volume of whole saliva in man. Arch Oral Biol. 1973;18:337–42.
2. van de Water TA, Bijl HP, Westerlaan HE, Langendijk JA. Delineation guidelines for organs at risk involved in radiation-induced salivary dysfunction and xerostomia. Radiother Oncol. 2009;93:545–52.
3. Brouwer CL, Steenbakkers RJ, Bourhis J, et al. CT-based delineation of organs at risk in the head and neck region: DAHANCA, EORTC, GORTEC, HKNPCSG, NCIC CTG, NCRI, NRG oncology and TROG consensus guidelines. Radiother Oncol. 2015;117:83–90.
4. Eisbruch A, Kim HM, Terrell JE, et al. Xerostomia and its predictors following parotid-sparing irradiation of head-and-neck cancer. Int J Radiat Oncol Biol Phys. 2001;50:695–704.
5. Blanco AI, Chao KS, El Naqa I, et al. Dose-volume modeling of salivary function in patients with head-and-neck cancer receiving radiotherapy. Int J Radiat Oncol Biol Phys. 2005;62:1055–69.
6. Li Y, Taylor JM, Ten Haken RK, Eisbruch A. The impact of dose on parotid salivary recovery in head and neck cancer patients treated with radiation therapy. Int J Radiat Oncol Biol Phys. 2007;67:660–9.
7. Robar JL, Day A, Clancey J, et al. Spatial and dosimetric variability of organs at risk in head-and-neck intensity-modulated radiotherapy. Int J Radiat Oncol Biol Phys. 2007;68:1121–30.
8. Chao KS, Deasy JO, Markman J, et al. A prospective study of salivary function sparing in patients with head-and-neck cancers receiving intensity-modulated or three-dimensional radiation therapy: initial results. Int J Radiat Oncol Biol Phys. 2001;49:907–16.
9. Saarilahti K, Kouri M, Collan J, et al. Sparing of the submandibular glands by intensity modulated radiotherapy in the treatment of head and neck cancer. Radiother Oncol. 2006;78:270–5.
10. Jen YM, Lin YC, Wang YB, Wu DM. Dramatic and prolonged decrease of whole salivary secretion in nasopharyngeal carcinoma patients treated with radiotherapy. Oral Surg Oral Med Oral Pathol Oral Radiol Endod. 2006;101:322–7.
11. Dijkema T, Raaijmakers CP, Ten Haken RK, et al. Parotid gland function after radiotherapy: the combined Michigan and Utrecht experience. Int J Radiat Oncol Biol Phys. 2010;78:449–53.
12. Lee N, Xia P, Quivey JM, et al. Intensity-modulated radiotherapy in the treatment of nasopharyngeal carcinoma: an update of the UCSF experience. Int J Radiat Oncol Biol Phys. 2002;53:12–22.
13. Kam MK, Leung SF, Zee B, et al. Prospective randomized study of intensity-modulated radiotherapy on salivary gland function in early-stage nasopharyngeal carcinoma patients. J Clin Oncol. 2007;25:4873–9.
14. Pow EH, Kwong DL, McMillan AS, et al. Xerostomia and quality of life after intensity-modulated radiotherapy vs. conventional radiotherapy for early-stage nasopharyngeal

carcinoma: initial report on a randomized controlled clinical trial. Int J Radiat Oncol Biol Phys. 2006;66:981–91.
15. Al-Mamgani A, van Rooij P, Verduijn GM, et al. Long-term outcomes and quality of life of 186 patients with primary parotid carcinoma treated with surgery and radiotherapy at the Daniel den Hoed Cancer Center. Int J Radiat Oncol Biol Phys. 2012;84:189–95.
16. Murdoch-Kinch CA, Kim HM, Vineberg KA, et al. Dose-effect relationships for the submandibular salivary glands and implications for their sparing by intensity modulated radiotherapy. Int J Radiat Oncol Biol Phys. 2008;72:373–82.
17. Jellema AP, Doornaert P, Slotman BJ, et al. Does radiation dose to the salivary glands and oral cavity predict patient-rated xerostomia and sticky saliva in head and neck cancer patients treated with curative radiotherapy? Radiother Oncol. 2005;77:164–71.
18. Seikaly H, Jha N, Harris JR, et al. Long-term outcomes of submandibular gland transfer for prevention of postradiation xerostomia. Arch Otolaryngol Head Neck Surg. 2004;130:956–61.
19. Meirovitz A, Murdoch-Kinch CA, Schipper M, et al. Grading xerostomia by physicians or by patients after intensity-modulated radiotherapy of head-and-neck cancer. Int J Radiat Oncol Biol Phys. 2006;66:445–53.
20. Deasy JO, Moiseenko V, Marks L, et al. Radiotherapy dose-volume effects on salivary gland function. Int J Radiat Oncol Biol Phys. 2010;76:S58–63.
21. Ortholan C, Benezery K, Bensadoun RJ. Normal tissue tolerance to external beam radiation therapy: salivary glands. Cancer Radiother. 2010;14:290–4.
22. Eisbruch A, Ten Haken RK, Kim HM, et al. Dose, volume, and function relationships in parotid salivary glands following conformal and intensity-modulated irradiation of head and neck cancer. Int J Radiat Oncol Biol Phys. 1999;45:577–87.
23. Noel G, Antoni D, Barillot I, Chauvet B. Delineation of organs at risk and dose constraints. Cancer Radiother. 2016;20:S36–60.
24. Cannon DM, Lee NY. Recurrence in region of spared parotid gland after definitive intensity-modulated radiotherapy for head and neck cancer. Int J Radiat Oncol Biol Phys. 2008;70:660–5.
25. Chambers MS, Garden AS, Kies MS, Martin JW. Radiation-induced xerostomia in patients with head and neck cancer: pathogenesis, impact on quality of life, and management. Head Neck. 2004;26:796–807.
26. Dirix P, Nuyts S, Van den Bogaert W. Radiation-induced xerostomia in patients with head and neck cancer: a literature review. Cancer. 2006;107:2525–34.
27. Brizel DM, Wasserman TH, Henke M, et al. Phase III randomized trial of amifostine as a radioprotector in head and neck cancer. J Clin Oncol. 2000;18:3339–45.
28. Munter MW, Hoffner S, Hof H, et al. Changes in salivary gland function after radiotherapy of head and neck tumors measured by quantitative pertechnetate scintigraphy: comparison of intensity-modulated radiotherapy and conventional radiation therapy with and without Amifostine. Int J Radiat Oncol Biol Phys. 2007;67:651–9.
29. Bourhis J, Blanchard P, Maillard E, et al. Effect of amifostine on survival among patients treated with radiotherapy: a meta-analysis of individual patient data. J Clin Oncol. 2011;29:2590–7.
30. Eisbruch A. Amifostine in the treatment of head and neck cancer: intravenous administration, subcutaneous administration, or none of the above. J Clin Oncol. 2011;29:119–21.
31. Eisbruch A, Ship JA, Dawson LA, et al. Salivary gland sparing and improved target irradiation by conformal and intensity modulated irradiation of head and neck cancer. World J Surg. 2003;27:832–7.
32. Nutting CM, Morden JP, Harrington KJ, et al. Parotid-sparing intensity modulated versus conventional radiotherapy in head and neck cancer (PARSPORT): a phase 3 multicentre randomised controlled trial. Lancet Oncol. 2011;12:127–36.
33. Lovelace TL, Fox NF, Sood AJ, et al. Management of radiotherapy-induced salivary hypofunction and consequent xerostomia in patients with oral or head and neck cancer: meta-analysis and literature review. Oral Surg Oral Med Oral Pathol Oral Radiol. 2014;117:595–607.
34. Pimentel MJ, Filho MM, Araujo M, et al. Evaluation of radioprotective effect of pilocarpine ingestion on salivary glands. Anticancer Res. 2014;34:1993–9.

35. Strojan P, Hutcheson KA, Eisbruch A, et al. Treatment of late sequelae after radiotherapy for head and neck cancer. Cancer Treat Rev. 2017;59:79–92.
36. Servagi-Vernat S, Ali D, Espinoza S, et al. Organs at risk in radiation therapy of head and neck tumors: practical aspects in their delineation and normal tissue tolerance. Cancer Radiother. 2013;17:695–704.
37. Teguh DN, Levendag PC, Voet P, et al. Trismus in patients with oropharyngeal cancer: relationship with dose in structures of mastication apparatus. Head Neck. 2008;30:622–30.
38. Dijkstra PU, Huisman PM, Roodenburg JL. Criteria for trismus in head and neck oncology. Int J Oral Maxillofac Surg. 2006;35:337–42.
39. Wang CJ, Huang EY, Hsu HC, et al. The degree and time-course assessment of radiation-induced trismus occurring after radiotherapy for nasopharyngeal cancer. Laryngoscope. 2005;115:1458–60.
40. Cefaro GA, Domenico G, Perez CA. Brain head, and neck. In: Delineating organs at risk in radiation therapy. Italia: Springer; 2013. p. 84–101.
41. Rapidis AD, Dijkstra PU, Roodenburg JL, et al. Trismus in patients with head and neck cancer: etiopathogenesis, diagnosis and management. Clin Otolaryngol. 2015;40:516–26.
42. Schwartz DL, Hutcheson K, Barringer D, et al. Candidate dosimetric predictors of long-term swallowing dysfunction after oropharyngeal intensity-modulated radiotherapy. Int J Radiat Oncol Biol Phys. 2010;78:1356–65.
43. Hoebers F, Yu E, Eisbruch A, et al. A pragmatic contouring guideline for salivary gland structures in head and neck radiation oncology: the MOIST target. Am J Clin Oncol. 2013;36:70–6.
44. Maria OM, Eliopoulos N, Muanza T. Radiation-induced oral mucositis. Front Oncol. 2017;7:89.
45. Lalla RV, Bowen J, Barasch A, et al. MASCC/ISOO clinical practice guidelines for the management of mucositis secondary to cancer therapy. Cancer. 2014;120:1453–61.
46. Blakaj A, Bonomi M, Gamez ME, Blakaj DM. Oral mucositis in head and neck cancer: evidence-based management and review of clinical trial data. Oral Oncol. 2019;95:29–34.
47. Bhandare N, Antonelli PJ, Morris CG, et al. Ototoxicity after radiotherapy for head and neck tumors. Int J Radiat Oncol Biol Phys. 2007;67:469–79.
48. Chan SH, Ng WT, Kam KL, et al. Sensorineural hearing loss after treatment of nasopharyngeal carcinoma: a longitudinal analysis. Int J Radiat Oncol Biol Phys. 2009;73:1335–42.
49. Pan CC, Eisbruch A, Lee JS, et al. Prospective study of inner ear radiation dose and hearing loss in head-and-neck cancer patients. Int J Radiat Oncol Biol Phys. 2005;61:1393–402.
50. van der Putten L, de Bree R, Plukker JT, et al. Permanent unilateral hearing loss after radiotherapy for parotid gland tumors. Head Neck. 2006;28:902–8.
51. Bhide SA, Harrington KJ, Nutting CM. Otological toxicity after postoperative radiotherapy for parotid tumours. Clin Oncol (R Coll Radiol). 2007;19:77–82.
52. Hitchcock YJ, Tward JD, Szabo A, et al. Relative contributions of radiation and cisplatin-based chemotherapy to sensorineural hearing loss in head-and-neck cancer patients. Int J Radiat Oncol Biol Phys. 2009;73:779–88.
53. Maingon P, Mammar V, Peignaux K, et al. Constraints to organs at risk for treatment of head and neck cancers by intensity modulated radiation therapy. Cancer Radiother. 2004;8:234–47.
54. Fleury B, Lapeyre M. Tolerance of normal tissues to radiation therapy: ear. Cancer Radiother. 2010;14:284–9.
55. Jereczek-Fossa BA, Zarowski A, Milani F, Orecchia R. Radiotherapy-induced ear toxicity. Cancer Treat Rev. 2003;29:417–30.
56. Benedict SH, Yenice KM, Followill D, et al. Stereotactic body radiation therapy: the report of AAPM task group 101. Med Phys. 2010;37:4078–101.
57. Grimm J, LaCouture T, Croce R, et al. Dose tolerance limits and dose volume histogram evaluation for stereotactic body radiotherapy. J Appl Clin Med Phys. 2011;12:3368.
58. Lee AW, Ng WT, Hung WM, et al. Major late toxicities after conformal radiotherapy for nasopharyngeal carcinoma-patient- and treatment-related risk factors. Int J Radiat Oncol Biol Phys. 2009;73:1121–8.

59. le Nobel GJ, Hwang E, Wu A, et al. Vestibular function following unilateral cochlear implantation for profound sensorineural hearing loss. J Otolaryngol Head Neck Surg. 2016;45:38.
60. Berger A, Bensadoun RJ. Normal tissue tolerance to external beam radiation therapy: the mandible. Cancer Radiother. 2010;14:295–300.
61. Cooper JS, Fu K, Marks J, Silverman S. Late effects of radiation therapy in the head and neck region. Int J Radiat Oncol Biol Phys. 1995;31:1141–64.
62. Marx RE. Osteoradionecrosis: a new concept of its pathophysiology. J Oral Maxillofac Surg. 1983;41:283–8.
63. Meyer I. Infectious diseases of the jaws. J Oral Surg. 1970;28:17–26.
64. Marx RE. A new concept in the treatment of osteoradionecrosis. J Oral Maxillofac Surg. 1983;41:351–7.
65. Ben-David MA, Diamante M, Radawski JD, et al. Lack of osteoradionecrosis of the mandible after intensity-modulated radiotherapy for head and neck cancer: likely contributions of both dental care and improved dose distributions. Int J Radiat Oncol Biol Phys. 2007;68:396–402.
66. Wahl MJ. Osteoradionecrosis prevention myths. Int J Radiat Oncol Biol Phys. 2006;64:661–9.
67. Tong AC, Leung AC, Cheng JC, Sham J. Incidence of complicated healing and osteoradionecrosis following tooth extraction in patients receiving radiotherapy for treatment of nasopharyngeal carcinoma. Aust Dent J. 1999;44:187–94.

Toxicity Management for Head and Neck Tumors in Radiation Oncology-II

3

Pervin Hurmuz

3.1 Pharyngeal Constrictor Muscles

3.1.1 Anatomy

The pharynx extends from the base of the skull to the cricoid cartilage. There are three pharyngeal constrictor muscles (PCM) delineated by their position relative to one another (superior, middle, and inferior) run both circularly on the outside and longitudinally on the inside. Their different attachment points and sequential, involuntary contraction allow the pharyngeal lumen to be closed in a cranial to caudal direction for peristalsis during swallowing, while alternately remaining open for breathing and speaking [1].

The superior pharyngeal constrictor muscle (SPCM) originates at the lateral base of tongue, medial pterygoid plate, pterygomandibular raphe, pterygoid hamulus, and the posterior end of the mylohyoid line. It inserts onto the pharyngeal raphe and contracts during deglutition to move the soft palate to the posterior pharyngeal wall, thus preventing the bolus from moving upward. The middle pharyngeal constrictor muscle (MPCM) originates from the stylohyoid ligament and the greater and lesser horns of the hyoid bone. It fans out to attach along the pharyngeal raphe, but this muscle rarely reaches the top of the pharynx (superiorly) or thyroid cartilage (inferiorly). The contraction of these fibers constricts and closes the pharynx during deglutition to propel the bolus downward. The inferior pharyngeal constrictor muscle (IPCM) originates from the cricoid and thyroid cartilages and crosses the cricothyroid muscle. It inserts onto the pharyngeal raphe and constricts in coordination with the SPCM and MPCM during deglutition to propel the bolus towards the

P. Hurmuz (✉)
Faculty of Medicine, Department of Radiation Oncology, Hacettepe University, Ankara, Turkey

© Springer Nature Switzerland AG 2020
G. Ozyigit, U. Selek (eds.), *Prevention and Management of Acute and Late Toxicities in Radiation Oncology*, https://doi.org/10.1007/978-3-030-37798-4_3

esophagus. Due to the finding that some of the inferior IPCM fibers merge with fibers of the cricothyroid muscle, the belief is that the IPCM serves as part of the functional upper esophageal sphincter [1–6].

The pharyngeal muscles receive their blood supply from branches of the external carotid artery according to their anatomic location. The ascending pharyngeal artery commonly supplies all of the pharyngeal muscles. Additionally, the constrictor muscles receive vascular supply from the tonsillar branch of the facial artery and the muscular branch of the inferior thyroid artery.

3.1.2 Contouring

There are several guidelines available that vary in cranial to caudal extension. For the sake of simplicity and reproducibility, PCM may be delineated as a single organ at risk (OAR) (Figs. 3.1, 3.2, and 3.3). The cranial border was defined as the caudal tip of pterygoid plates [7], occipital condyle [8], or the level of C1–C2 interspace and the caudal border as the lower edge of the cricoid cartilage. Table 3.1 summarizes the anatomic boundaries of PCMs.

3.1.3 Dose Constraints

Except cases with gross positive retropharyngeal LNs and/or posterior pharyngeal wall involvement it is recommended to keep the mean dose to uninvolved pharynx to be less than 40 Gy. Evidence based literature summary with a final dose constraints on PCM is presented in Table 3.2. Based on this data, limiting the mean dose to <55 Gy for the PCMs should safely and effectively reduce the risk for long-term dysphagia.

3.1.4 Pathophysiology

Dysphagia is defined as difficulty in swallowing. Although most head and neck cancer patients present with pretreatment dysphagia due to local effects of tumor some develop worsening of swallowing functions after radiotherapy ± chemotherapy. Some patients develop aspiration pneumonia later in the follow up if the dose constraints for larynx and pharyngeal constrictor muscles are not taken into account.

Dysphagia may develop due to radiation-induced normal tissue changes including edema, neuropathy, and fibrosis. Acute toxicities such as mucositis and edema commonly disturb normal swallowing during treatment, but improve substantially following treatment in majority of patients in months. However, neuropathy and fibrosis of the pharyngeal musculature may develop or persist long after the completion of treatment and impair the swallowing functions permanently [15].

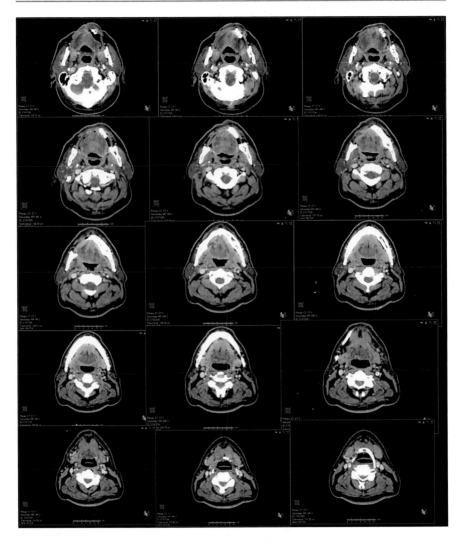

Fig. 3.1 Delineation of superior pharyngeal constrictor muscle

3.1.5   Treatment

Prevention is the most effective approach and is achieved with careful treatment planning. Supraglottic and glottis larynx should be contoured as organ at risk if not involved by the tumor. Mean laryngeal dose should be kept below 35 Gy in case of bilateral neck irradiation. Patients should be evaluated if possible with a speech language pathologist.

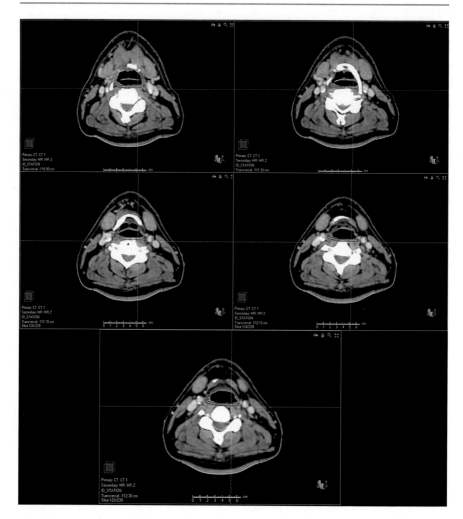

Fig. 3.2 Delineation of middle pharyngeal constrictor muscle

3.2 Larynx

3.2.1 Anatomy

Larynx is a midline structure located in the neck region anterior to the esophagus and cervical vertebrae. It is comprised of a mucosal lining covered by cartilaginous skeleton, and extrinsic and intrinsic muscles. The larynx is suspended from the hyoid bone in the anterior neck by soft tissue attachments. The laryngeal skeleton consists of nine cartilages; paired arytenoid, corniculate, cuneiform cartilages and unpaired thyroid, cricoid, and epiglottis.

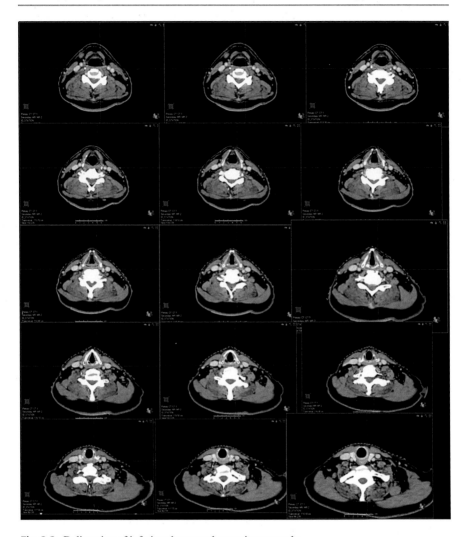

Fig. 3.3 Delineation of inferior pharyngeal constrictor muscle

During the process of swallowing, the epiglottis folds over to cover the glottis and prevents food from blocking the airway. The true vocal folds are bands of tissue comprised of muscle, fibrous ligament, and mucosa extending from the arytenoids posteriorly to the midline thyroid cartilage anteriorly. The false (ventricular) vocal folds are located superior to the true vocal folds and are separated from them by a lateral recess termed the laryngeal ventricle. The ventricle contains mucus-producing glands that provide lubrication for the true vocal folds, which are themselves devoid of glandular elements.

The larynx is subdivided into three regions: the supraglottis, glottis, and subglottis. The supraglottis covers the area above the true vocal folds (including epiglottis,

Table 3.1 Anatomic boundaries of pharyngeal constrictor muscles [9]

Organ	Cranial	Caudal	Anterior	Posterior	Lateral
Superior pharyngeal constrictor muscle	Caudal edge of pterygoid plates	Cranial edge of hyoid bone	Nasopharynx, oropharynx, laryngopharynx, base of tongue	Longus capitis m., longus colli m., body of cervical vertebra	Carotid sheath
Middle pharyngeal constrictor muscle	Cranial edge of hyoid bone	Caudal edge of hyoid bone	Laryngopharynx	Longus capitis m., longus colli m., body of cervical vertebra	Hyoid bone
Inferior pharyngeal constrictor muscle	Caudal edge of hyoid bone	Caudal edge of cricoid cartilage	Laryngopharynx or cricoids cartilage	Longus capitis m., longus colli m., body of cervical vertebra	Thyroid cartilage or thyroid gland

Table 3.2 Summary of dose constraints on pharyngeal constrictor muscles

Study	Patient number	Study type	Follow up, months	PCM dose	Endpoint
Schwartz et al. [10]	33	Prospective, oropharyngeal ca	6–24	*Superior PCM* V55 < 80% V65 < 30%	Swallowing dysfunction
Caglar et al. [11]	96	Retrospective, oropharyngeal ca (44%) Hypopharynx/ larynx (17%)	10 (median)	*Inferior PCM* Mean < 54 Gy D60 < 52 Gy V50 < 51% *Superior PCM* Mean < 63 Gy (aspiration)	Aspiration, stricture
Caudell et al. [12]	83	Retrospective, oropharyngeal ca (53%) Hypopharynx/ larynx (28%)	12 (minimum)	*Inferior PCM* V60 < 12%	PEG tube dependence, aspiration
				Superior PCM V65 < 33% Middle PCM: V65 < 75%	Pharyngoesophageal stricture requiring dilation
Eisbruch et al. [13]	73	Prospective, oropharynx (100%)	36 (median)	*PCM* Mean = 63 Gy (TD50) mean = 56 Gy (TD25)	Aspiration
Li et al. [14]	39	Retrospective, oropharynx (64%) Hypopharynx/ larynx (23%)	16 (mean)	*Inferior PCM* Dmean <55 Gy, V65 < 15%, V60 < 40%,	Gastrostomy tube dependence

false vocal folds, aryepiglottic folds, and arytenoids). The glottis consists of the true vocal folds and the immediate subjacent area extending 1 cm inferiorly. The subglottis refers to the region beginning at the inferior edge of the glottis and extending down to the inferior border of the cricoid cartilage. Vagus nerve innervates the laryngopharynx. Recurrent laryngeal nerve (branch of vagus nerve) innervates all intrinsic muscles except for the cricothyroid muscle, which is innervated by the external branch of the superior laryngeal nerve. A mass lesion along the course of these nerves can result in vocal fold paralysis.

3.2.2 Contouring

Except RTOG 1016 study for oropharynx cancer there has been no validated standardized approach for contouring the larynx for radiotherapy treatment planning. In this study larynx was defined as a "triangular prism-shaped" volume that begins just inferior to the hyoid bone and extends to the cricoid cartilage inferiorly and extends from the anterior commissure to include the arytenoids. This includes the infrahyoid but not the suprahyoid epiglottis. Choi et al. developed a standardized laryngeal contouring atlas which is summarized below [16]. The volumes are defined in bone and soft tissue window (Fig. 3.4).

Bone Window
- *Thyroid cartilage*: The two ala of the thyroid cartilage fuse anteriorly to form a V-shaped shield. The superior and inferior cornua project from the posterior free edges of the thyroid cartilage.
- *Cricoid cartilage*: The cricoid cartilage forms a complete ring to form the base and back of the larynx; it forms a narrow rim anteriorly and a broad lamina posteriorly. Superiorly, it begins just below the arytenoid cartilages. Inferiorly, it ends just above the first tracheal ring.
- *Arytenoid cartilages*: This pair of pyramid-shaped cartilages sits directly on the posterior rim of the cricoid cartilage and posteromedial to the thyroid cartilage.
- *Glottic larynx*: Sits on the same axial plane as the inferior edge of the arytenoid cartilages. Anteriorly and laterally, the glottic larynx is bound by the posteromedial edge of the thyroid cartilage. Posteriorly, it is bound by the anterior edge of the arytenoid cartilages.
- *Subglottic larynx*: This area is composed of the airspace and mucosa housed by the cricoid cartilage. Superiorly, it begins at the slice below the glottic larynx. Inferiorly, it ends at the same level as the most inferior slice of the cricoid cartilage.

Soft Tissue Window
- *Suprahyoid portion of the epiglottis*: A leaf-like cartilage that hovers over the glottic inlet at and above the level of the hyoid bone. Superiorly, it sits in air within the inferior oropharynx and extends inferiorly to the level of the bottom slice of the hyoid bone. The epiglottis forms the anterior wall of the laryngeal

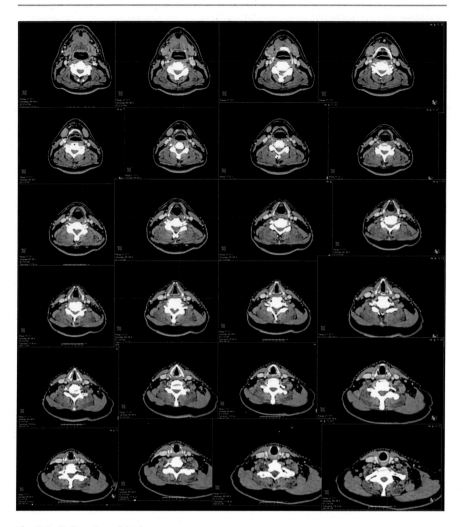

Fig. 3.4 Delineation of the larynx

vestibule. Typically, a clear fat plane can be seen wrapping antero-laterally around the epiglottis and should not be included.

- *Infrahyoid epiglottis*: This structure begins below the inferior aspect of the supra-hyoid epiglottis. Inferiorly, the epiglottis forms a narrow stem that attaches to the posterior surface of the angle of the thyroid cartilage and ends just above the glottic larynx.
- *Aryepiglottic folds and false vocal folds*: Because they are difficult to differentiate from one another without direct visualization, identify and contour the aryepiglottic folds and false vocal folds as a single structure. Superiorly, the structure begins at the superior aspect of the valleculae, forming the lateral walls of this structure. Inferiorly, the structure forms the lateral wall of the supraglottic larynx and medial wall of the pyriform sinuses.

- *Epiglottis*: Combine the contours of the suprahyoid epiglottis and infrahyoid epiglottis.
- *Supraglottic larynx*: Combine the contours for the epiglottis, arytenoids, and the antero-medial wall of the aryepiglottic folds and false vocal folds. The postero-lateral wall of the aryepiglottic folds forms the medial wall of the pyriform sinuses and is part of the hypopharynx.

It is recommended to create the larynx OAR by combining the supraglottic larynx, glottic larynx, subglottic larynx, thyroid cartilage, and cricoid cartilage contours.

3.2.3 Dose Constraints

Laryngeal edema, aspiration, and vocal dysfunction are the endpoints of laryngeal irradiation. Voice changes following radiotherapy may include reduced vocal loudness, low modal speaking pitch, reduced phonic breath support, vocal roughness, hoarseness, and vocal fatigue [17]. Table 3.3 represents the currently used dose constraints for radiotherapy.

3.2.4 Pathophysiology

Radiotherapy induces sterile inflammation. Acute-responding tissues like mucosa of the head and neck region have high stem cell activity and high regenerative capacity [21]. In these tissues, radiation induces rapid p53-mediated primary apoptosis and delayed secondary apoptosis to eliminate severely damaged cells. These processes cause inflammation, hyperemia, and erythema of the laryngeal mucosa [22]. Acute radiation toxicity is reversible if managed properly.

Table 3.3 Dose constraints and endpoints for treatment

Study	Organ	Dose limit	Endpoint
QUANTEC [18]	Larynx	Maximum dose <63–66 Gy	Voice dysfunction
		V50 < 27%; mean dose <44 Gy EUD <30–35 Gy ($n = 0.45$)	Laryngeal edema
Eisbruch et al. [19]	Larynx	V50 < 50%	Aspiration
	Pharyngeal constrictor	Mean < 60 Gy V50 < 80% V60 < 70% V65 < 50%	
Jensen et al. [20]	Larynxs Upper Esophageal Sphincter	Mean < 60 Gy	Aspiration

EUD equivalent uniform dose

Late radiation toxicity may be caused by a persistent and exaggerated wound healing response that leads to excessive fibroblast replication and matrix deposition leading to extensive fibrogenesis. Other late effects include vascular damage, neural damage, tissue atrophy, and necrosis as well as radiation-induced second malignancies [23, 24].

Voice problems after radiotherapy may be attributed to hyperemia, erythema, dryness of the laryngeal mucosa, muscle atrophy, and fibrosis. The larynx has many mixed serous-mucinous-type glands that is essential to phonation by lubrication of the larynx. Due to radiation-induced atrophic changes in laryngeal glands, the quantity and quality of secretions change leading to poor lubrication of the vocal folds, and subsequent voice problems [22].

3.2.5   Treatment

Mucositis due to radiation leads to pain; thus, the exposure of the affected mucosa to irritants such as alcohol and smoking should be avoided and maintaining adequate pain management should be achieved. Mucosal healing usually occurs rapidly after completing radiation treatment.

Edema of the arytenoids may occur due to laryngeal irradiation during the first 2–3 weeks of radiation therapy with continuous increase to the end of treatment. The incidence of laryngeal edema increases with total radiation dose, field size, tumor stage, smoking, and chemotherapy administration [22]. Usually recovery begins 3 weeks after treatment and may require 6–12 months to subside. Conservative management includes voice rest, the use of antibiotics for ulceration and possibly steroids. Persistence of edema longer than 3 months after radiotherapy is an indicative of recurrent or persistent tumor. Laryngectomy may be needed for management of laryngeal edema for these patients. Voice therapy following chemoradiotherapy focuses on vocal hygiene, direct voice therapy, and helping the patient to produce voice without using inefficient compensatory behaviors such as increased laryngeal strain and supraglottic constriction [17].

3.2.6   Rx: Sample Prescriptions

- *Pain*: NSAIDs, opiates.
    - Mild:
        Ibuprofen. 200–800 mg po q4–6 h prn. Max 3200 mg/day.
        Naproxen. 250–500 mg po bid. Max 1500 mg/day.
    - Severe:
        Oxycodone. 5–30 mg po q4h prn. 5, 15, 30 mg tablets.
        Fentanyl transdermal. 25–100 µg/h patch q72 h
- *Laryngeal edema*: Dexamethasone, 2–4 mg/day PO.

3.3   Thyroid Gland

3.3.1   Anatomy

The thyroid gland is a midline structure located inferior to the laryngeal thyroid cartilage typically corresponding to the vertebral levels of C3–C6. It is divided into two lobes that are connected by isthmus. The gland lies posterior to the sternothyroid and sternohyoid muscles, wrapping around the thyroid cartilage. The parathyroid glands are embedded within it and the carotid arteries are located posterolateral to the gland.

Thyroid gland is a highly vascular organ that receives blood from the superior and inferior thyroid arteries. The superior thyroid artery is the first branch of the external carotid artery as it arises near the level of the superior horn of the thyroid cartilage. The inferior thyroid artery branches from the thyrocervical trunk at the inner border of the anterior scalene muscle and advances medially to the thyroid gland. The thyroid gland is drained via the superior, middle, and inferior thyroid veins. The middle and superior thyroid veins eventually drain into the internal jugular vein on either side of the neck. The drainage of the inferior thyroid vein may enter either the subclavian or brachiocephalic veins, located just posterior to the manubrium.

Lymphatic drainage of the thyroid gland involves the lower deep cervical, prelaryngeal, pretracheal, and paratracheal nodes. The paratracheal and lower deep cervical nodes, specifically, receive lymphatic drainage from the isthmus and the inferior lateral lobes. The superior portions of the thyroid gland drain into the superior pretracheal and cervical nodes. The vagus nerve provides the main parasympathetic fibers, while sympathetic fibers originate from the inferior, middle, and superior ganglia of the sympathetic trunk.

3.3.2   Contouring

Delineation of thyroid gland is shown in Fig. 3.5. The anatomical boundaries for thyroid gland are shown in Table 3.4.

3.3.3   Dose Constraints

Dose constraints for thyroid gland and the risk of hypothyroidism are shown in Table 3.5.

3.3.4   Pathophysiology

Thyroid gland is an endocrine organ which produces thyroid hormones that is essential for maintaining normal metabolism. Thyroid disorders such as thyroiditis

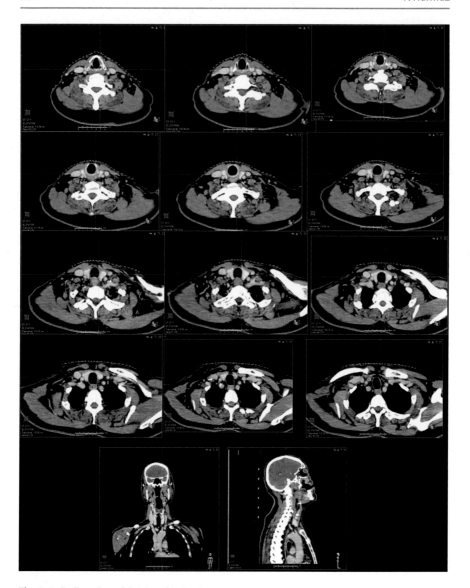

Fig. 3.5 Delineation of the thyroid gland

Table 3.4 The anatomical boundaries for thyroid gland

Cranial	Caudal	Anterior	Posterior	Lateral	Medial
Caudal edge of pyriform sinus or midpoint of thyroid cartilage	Body of fifth to seventh cervical vertebra	Sternohyoid or sternocleidomastoid	Cervical vessels or longus colli m	Cervical vessels or sternocleidomastoid	Thyroid cartilage or cricoids cartilage or esophagus or pharyngeal constrictor

Table 3.5 Dose constraints for thyroid gland and the risk of hypothyroidism

Literature	Dose	Risk of hypothyroidism (%)
Emami et al. [25]	<45 Gy	8
Grande [26]	<60 Gy	22.4
Kim et al. [27]	V45 < 50%	22.8
Cella et al. [28]	V30 ≤ 62.5%	11.5
Fujiwara et al. [29]	Mean < 30 Gy	10

and hypothyroidism leading to metabolic effects have been reported after radiotherapy of head and neck region. Radiation-induced thyroiditis is considered as the primary damage to the thyroid gland when the follicular epithelial cells and blood vessels are damaged leading to hypothyroidism as a late effect [30]. Autoimmune reactions and parenchymal cell damages after radiotherapy have also been reported as a cause of thyroid damage [31, 32]. Common symptoms of hypothyroidism are fatigue, weakness, cold intolerance, cognitive dysfunction, dry skin, constipation, and depression [33].

Radiation-induced hypothyroidism (RIH) is the most common thyroid disorder after radiotherapy to head and neck with an average incidence of 20–45% [32, 34, 35]. Most of RIHs are subclinical which are asymptomatic and can only be detected by elevated thyroid stimulating hormone (TSH) level. RIH is often diagnosed within 5 years after radiotherapy; however, late onset might also be seen [36, 37]. Exposure of thyroid gland to a dose above 40 Gy is associated with significant increase in TSH level. Additionally combination of surgery with radiotherapy, age, gender, radiation field, chemotherapy, smoking also affects the development of hypothyroidism.

Main mechanisms of damage to thyroid gland include vascular effects in the epithelium of small vessels and the development of fibrosis of capsular structures and the damage to the follicular epithelial cells [37, 38]. It has been shown that changes in both the blood vessels and the gland echogenicity occur during RT, and subsequent development of acute thyroiditis was correlated to vessel changes [39]. The predominant late morphological changes consist of atrophy, chronic inflammation (thyroiditis) with lymphocytic infiltration, vascular fibrosis, and focal and irregular follicular hyperplasia. Low doses of irradiation may result in focal and irregular follicular hyperplasia, hyalinization and fibrosis beneath the vascular endothelium, lymphocytic infiltration, single and multiple adenomas, and thyroid carcinomas [38].

3.3.5 Treatment

Hypothyroidism is biochemically characterized by high serum TSH and low serum free thyroxine (fT4) concentration. Subclinical hypothyroidism is characterized by high serum TSH and normal fT4 and is usually asymptomatic. Anti-thyroid peroxidase antibody (TPOAb) measurements should be considered when evaluating patients with subclinical hypothyroidism.

Guidelines generally recommend lifelong hormone replacement therapy (levothyroxine), therapy is indicated for hypothyroidism if TSH level is above 10 mIU/L after at least two consecutive thyroid function tests [40]. The current recommendations for starting treatment for hypothyroidism are shown in Table 3.6. Serum TSH and fT4 should be monitored regularly for diagnosis of subclinical hypothyroidism and follow up of replacement therapy effectiveness [37, 38].

3.3.6 Rx: Sample Prescriptions

The objectives of therapy are amelioration of hypothyroid symptoms, normalization of TSH levels, treatment of goiter (if present) without leading to iatrogenic

Table 3.6 Current recommendations on thyroid hormone replacement therapy for hypothyroidism

Organization	Recommendation	Treatment
American Thyroid Association (ATA) [41]	• TSH >10 mIU/L, consider treatment • TSH <10 mIU/L, consider treatment if symptoms suggestive of hypothyroidism, positive antibodies to thyroid peroxidase, or evidence of atherosclerotic cardiovascular disease, heart failure, or risk factors for these diseases	When initiating therapy in young healthy adults with overt hypothyroidism, beginning treatment with full replacement doses should be considered. When initiating therapy in patients older than 50–60 years with overt hypothyroidism, without evidence of coronary heart disease, an L-thyroxine dose of 50 µg daily should be considered in patients with subclinical hypothyroidism initial L-thyroxine dosing is generally lower than what is required in the treatment of overt hypothyroidism. A daily dose of 25–75 µg should be considered, depending on the degree of TSH elevation. Further adjustments should be guided by clinical response and follow up laboratory determinations including TSH values
European thyroid association (ETA) [42]	• Age ≤70 years – TSH ≥10 mIU/L, treat with LT4 – TSH <10 mIU/L with symptoms, start 3 month trial of LT4, then assess response to treatment – TSH <10 mIU/L without symptoms, observe and repeat TFT in 6 months • Age >70 years – TSH <10 mIU/L, observe and repeat TFT in 6 months – TSH ≥10 mIU/L, consider LT4 if clear symptoms or high cardiovascular risk	Typical L-thyroxine treatment regimens have started with 25 or 50 µg daily, with subsequent monthly or 2-monthly dose adjustment to maintain serum TSH within reference range (0.4–2.5 mU/l)

thyrotoxicosis. Serum TSH is expected to be kept within the normal reference range (usually, 0.5–5.0 mU/L).

For patients without cardiac disease, a weight-related dose of L-thyroxine should be used, approximating to 1.5 µg/kg/day (e.g., 75 or 100 µg/day for a woman, 100 or 125 µg for a man). For patients with cardiac disease and in the elderly, a small dose of L-thyroxine should be started, 25 or 50 µg daily. The dose of L-thyroxine should be increased by 25 µg/day every 14–21 days until a full replacement dose is reached. L-Thyroxine should be taken on an empty stomach, either first thing in the morning, an hour before food, or at bedtime, 2 h or more after the last food. Medications causing interference with L-thyroxine absorption (calcium and iron salts, proton pump inhibitors, etc.) should be avoided, or taken 4 h or more after L-thyroxine ingestion. The serum TSH should be re-checked 2 months after starting L-thyroxine therapy, and dosage adjustments made accordingly. In the elderly, any treatment should be individualized. For patients with mild subclinical hypothyroidism (serum TSH <10 mU/l) response to treatment should be reviewed 3 or 4 months after a serum TSH within the reference range is reached. If there is no improvement in symptoms, L-thyroxine therapy should generally be stopped [42].

3.4 Brachial Plexus

3.4.1 Anatomy

The cervical plexus is a complex neurologic structure located within the head and neck. It is formed by the anterior divisions of the upper four cervical nerves; each nerve, except the first, divides into an upper and a lower branch, and the branches unite to form three loops. The plexus is situated opposite the upper four cervical vertebrae, in front of the levator scapula and scalenus medius, and covered by the sternocleidomastoid muscles.

3.4.2 Contouring

The Radiation Therapy Oncology Group (RTOG) has endorsed an atlas that has been developed and validated for delineating the brachial plexus (BP). The following step-by-step technique for contouring the brachial plexus on axial non-contrast CT was devised [43] (Fig. 3.6):

- Identify and contour C5, T1, and T2.
- Identify and contour the subclavian and axillary neurovascular bundle.
- Identify and contour anterior and middle scalene muscles from C5 to insertion onto the first rib.
- To contour the brachial plexus OAR use a 5-mm diameter paint tool.
- Start at the neural foramina from C5 to T1; this should extend from the lateral aspect of the spinal canal to the small space between the anterior and middle scalene muscles.

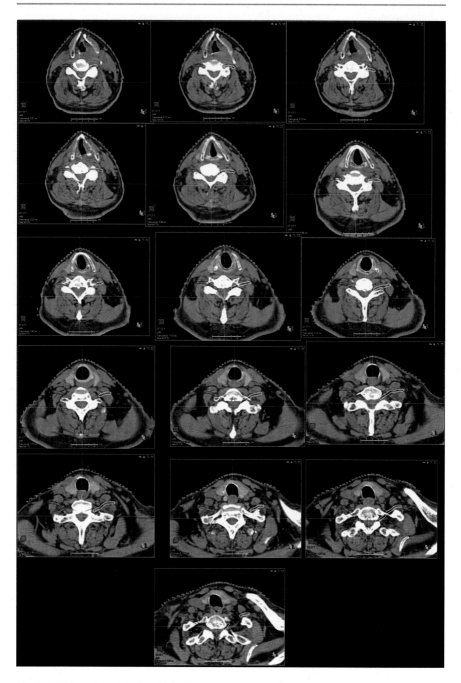

Fig. 3.6 Delineation of the brachial plexus

- For CT slices, where no neural foramen is present, contour only the space between the anterior and middle scalene muscles.
- Continue to contour the space between the anterior and middle scalene muscles; eventually the middle scalene will end in the region of the subclavian neurovascular bundle.
- Contour the brachial plexus as the posterior aspect of the neurovascular bundle inferiorly and laterally to one to two CT slices below the clavicular head.
- The first and second ribs serve as the medial limit of the OAR contour.

3.4.3 Dose Constraints

Brachial plexus dose constraints on Radiation Therapy Oncology Group (RTOG) head and neck cancer protocols are summarized in Table 3.7.

3.4.4 Pathophysiology

The brachial plexus innervates the sensory and motor function of upper limb and may be affected by treatment of the positive LNs of the head and neck region. Radiotherapy induced brachial plexopathy may vary depending on dose per fraction, total dose, volume of BP exposed to radiation, and the use of concomitant chemotherapy [44].

Bowen divided radiation-induced BP into acute plexopathy and classic delayed injury. Acute injury develops several days to 6 months after the completion of radiotherapy. The main pathological of acute injury is inflammatory edema due to the direct neurotoxicity of radiation. Delayed injury occurs 6 months or later. The vascular lesions and fibrosis of connective tissues surrounding the brachial plexus may ultimately result in ischemia as well as nerve demyelination [45]. This type of radiation injury is thought to be a consequence of late fibrotic changes, where muscle fibers are persistently replaced with fibrotic tissue, subsequently reducing their motility as they become weakened and atrophied. Fibrosis is characterized by a loss

Table 3.7 Brachial plexus dose constraints on Radiation Therapy Oncology Group (RTOG) head and neck cancer protocols

Study	Dose constraint
RTOG 0435	$D_{max} \leq 60$ Gy
RTOG 0522	$D_{max} \leq 60$ Gy
RTOG 0615	$D_{max} \leq 66$ Gy
RTOG 0619	$D_{max} \leq 66$ Gy, D05 ≤ 60 Gy
RTOG 0912	$D_{max} \leq 66$ Gy to point source at least 0.03 cm^3
RTOG 1008	$D_{max} <60$ Gy if no involved low neck nodes; <66 Gy if low neck nodes involved

of vascularity and matrix disorganization, which disrupts well-defined compartmentalized structures. The excessive collagen deposits can eventually entrap nerve trunks or alter the vascular networks between or within the nerve tracts, leading to neurologic deficits (i.e., neuropathy, myopathy) [46, 47].

3.4.5 Treatment

Radiation-induced brachial plexopathy is a concerning adverse event among HNC patients defined as transient or permanent neurologic impairment of affected nerves. Symptoms are paresthesia, pain, weakness, and motor dysfunction affecting the chest, shoulder, and upper extremity [44]. The treatment is symptomatic. The best approach is always prevention in respect of RT limits by reducing total RT dose, dose per fraction, and RT volume and identifying patients with serious comorbidities. Management of the symptoms is shown in Table 3.8.

Vitamins B1–B6 are often used routinely, but detailed data are lacking. Physical therapy is valuable in maintaining function and preventing joint complications. It is important to prevent any stretching of a plexus immobilized by fibrosis by avoiding the carrying of heavy loads and extensive movements, which are likely to cause sudden neurological decompensation [48].

Removal of inciting stimuli is helpful in controlling the progression of neuropathy [49]. First, removing co-morbidity factors by general measures as controlling diabetes and high blood pressure; stopping alcohol abuse, avoiding fibrogenic drugs and statins (potential neuromuscular toxicity); and by local measures consisting in avoiding any local trauma in the irradiated volume, such as new surgery or biopsy (hematoma, infection). Second, controlling acute inflammation with corticosteroids, which are of value in reducing the acute inflammation associated with RIF and should first be used to circumscribe the fibrotic volume and density, despite lack of any objective efficacy in reduction of fibrosis and nerve lesions [49].

Evidence for the benefit of hyperbaric oxygen (HBO) in fibrosis is not clear. HBO reduces tissue edema and stimulates angiogenesis, fibroblast proliferation, and collagen formation in irradiated hypoxic tissue, which paradoxically may enhance fibrotic properties [48]. Because of vascular changes and ischemia, heparin and warfarin have been used in an attempt to halt progression of radiation necrosis [50].

Table 3.8 Management of symptoms

Symptom	Management
Pain	Non-opioid analgesics, benzodiazepines, tricyclic antidepressants and anti-epileptics
Paresthesia	Benzodiazepines
Cramps	Quinine
Nerve hyperexcitability	Membrane-stabilizing drugs (carbamazepine)
Nerve entrapment related pain	Surgery (mechanical separation)

Although pathogenesis of RIPN initially involves vascular mechanisms, fibrosis and atrophy are the main targets for therapeutic interventions. It has been known for two decades now that combined pentoxifylline-tocopherol (PE) significantly reduces RIF due to their synergistic clinical and biological properties [51, 52].

3.4.6 Rx: Sample Prescriptions

- Gabapentin (Neurontin): An anticonvulsant with antineuralgic effects. Titration of the dose over several days is required (300 mg on day 1, 300 mg bid on day 2, and 300 mg tid on day 3).
- Pregabalin (Lyrica): Initial: 75 mg PO q12 h (150 mg/day); may increase within 1 week to 300 mg/day PO divided q12 h. If there is insufficient pain relief after 2–3 weeks and 300 mg/day dose is tolerated, may increase dose again up to 600 mg/day PO divided q12 h.
- Tricyclic antidepressants: Amitriptyline is indicated as an analgesic for certain types of chronic and neuropathic pain. 65–100 mg PO qDay for at least 3 weeks.
- Selective serotonin/norepinephrine reuptake inhibitor: (Duloxetine-Cymbalta): 60 mg/day PO initially (in single daily dose or divided q12 h); consider lowering dosage if tolerability is concern. Do not exceed 60 mg/day.

References

1. Heyd C, Yellon R. Anatomy head and neck, pharynx muscles. Treasure Island: StatPearls; 2019.
2. Sakamoto Y. Gross anatomical observations of attachments of the middle pharyngeal constrictor. Clin Anat. 2014;27(4):603–9.
3. Lengele B, Hamoir M, Scalliet P, Gregoire V. Anatomical bases for the radiological delineation of lymph node areas. Major collecting trunks, head and neck. Radiother Oncol. 2007;85(1):146–55.
4. Shaw SM, Martino R. The normal swallow: muscular and neurophysiological control. Otolaryngol Clin North Am. 2013;46(6):937–56.
5. Mu L, Sanders I. Neuromuscular compartments and fiber-type regionalization in the human inferior pharyngeal constrictor muscle. Anat Rec. 2001;264(4):367–77.
6. Tsumori N, Abe S, Agematsu H, Hashimoto M, Ide Y. Morphologic characteristics of the superior pharyngeal constrictor muscle in relation to the function during swallowing. Dysphagia. 2007;22(2):122–9.
7. Brouwer CL, Steenbakkers RJ, Bourhis J, et al. CT-based delineation of organs at risk in the head and neck region: DAHANCA, EORTC, GORTEC, HKNPCSG, NCIC CTG, NCRI, NRG oncology and TROG consensus guidelines. Radiother Oncol. 2015;117(1):83–90.
8. Genovesi D, Perrotti F, Trignani M, et al. Delineating brachial plexus, cochlea, pharyngeal constrictor muscles and optic chiasm in head and neck radiotherapy: a CT-based model atlas. Radiol Med. 2015;120(4):352–60.
9. Harari PM, Song S, Tome WA. Emphasizing conformal avoidance versus target definition for IMRT planning in head-and-neck cancer. Int J Radiat Oncol Biol Phys. 2010;77(3):950–8.
10. Schwartz DL, Hutcheson K, Barringer D, et al. Candidate dosimetric predictors of long-term swallowing dysfunction after oropharyngeal intensity-modulated radiotherapy. Int J Radiat Oncol Biol Phys. 2010;78(5):1356–65.

11. Caglar HB, Tishler RB, Othus M, et al. Dose to larynx predicts for swallowing complications after intensity-modulated radiotherapy. Int J Radiat Oncol Biol Phys. 2008;72(4):1110–8.

12. Caudell JJ, Schaner PE, Desmond RA, Meredith RF, Spencer SA, Bonner JA. Dosimetric factors associated with long-term dysphagia after definitive radiotherapy for squamous cell carcinoma of the head and neck. Int J Radiat Oncol Biol Phys. 2010;76(2):403–9.

13. Eisbruch A, Kim HM, Feng FY, et al. Chemo-IMRT of oropharyngeal cancer aiming to reduce dysphagia: swallowing organs late complication probabilities and dosimetric correlates. Int J Radiat Oncol Biol Phys. 2011;81(3):e93–9.

14. Li B, Li D, Lau DH, et al. Clinical-dosimetric analysis of measures of dysphagia including gastrostomy-tube dependence among head and neck cancer patients treated definitively by intensity-modulated radiotherapy with concurrent chemotherapy. Radiat Oncol. 2009;4(1):52.

15. Hutcheson KA, Lewin JS, Barringer DA, et al. Late dysphagia after radiotherapy-based treatment of head and neck cancer. Cancer. 2012;118(23):5793–9.

16. Choi M, Refaat T, Lester MS, Bacchus I, Rademaker AW, Mittal BB. Development of a standardized method for contouring the larynx and its substructures. Radiat Oncol. 2014;9:285.

17. Lazarus CL. Effects of chemoradiotherapy on voice and swallowing. Curr Opin Otolaryngol Head Neck Surg. 2009;17(3):172–8.

18. Rancati T, Schwarz M, Allen AM, et al. Radiation dose-volume effects in the larynx and pharynx. Int J Radiat Oncol Biol Phys. 2010;76(Suppl 3):S64–9.

19. Eisbruch A, Schwartz M, Rasch C, et al. Dysphagia and aspiration after chemoradiotherapy for head-and-neck cancer: which anatomic structures are affected and can they be spared by IMRT? Int J Radiat Oncol Biol Phys. 2004;60(5):1425–39.

20. Jensen K, Lambertsen K, Grau C. Late swallowing dysfunction and dysphagia after radiotherapy for pharynx cancer: frequency, intensity and correlation with dose and volume parameters. Radiother Oncol. 2007;85(1):74–82.

21. De Ruysscher D, Niedermann G, Burnet NG, Siva S, Lee AWM, Hegi-Johnson F. Radiotherapy toxicity. Nat Rev Dis Primers. 2019;5(1):13.

22. Sourati AAA, Malekzadeh M. Laryngeal edema. In: Acute side effects of radiation therapy. Cham: Springer; 2017.

23. Bentzen SM. Preventing or reducing late side effects of radiation therapy: radiobiology meets molecular pathology. Nat Rev Cancer. 2006;6(9):702–13.

24. Khanna A. DNA damage in cancer therapeutics: a boon or a curse? Cancer Res. 2015;75(11):2133–8.

25. Emami B, Lyman J, Brown A, et al. Tolerance of normal tissue to therapeutic irradiation. Int J Radiat Oncol Biol Phys. 1991;21(1):109–22.

26. Grande C. Hypothyroidism following radiotherapy for head and neck cancer: multivariate analysis of risk factors. Radiother Oncol. 1992;25(1):31–6.

27. Kim MY, Yu T, Wu H-G. Dose-volumetric parameters for predicting hypothyroidism after radiotherapy for head and neck cancer. Jpn J Clin Oncol. 2014;44(4):331–7.

28. Cella L, Conson M, Caterino M, et al. Thyroid V30 predicts radiation-induced hypothyroidism in patients treated with sequential chemo-radiotherapy for Hodgkin's lymphoma. Int J Radiat Oncol Biol Phys. 2012;82(5):1802–8.

29. Fujiwara M, Kamikonya N, Odawara S, et al. The threshold of hypothyroidism after radiation therapy for head and neck cancer: a retrospective analysis of 116 cases. J Radiat Res. 2015;56(3):577–82.

30. Alterio D, Jereczek-Fossa BA, Franchi B, et al. Thyroid disorders in patients treated with radiotherapy for head-and-neck cancer: a retrospective analysis of seventy-three patients. Int J Radiat Oncol Biol Phys. 2007;67(1):144–50.

31. Miller MC, Agrawal A. Hypothyroidism in postradiation head and neck cancer patients: incidence, complications, and management. Curr Opin Otolaryngol Head Neck Surg. 2009;17(2):111–5.

32. Nishiyama K, Tanaka E, Tarui Y, Miyauchi K, Okagawa K. A prospective analysis of subacute thyroid dysfunction after neck irradiation. Int J Radiat Oncol Biol Phys. 1996;34(2):439–44.

33. Khandelwal D, Tandon N. Overt and subclinical hypothyroidism. Drugs. 2012;72(1):17–33.

34. Bhandare N, Kennedy L, Malyapa RS, Morris CG, Mendenhall WM. Primary and central hypothyroidism after radiotherapy for head-and-neck tumors. Int J Radiat Oncol Biol Phys. 2007;68(4):1131–9.

35. Ozawa H, Saitou H, Mizutari K, Takata Y, Ogawa K. Hypothyroidism after radiotherapy for patients with head and neck cancer. Am J Otolaryngol. 2007;28(1):46–9.

36. Murtha AD, Knox SJ, Hoppe RT, Rupnow BA, Hanson J. Long-term follow-up of patients with stage III follicular lymphoma treated with primary radiotherapy at Stanford University. Int J Radiat Oncol Biol Phys. 2001;49(1):3–15.

37. Hancock SL, Cox RS, McDougall IR. Thyroid diseases after treatment of Hodgkin's disease. N Engl J Med. 1991;325(9):599–605.

38. Jereczek-Fossa BA, Alterio D, Jassem J, Gibelli B, Tradati N, Orecchia R. Radiotherapy-induced thyroid disorders. Cancer Treat Rev. 2004;30(4):369–84.

39. Bakhshandeh M, Hashemi B, Mahdavi SR, Nikoofar A, Edraki HR, Kazemnejad A. Evaluation of thyroid disorders during head-and-neck radiotherapy by using functional analysis and ultrasonography. Int J Radiat Oncol Biol Phys. 2012;83(1):198–203.

40. Bekkering GE, Agoritsas T, Lytvyn L, et al. Thyroid hormones treatment for subclinical hypothyroidism: a clinical practice guideline. BMJ. 2019;365:l2006.

41. Garber JR, Cobin RH, Gharib H, et al. Clinical practice guidelines for hypothyroidism in adults: cosponsored by the American Association of Clinical Endocrinologists and the American Thyroid Association. Endocr Pract. 2012;18(6):988–1028.

42. Pearce SH, Brabant G, Duntas LH, et al. 2013 ETA guideline: management of subclinical hypothyroidism. Eur Thyroid J. 2013;2(4):215–28.

43. Hall WH, Guiou M, Lee NY, et al. Development and validation of a standardized method for contouring the brachial plexus: preliminary dosimetric analysis among patients treated with IMRT for head-and-neck cancer. Int J Radiat Oncol Biol Phys. 2008;72(5):1362–7.

44. Thomas TO, Refaat T, Choi M, et al. Brachial plexus dose tolerance in head and neck cancer patients treated with sequential intensity modulated radiation therapy. Radiat Oncol. 2015;10(1):94.

45. Bowen BC, Verma A, Brandon AH, Fiedler JA. Radiation-induced brachial plexopathy: MR and clinical findings. Am J Neuroradiol. 1996;17(10):1932–6.

46. Gillette EL, Mahler PA, Powers BE, Gillette SM, Vujaskovic Z. Late radiation injury to muscle and peripheral nerves. Int J Radiat Oncol Biol Phys. 1995;31(5):1309–18.

47. King SN, Dunlap NE, Tennant PA, Pitts T. Pathophysiology of radiation-induced dysphagia in head and neck cancer. Dysphagia. 2016;31(3):339–51.

48. Delanian S, Lefaix JL, Pradat PF. Radiation-induced neuropathy in cancer survivors. Radiother Oncol. 2012;105(3):273–82.

49. Delanian S, Lefaix JL. Current management for late normal tissue injury: radiation-induced fibrosis and necrosis. Semin Radiat Oncol. 2007;17(2):99–107.

50. Glantz MJ, Burger PC, Friedman AH, Radtke RA, Massey EW, Schold SC. Treatment of radiation-induced nervous system injury with heparin and warfarin. Neurology. 1994;44(11):2020.

51. Delanian S, Porcher R, Balla-Mekias S, Lefaix JL. Randomized, placebo-controlled trial of combined pentoxifylline and tocopherol for regression of superficial radiation-induced fibrosis. J Clin Oncol Off J Am Soc Clin Oncol. 2003;21(13):2545–50.

52. Hamama S, Gilbert-Sirieix M, Vozenin MC, Delanian S. Radiation-induced enteropathy: molecular basis of pentoxifylline-vitamin E anti-fibrotic effect involved TGF-beta1 cascade inhibition. Radiother Oncol. 2012;105(3):305–12.

Toxicity Management for Thorax Tumors in Radiation Oncology

4

Teuta Zoto Mustafayev and Banu Atalar

4.1 Lung

4.1.1 Anatomy

Lungs are the two spongy structure filling most of the thoracic cavity. They constitute the parenchymal part of the respiratory system, as opposed to the trachea and main bronchi which form the airways. Anatomically lungs are described as having an apex (part of lung lying above the first rib), three borders, and three surfaces. Right and left lung anatomy is asymmetrical; right lung is usually larger and consists of three lobes (upper, middle, and lower), and left lung consists of two lobes (upper and lower). Lobes are further divided into segments. Hilum, lying at the T5–T7 vertebra level, is the point where vasculature, bronchi, lymphatics, and nerves enter and exit the lung [1].

Due to the type and severity of toxicities noticed in SABR, beside describing lesions' position according to the aforementioned anatomical divisions, central and peripheral location of the tumor is also important. While definition of central lesion varied in different studies, International Association for the Study of Lung Cancer (IASLC) definition might be the more appropriate. Accordingly, central lesion is considered as a tumor within 2 cm in all directions from airways (bronchial tree), esophagus, brachial plexus, spinal cord, phrenic nerve, recurrent laryngeal nerve, major vessels, and heart (Fig. 4.1) [2]. While there is no clear definition for peripheral lung, it is considered as the part of lung residing outside the central area.

From a radiation oncologist point of view lungs are considered as parallel organs, where each subunit can function independently and rather than maximum dose, mean dose and dose to specific volume are determinant for toxicity.

T. Zoto Mustafayev
Acibadem Maslak Hospital, Department of Radiation Oncology, Istanbul, Turkey

B. Atalar (✉)
Acibadem University, Faculty of Medicine, Department of Radiation Oncology,
Istanbul, Turkey

© Springer Nature Switzerland AG 2020
G. Ozyigit, U. Selek (eds.), *Prevention and Management of Acute and Late Toxicities in Radiation Oncology*, https://doi.org/10.1007/978-3-030-37798-4_4

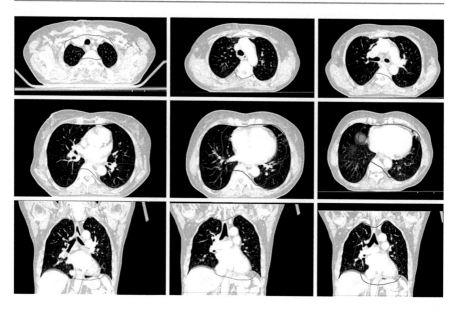

Fig. 4.1 Delineation of central zone (purple)

4.1.2 Contouring

The RTOG contouring guideline [3] used in lung cancer trial protocols stresses some important points in lung contouring:

1. *Both lungs should be contoured using pulmonary windows.* It decreases variation since segmentation in different window may change lung edges.
2. *The right and left lungs can be contoured separately, but they should be considered as one structure for lung dosimetry.* While total lung volume is used for dosimetry in primary lung cancer, breast treatments require ipsilateral lung volume as well.
3. *All inflated and collapsed (atelectatic), fibrotic, and emphysematic lungs should be contoured as lung.* Contouring lung manually may be time-consuming and since it has a homogenous density it is well suited for auto-segmentation. However, auto-segmentation cannot distinguish unaerated area from soft tissue thus these areas should be checked and added manually. In one study exclusion of emphysematic lung was a better predictor of radiation pneumonitis [4]
4. *Small vessels extending beyond the hilar regions should be included.* Similarly, due to difference in density these structures are usually not included during auto-segmentation. Adding small vessels can be done manually or through "filling the gaps" in some systems.
5. *GTV, hilars, and trachea/main bronchus should not be included in this structure.* As mentioned in the "Anatomy" section, trachea and main bronchi form the airway part of respiratory system, they have different toxicity profile and different dose constraints and they should not be included in the lungs. GTV, but not

whole PTV, should be excluded from lungs [5]. If PTV is excluded, the apparent lung exposure may be reduced (since normal lung within PTV will be excluded). However, in a small study dosimetric data related to lung were more predictive of RP when PTV, rather than GTV, was excluded from total lung volume in patients treated with intensity modulated radiation therapy for lung cancer [6]. Figure 4.2 shows normal lung tissue contouring according to the abovementioned guidelines.

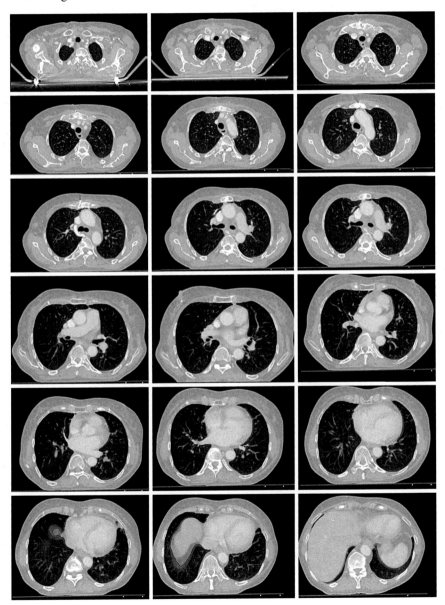

Fig. 4.2 Delineation of lungs (blue)

4.1.3 Pathophysiology

Relation between radiation and some of its toxicities in the lungs and division of lung injury into acute radiation pneumonitis-RP (usually occurring within 6 months after RT) and the following chronic stage radiation pulmonary fibrosis-RPF (mostly occuring1 year after RT) has been described almost a century ago [7]. However, with the advances in histology, biochemistry, and immunology mechanisms underlying some of the radiation induced lung injury could be discovered [8].

Radiation Pneumonitis RP starts 1–6 months after radiation exposure. Radiographically it is defined as straight edged parenchymal opacities that conform to the radiation port and traction bronchiectasis [9]. Most patients have asymptomatic radiological pneumonitis; however, symptomatic patients may have dyspnea, non-productive cough, or low-grade fever. On physical examination no findings are noticed though less commonly rales and friction rub are seen. It can spontaneously resolute within 1 month or progress to fibrosis [10]. Grading of radiation pneumonitis according to different oncology groups is summarized in Table 4.1.

Table 4.1 Grading of Radiation Pneumonitis according to different oncology groups

	Grade 1	Grade 2	Grade 3	Grade 4	Grade 5
CTCAE v5.0	Asymptomatic; clinical or diagnostic observations only; intervention not indicated	Symptomatic; medical intervention indicated; limiting instrumental ADL	Severe symptoms; limiting self-care ADL; oxygen indicated	Life-threatening respiratory compromise; urgent intervention indicated (e.g., tracheotomy or intubation)	Death
RTOG	Mild symptoms of dry cough or dyspnea on exertion	Persistent cough requiring narcotic, antitussive agents/dyspnea with minimal effort but not at rest	Severe symptoms, possibly requiring intermittent O2 or steroids may be required	Severe respiratory insufficiency/continuous O2 or assisted ventilation	Death
EORTC	Asymptomatic or mild symptoms; slight imaging changes	Moderate symptoms; patchy imaging changes	Severe symptoms; increased density imaging changes	Severe symptoms requiring continuous O2 or assisted ventilation	Death
SWOG	Imaging changes; mild symptoms without steroids	Symptoms requiring steroids or tap for effusion	Symptoms requiring oxygen	Symptoms requiring assisted ventilation	Death

Table 4.1 (continued)

	Grade 1	Grade 2	Grade 3	Grade 4	Grade 5
LENT/ SOMA	Asymptomatic or mild signs (cough). Discrete radiological signs	Symptomatic moderate fibrosis. Non-radiologically confluent opacities, O2 discontinuous	Symptomatic fibrosis or severe lung disease, radiological confluent opacities, O2 continuous, steroid use intermittent	Severe respiratory failure. Assisted ventilation, use of steroids continuous	

CTCAE (Common Terminology Criteria for adverse events), *RTOG* (Radiation Therapy Oncology Group), *EORTC* (European Organization for Research and Treatment of Cancer), *SWOG* (Southwest Oncology Group), *SOMA-LENTE* (The Late Effects Normal Tissue/Subjective Objective Management Analytic)

Injury to type I and II pneumocytes residing in the alveoli and endothelial cells in the adjacent vasculature results in disruption of connections between cells and decrease in surfactant production. Simultaneously these damaged cells start secreting proinflammatory cytokines. Increased permeability and dilation of blood vessels together with high level of cytokines allow for abundant accumulation of exudate and inflammatory cells in the irradiated area.

In the acute phase T helper type 1 (Th1) cells secrete IFN which has an anti-fibrotic and immunomodulatory effect; it inhibits the differentiation, function, and cytokines produced by Th2. This phase correlates with radiation pneumonitis or the acute phase [11, 12].

The prediction of RP after radiotherapy has not been clearly defined until the 3D era. The classical or "in-field" RP can be described as damage after irradiation of "large lung volumes." However it was not possible to define for sure what can be considered as "large" until volumetric has been introduced to our practice, and from a long history of radiobiological studies, dosimetric studies, retrospective data and experimental models it can be concluded that when more than a specific ratio of lung receives more than a specific dose then it can be considered as large volume, i.e., volume of lung receiving doses of 20 Gy (V_{20}) or higher is more than 30% of total lung volume or volume of lung receiving doses of 5 Gy (V_5) or higher is more than 60% of total lung volume in conventional fractionation. It is basically a dose–volume relation to define the risk of RP. It is considered that when V_{20} is higher than 30% then the risk of RP is over 30% [13].

Radiation Induced Pulmonary Fibrosis RPF starts 6–24 months after exposure. On radiologic examination it is observed as an ill-defined or straight edged fibrosis, scarring with or without traction bronchiectasis. Respiratory examination findings and symptoms are similar to RP, depending on severity. In severe cases it may cause pulmonary hypertension resulting in cor pulmonale, cyanosis, clubbing, and hepatomegaly. RPF is a permanent parenchymal damage that stabilizes within 2 years after exposure [11, 12].

Gradually T helper type 2 (Th2) cells replace Th1 in sustained injury and pro-fibrotic IL-4, IL-13 are released. IL-4 specifically inhibits Th1 and is found to be increased in patients with RILI and IPF by stimulating fibroblast to increase expression of type I, type III collagen, and fibronectin, while IL-13 is known to increase fibrosis in liver, lung, and skin [11, 12].

Increased interleukins, TNF, PDGF, and TGF result in activation of macrophages and fibroblasts. Similarly activated alveolar macrophages increase production of TGF beta 1 which is one of the main mediators of fibrosis in the lung. Thus, activation and proliferation of fibroblasts and myofibroblasts, epithelial or endothelial-to-mesenchymal transformation leads to accumulation of pro-fibrotic cells, which result in uncontrolled extracellular matrix deposition, fibrosis, and disruption of lung architecture and function. This is the spontaneously irreversible chronic pulmonary fibrosis [12].

Fatal Acute Radiation Pneumonitis Sometimes referred to as "sporadic" is a rare though fatal complication of radiotherapy. While the "classic" RP needs a latent period to develop and is limited to the area irradiated, this type of RP develops much earlier and precipitates rapidly into the fibrosis stage, which unfortunately is not confined to the treated area but can sometimes spread to both lungs. Its mechanism is not clear yet though retrospective data and case reports suggest that idiopathic pulmonary fibrosis or pulmonary interstitial disease is one of the main predisposition factors of FARP for both stereotactic and conventionally fractionated treatments [14–18]. A chronic inflammatory state (such as in chronic heart diseases) or genetic abnormalities in cytokines or genes related to the immune response and fibrosis might play a role [19–21].

4.1.4   Dose Constraints

In order to investigate the effect and distinguish a cut-off dose for RP/RPF a clear definition of the disease is required. As noticed in Table 4.1 there are many grades of disease and in order to characterize a reasonable constraint, a cut-off toxicity should be made too. Arbitrarily, in many studies a clinically significant RP/RPF is considered as grade 2–3 or higher. Severity of symptoms is similarly graded by most scales. Clinically significant symptomatic RP is highest for lung cancer (5–50%, fatal 1.9%) followed by mediastinal irradiation due to other malignancies (5–10% esophageal cancer 6.6%) and breast cancer (1–5%) as roughly reported in reviews and meta-analysis [22, 23].

4.1.4.1 The Literature Review of Conventional Fractionated Radiotherapy for Lung Toxicity

Many retrospective data and prospective analysis in clinical trials can be found in the literature regarding the effect of dosimetric data on incidence of RP and RPF for definitive irradiation of primary lung cancer [13, 24–29], esophageal cancer [23], and breast cancer [30–35].

Lung Cancer Radiotherapy RP after radiotherapy for NSCLC is a dose limiting toxicity and extensively studied. While it would be difficult to review all pertinent literature, we would focus on some of the most important studies regarding the topic.

In 2013 Palma et al. reported the result of an international individual patient data meta-analysis regarding the factors predicting RP after chemoradiotherapy for lung cancer. In the study 836 patients treated with median 60 Gy (given in mostly 2 Gy/fraction) and concurrent chemotherapy (cisplatin-etoposide or carboplatin-paclitaxel) were included. After a median follow-up of 2.3 years the overall rate of symptomatic pneumonitis (grade >2) was 29.8%, fatal pneumonitis 1.9%. Higher rate of grade >2 pneumonitis was noticed in patients >65 years of age and carboplatin-paclitaxel use (risk >50%). Fatal pneumonitis correlated with V_{20} and lower lobe location [13].

In the study by Marks et al. in 2010, where meta-analysis and model-based prediction of pneumonitis were used, no clear threshold could be defined due to heterogeneity of studies included. However, they suggested to limit V_{20} to <30–35 Gy, MLD <20–23 Gy, in order to limit risk of RP below 20% [27].

In the meta-analysis by Vogelius and Bentzen other risk factors besides dosimetric parameters were investigated. They identified 31 studies for at least one candidate risk factor. Location in the mid or inferior lobes, presence of comorbidity, and older age increased the risk of developing RP while smoking protected against RP. Higher RP was noticed in sequential versus concomitant chemotherapy, though the authors argue this was due to bias [34].

In the systematic review by Zhang et al. 2012 similar risk factors were noticed: For RP grade >2, no surgery before RT, mid-lower lobe location, COPD, concomitant chemotherapy end/pre-RT TGF beta 1 ratio >1 and gross tumor volume. For RP of all grade: beside the aforementioned factors, dosimetric data including V_{10} >34 Gy, V_{20} >25 Gy, V_{30} >18 Gy, V_5, and MLD were predictive [24].

Breast Cancer As the most frequent cancer in women and with a high probability of receiving radiotherapy due to extensive use of breast conserving surgery and better identification of its benefits in lymphatic involvement, together with high overall survivals makes RP after breast RT an important concern that should be addressed. Fortunately, RP frequency is much less when compared to RT for primary lung cancer [36].

In the 2-D era of RT a study which included 613 patients showed that regional irradiation caused higher RP (4.1%) as compared to local RT alone (0.9%). Although not significant in the multivariate analysis, chemotherapy use is related to higher rates of RP (3.9%) as compared to treatment without chemotherapy (1.4%) [36]. In 2001 the same group identified ipsilateral lung V_{20} as an important parameter in 3-D planning DVH that correlated with higher rate of RP, together with regional irradiation (11%) vs. <1% in local RT only [37]. They also identified older age and reduced pre-RT lung functional level as risk factors for RP. They followed by prospectively limiting the dose to ipsilateral lung V_{20} < 30%, which holds its importance to this day [30]. This resulted in 3 mild and one moderate RP out of 66 patients. Mean V_{20} was 29% for RP and 24% in the non-RP population.

Table 4.2 Normal lung tissue dose constraints for conventional fractionated radiotherapy

Structure	Dose/fraction	Dose	Volume	Symptomatic RP	Fatal RP
Bilateral lung	2 Gy	>20 Gy	<20%	18.4%	0%∗
Bilateral lung	2 Gy	>20 Gy	20–30%	30.3%	1%
Bilateral lung	2 Gy	>20 Gy	30–40%	32.6%	2.9%
Bilateral lung	2 Gy	>20 Gy	>40%	35.9%	3.5%
Bilateral lung	2 Gy	>5 Gy	60%		
Bilateral lung	2 Gy	>10 Gy	30%		
Bilateral lung	2 Gy	>30 Gy	18%		
Bilateral lung	2 Gy	>18Gy	MLD		
Ipsilateral lung (breast cancer)	2 Gy	>20 Gy	30%		
Unilateral lung (post-pneumonectomy in mesothelioma	2 Gy	>5 Gy	60%		
Unilateral lung (post-pneumonectomy in mesothelioma	2 Gy	>20 Gy	10%		
Unilateral lung (post-pneumonectomy in mesothelioma	2 Gy	<8 Gy	MLD		

MLD (Mean Lung Dose), Radiation Pneumonitis (RP)

IMRT is not routinely recommended for breast cancer; however, with the inclusion of internal mammary nodes (IMN) to the irradiated area it has been difficult to obtain both good coverage and respect the lung and heart constraints. Lately, in a study of 113 node positive patients treated with inverse planning IMRT, beside showing a good coverage of IMN, the incidence of grade 3 RP was 0.96% after a 53.4 years of follow-up [38].

By using Lyman normal-tissue complication (NTCP) model similar cut-off was found for IMRT patients in another study $V_{20} = 29.03\%$ [35].

Hypofractionation as used in the START A and START B trials where standard dose of 50 Gy in 25 fractions was compared with 41.6 Gy or 39 in 13 fractions and 40 Gy in 15, respectively, showed that reported and confirmed RT were less than 1.7% and 0.7% [39].

Table 4.2 shows the dosimetric data of normal lung tissue related with symptomatic and fatal RP.

4.1.4.2 The Literature Review of Stereotactic Ablative (SABR) Radiotherapy for Lung Toxicity

Established treatment of choice in inoperable stage I NSCLC and comparable with surgery in operable patients, SBRT use has spread successfully to oligometastatic treatments as well [40–42].

In the study by Zhao et al. 2016, data from 88 studies were pooled in order to distinguish factors associated with RP and RPF [43]. They noticed an increased rate of grade 2 and 3 toxicity in older patients and larger tumors, and significant higher MLD and V_{20} in grade >2 patients.

Table 4.3 Normal lung tissue dose constraints for SABR

	Constraint	1 frx	3 frx-60 Gy	4 frx-50Gy	5 frx 50–55 Gy	8 frx-60 Gy	Endpoint
Bilateral Lungs	V_{20}		<10%	<12%	<10%	<10%	Grade >3 pneumonitis
Bilateral Lungs	V_{25}			<4.2%			Gr2 14.8%
Lungs	V_{25}		<4%				Gr2 7% Gr3 2% Gr4 0.4%
Lungs	MLD			6Gy			Gr2 11% Gr3 1% Gr4–5 0%
Lungs	MLD		4 Gy				Gr2 7% Gr3 2% Gr4 0.4%
Lungs	MLD	4.7Gy	Gr ≥2				
Lungs	V_5	26.8%	Gr ≥2				
	V_{10}	12%	Gr ≥2				
	V_{20}	5.8%	Gr ≥2				
Lungs	1500 cc	7 Gy	10.5 Gy	11.6 Gy	12.5 Gy	Lung function	
Lungs	1000 cc	7.4 Gy	11. 4 Gy	12.4 Gy	15.5 Gy	Pneumonitis	

Fractions (frx), Volume of lung receiving 20 Gy (V_{20}), Volume of lung receiving 25 Gy (V_{25}), Volume of lung receiving 10 Gy (V_{10}), Volume of lung receiving 5 Gy (V_5), MLD (Mean Lung Dose)

Constraints regarding RP in SBRT from prospective RTOG trials and retrospective data are reviewed in many studies and guidelines [44–46]; there is a summary of most recent published dose constraints for lung tissue when treated with SABR in Table 4.3.

4.1.5 Treatment

Prevention and choosing the least toxic option are more effective than any treatment. Thus, respecting the dose constraints is the first step for reducing radiation toxicity burden, since it is the proven, consistent cause for RP. However, patient and disease characteristic should be taken into account before treatment and if needed harder constraints should be chosen or, if risk exceeds benefit, radiotherapy should be avoided altogether.

1. Use of IMRT instead of 3D and respiratory gating/breath hold technique is encouraged and they should be used when feasible since they are related with decreased rate of RP [47–49].
2. Changes in the lung and GTV during treatment and re-planning should be considered in patients where atelectatic region inflates during the course of the treatment [50].

3. Lower lobe location, chemotherapy use, and older age are known factors that are related to higher RP [13, 24, 34]. Other characteristics such as smoking status, surgery before RT, pre-RT pulmonary function, COPD, chronic heart disease, diabetes mellitus, gender, performance status, ratio of TGFbeta1 pre and post RT, weight loss, and histological type are shown to be risk factors in some but not all studies [24].

Special consideration:

1. Whichever RT modality is chosen (conventional or SBRT) radiotherapy is related to extremely high rates of clinically significant RP in Interstitial Pulmonary Fibrosis (IPF) patients. No dose constraint can be considered safe in these patients and discussion in a multidisciplinary tumor board may be required to decide the best option for these patients, since radiotherapy is not recommended [51]. Proton therapy may be a safer option if RT is required [52].
2. Similarly, although reirradiation is relatively safe in peripheral lung, reirradiation in central lesions may be associated with high rates of toxicity thus prompting a more careful approach.
3. Recall pneumonitis: Immunotherapy, targeted therapy (erlotinib, osimertinib), and some drugs that are known to increase radiation toxicity (paclitaxel, adriamycin, gemcitabine, mTOR inhibitors) can have the potential to increase severity or cause reactivation of RP [53–58].

Preventive drugs: Chemical drugs used during radiotherapy with the intention to reduce occurrence and severity of RP.

1. Amifostine: It is the only drug approved to prevent radiation induced side effects. In a study by Antonadou et al. amifostine use was associated with lower rates of grade 2 or higher pneumonitis in patients with advanced-stage lung cancer receiving radiation [59]. However, its side effect profile makes it very difficult to administer in patients which already have similar complaints due to radio-chemotherapy (i.e., nausea, vomiting, and hypotension).
2. Pentoxifylline: Pentoxifylline is known to prevent pneumonitis in breast and lung patients when given prophylactically 400 mg three times a day [60].

Other considered drugs such as corticosteroids and azathioprine did not show any preventive effect [61].

Beside conventional drugs, herbal treatments have been studied for the prevention of RP. In a meta-analysis of studies investigating the effect of herbal formula, lower rate of both overall and severe RP as well as better quality of life was reported for the RT + herbal formula arm. It was concluded that due to the insufficient quality of the methods used no clear conclusions could be drawn [62].

Treatment: When a patient with a history of radiation to the chest develops dyspnea, dry cough, and the aforementioned radiological features, radiation pneumonitis should be considered in the differential diagnosis. Other conditions such as disease progression, infection, exacerbation of COPD, and chemotherapy induced pneumonitis can be confounded and their presence should be ruled out.

1. Corticosteroids Once infection or tumor progression is ruled out symptomatic RP can be successfully treated with 1 mg/kg of prednisone for 2–4 weeks. Then the dose should be decreased gradually in the sequent 6–12 weeks. Monitoring after discontinuation is required since exacerbation of RP can happen.

Nevertheless, supportive care and symptom relief according to grade, as well as careful follow-up by a specialized pulmonologist is required.

Preclinical studies: After elucidating at least part of the pathophysiology of RP, molecules that target elements in the cascade of events that lead to RP formation have been studied. Superoxide dismutase (SOD), glutathione, genistein (a soy isoflavone), cyclo-oxygenase-2 inhibitors, statins, angiotensin converting enzyme (ACE) inhibitors [63], proton pump inhibitors, drugs that stimulate the innate immunity, drugs that target IL-1, IL-13, IL-17, STAT3,TNF, TGF beta have all been studied in preclinical setting and maybe in combination may one day be able to mitigate RP [64, 65].

Ongoing studies:

1. Nintedanib, intracellular inhibitor of tyrosine kinases, was shown to have the potential to decrease incidence and prevent RP and RPF [66]. It is approved for treatment of IPF and due to its effect to inhibit the initiation and progression of fibrosis such as inflammation, activation of fibroblasts, and deposition of extracellular matrix [67]

   Two ongoing studies are comparing its efficacy in reducing Radiation-Induced Pneumonitis ClinicalTrials.gov. NCT02452463. Nintedanib Compared with Placebo in Treating Against Radiation-Induced Pneumonitis in Patients with Non-small Cell Lung Cancer That Cannot Be Removed by Surgery and Are Undergoing Chemoradiation Therapy, https://clinicaltrials.gov/ct2/show/NCT02452463 and ClinicalTrials.gov. NCT02496585. Study to Evaluate the Efficacy and Safety of Nintedanib (BIBF 1120) þ Prednisone Taper in Patients with Radiation Pneumonitis, https://clinicaltrials.gov/ct2/show/NCT02496585

2. Pirfenidone, an oral anti-fibrotic agent confirmed its potential for treatment of radiation induced fibrosis in one pilot study, where 7 patients who were irradiated predominantly to the head and neck region showed an improvement of 25% [68].

Both drugs, nintedanib and pirfenidone, are used in IPF. In a study regarding their mechanism of action, fibroblasts where treated with each of the drugs, in the presence or absence of transforming growth factor-β1. It was shown that both of them are able to inhibit collagen I formation, with nintedanib being more effective in down-regulating pro-fibrotic gene expression, collagen I and V, fibronectin, and FKBP10 [69].

4.1.6 Rx: Prescription Samples

A 74-year-old male patient with a 50 packs/year cigarette smoking history, coronary heart, and COPD diagnosed with limited stage SCLC was treated with CRT. V_{20} was 29% and MLD was 18 Gy. He had an excellent response and on the last week of CRT CBCT showed a 70% decrease in GTV. CRT was followed by chemotherapy and PCI. 9 months after RT treatment the patient developed unproductive cough and dyspnea. On thorax CT isolated pleural effusion and opacities corresponding to the high dose area were noticed. He had no other symptoms and to rule out disease progression PET-CT was done and minimal increase in FDG uptake was noticed in the local pleural effusion and in the opacities, no recurrent mass or metastasis was observed. Patient was given 48 mg of methylprednisolone/day (which corresponds to 60 mg of prednisone, the weight of the patient at that time) for 2 weeks which was tapered in 4 weeks. He had clinical improvement after 5 days. After 6 weeks he had a thorax CT which showed resolution of the pleural effusion and decrease in the lung opacities.

Mildly symptomatic grade 2: Antitussive if necessary.

Moderately symptomatic grade 3: prednisone 1 mg/kg/day for 2 weeks than slowly taper over 1–3 months, antitussive accordingly.

Grade 4: Refer to pulmonologist for hospitalization, treatment, and follow-up.

4.2 Heart

4.2.1 Anatomy

Heart is a muscular organ residing in the mediastinum with two thirds of the mass to the left of midline. It is composed of three layers: pericardium—the serous membranes enclosing the heart (parietal and visceral-epicardium), myocardium—the muscular part, and the endocardium. The four chambers of the heart: right atrium (RA) and ventricle (RV) and left atrium (LA) and ventricle (LV); the four valves: tricuspid valve (between right atrium and ventricle), mitral valve (between left atrium and ventricle), aortic semilunar valve (between left ventricle and aorta), and pulmonary semilunar valve (between right ventricle and pulmonary trunk) are the main components. Coronary arteries (CA) originating from ascending aorta are the right CA (RCA) and left main CA. Left CA then branches into left anterior descending (LAD) and circumflex CA (Cx).

Treatment planning for radiotherapy is done by the help of tomographic images; for this reason a mere description of heart according to its true anatomical division might not be sufficient and definition of sectional radiographic divisions is needed. In order to unify nomenclature regarding heart anatomy, a standardized myocardial segmentation was proposed by Cardiac Imaging Committee of the Council on Clinical Cardiology of the American Heart Association in 2002 [70]. According to their description, the heart is divided into 17 segments for assessment of the myocardium and the left ventricular cavity and blood supply for each segment is identified.

4.2.2   Contouring

For contouring of the heart in lung cancer the contouring recommendation of RTOG 11-06 trial protocol can be followed. It is stated that heart should be contoured together with the pericardial sac extending from the base (the inferior part of pulmonary artery passing the midline) to the apex. The contouring of heart according to this definition is shown in Fig. 4.3. For breast cancer radiotherapy, a detailed heart contouring was suggested by Feng et al. [71]. In 2017 Duane et al. developed an atlas of the heart for radiotherapy in which a more detailed description and contouring of heart and its components are shown in Fig. 4.4 [72]. In the atlas 5 left ventricle (anterior, inferior, lateral, septal, and apical) and 10 coronary artery segments (1. left main coronary artery, 2. proximal LAD, 3. mid LAD, 4. distal LAD, 5. proximal Cx, 6. distal Cx, 7. proximal RCA, 8. mid RCA, 9. distal RCA, and 10. posterior descending) are identified, beside RA, LA, RV, and LV.

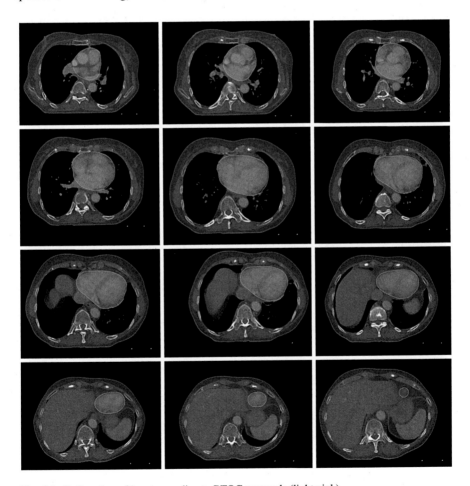

Fig. 4.3 Delineation of heart according to RTOG protocols (light pink)

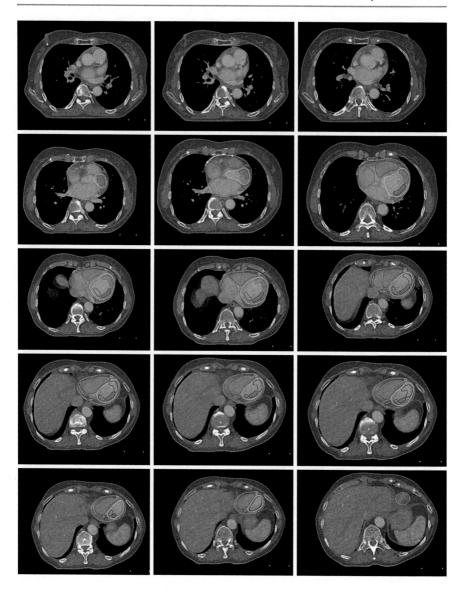

Fig. 4.4 Delineation of heart according to Duane. Sections of heart; Ascending Aorta: Green, Pulmonary artery: light blue, Left atrium: army green, Right atrium: light purple, Distal Circumflex coronary artery: light green, Proximal Circumflex coronary artery: light cyan, Distal Left anterior descending coronary artery: lemon, Mid Left anterior descending coronary artery: light purple, Proximal Left anterior descending coronary artery: yellow, Left main artery: dark pink, Left ventricle: dark yellow, Right coronary artery: distal: Bordeaux, Mid Right coronary artery: brown, Right coronary artery-posterior descending: dark pink, Proximal Right coronary artery: light pink, Right ventricle: opaque bluish green, Vena Cava Inferior: orange, Vena Cava Superior: dark blue, Anterior ventricle: opaque dark green, Apical Left ventricle: dark Bordeaux, Inferior Left ventricle: Transparent dark green, Lateral Left ventricle: blue, Septal Left ventricle: light blue

4.2.3   Pathophysiology

Radiation induced cardiovascular disease (RICVD) comprises different disease entities such as pericarditis, cardiomyopathy, valvular heart disease, and coronary heart disease. The grading of RICVD is seen in Table 4.4. Despite their different clinical, prognostic, and treatment strategies the main culprit of their development being radiotherapy, pathophysiological changes follow the same path; acute inflammation is followed by noncontrolled fibrosis.

- *Acute inflammation and oxidative stress:* Immediately after RT the first recognizable changes occur at the endothelium, within minutes it becomes hyperpermeable, starts displaying chemokines and molecules that attract immune cell, and allows for their transmigration. The recruited neutrophils secrete proinflammatory mediators such as IL-8, TNF, and together with chemokines from endothelium itself, they form an acute inflammatory response. At the same time oxidative stress caused by radiation also influences macrophages which in turn increase the production of proinflammatory mediators. Free radicals increase is associated with a specific type of inflammation where T helper cell type 2 are over stimulated and preferentially secrete IL-4, IL-13, TGF beta, chemical signals that are known to stimulate fibroblasts and fibrosis [73, 74].
- *Fibrosis:* Increase in pro-fibrotic cytokines causes production of connective tissue growth factor (CTGF) which induces transformation of fibroblasts into myofibroblasts [75]. It is also able to simulate production of extracellular matrix (ECM) even when TGF beta is not present anymore [76]. The transformed myofibroblasts, in contrast to normal wound healing, do not undergo apoptosis after irradiation and their persistent presence causes progression of fibrosis. The mechanism of fibroblast persistence might be due to epigenetic changes that occur during RT [77].

4.2.4   Dose Constraints

Cardiac toxicity was generally thought to be a late sequela of radiotherapy. Its incidence, therefore, was mostly recognized in patients with cancers showing relatively long survival such as breast and Hodgkin disease. However, its detrimental effects in lung cancer patients are also known to be a factor for decreased survival within 2 years after radiotherapy. Due to poor prognosis of the cancer, more loose constraints have been used for NSCLC radiotherapy, when compared to breast cancer. It should be kept in mind that lung cancer has same risk factor as heart disease, thus making these patients already more susceptible to heart related morbidity. Violating heart constraints, even in lung cancer, is not justifiable anymore since its toxicity is now recognized as an important cause of mortality.

Table 4.4 Toxicity grading for radiation induced cardiovascular disease (RICVD)

CTCAE v5	Grade 1	Grade 2	Grade 3	Grade 4	Grade 5
Pericarditis	Asymptomatic, ECG or physical findings (e.g., rub) consistent with pericarditis	Symptomatic pericarditis (e.g., chest pain)	Pericarditis with physiologic consequences (e.g., pericardial constriction)	Life-threatening consequences; urgentintervention indicated	Death
Valve disease	Asymptomatic valvular thickening with or without mild valvular regurgitation or stenosis by imaging	Asymptomatic; moderate regurgitation or stenosis by imaging	Symptomatic; severe regurgitation or stenosis by imaging; symptoms controlled with medical intervention	Life-threatening consequences; urgent intervention indicated (e.g., valve replacement, valvuloplasty)	Death
Restrictive cardiomyopathy	Imaging findings only	Symptomatic without signs of heart failure	Symptomatic heart failure or other cardiac symptoms, responsive to intervention; new onset of symptoms	Refractory heart failure or other poorly controlled cardiac symptoms	Death

4.2.4.1 The Literature Review of Conventional Fractionated Radiotherapy for Radiation Induced Cardiovascular Disease (RICVD)

Lung Cancer

RTOG 0617 trail is the most eye opener study in regard to radiotherapy induced heart toxicity [78]. The trail was designed as two-by-two factorial, randomize phase 3 study which would compare standard dose (60 Gy) and high dose (74 Gy) radiotherapy given concurrently with carboplatin/paclitaxel, with or without cetuximab [78]. The result of the trial was not as expected and standard dose appeared to be better than high dose in terms of overall survival (28.7 vs. 20.3 months). The explanation given by the investigators was that heart doses were much higher (specifically V_5 and V_{30}) in the high dose group, leading to cardiac related toxicity and death. In subsequent analysis of the cohort it was noticed that V_{40} is one of the factors influencing overall survival [47] and IMRT can lower it significantly when compared to 3D conformal RT. In the years that followed other studies start taking into account heart dose and in the RTOG 1106 trial dose limits to the heart are: D_{max} <70 Gy, D_{mean} <30 Gy, V_{30} Gy <50%, and V_{40} <35%. A similar single arm phase 2 trial from the same group showed that mid-treatment adaptation of RT according to metabolic response (by PET-CT) increases local control [79]. They accrued 42 patients with more advanced disease, worst performance, and more comorbidity than the RTOG 0617 trial, and the cardiac related toxicity was 28%. Though no cardiac related death was noticed, invasion of great vessels could be related to 4 deaths through massive bleeding (two from lung, one during endoscopy, and one unknown). In one study V_{50} correlated with RICDV, patients with V_{50} >25% had 2 year OS of 26% as compared to 45.9% OS in patients having V_{50} <25% [80]. Mean heart dose was found to relate to grade >3 heart toxicity in another study [81]. Specific dose to a specific compartment of the heart correlated with different types of toxicity: V_{30} of whole heart, RA and LA correlated with pericarditis, LV and whole heart V_{30} correlated with ischemic attack [82]. Similarly, in a small cohort of patient, 63 and 69 Gy doses to the left atrium significantly associated with death rate [83].

Breast Cancer

Cardiac toxicity has been recognized as an important factor affecting mortality in surviving breast cancer patients, especially in left breast irradiation [84–87]. From different studies conducted through the years effect of RT to breast and it components has been reviewed in a recent guideline [88]. Worth mentioning are the studies by Darby et al. 2013, van den Bogaard et al. 2017, Marks et al. 2005, Nilsson et al. 2012, Moignier et al. 2015, Erven et al. 2011 [89–93]. The results of their studies and the constraints that are found important in heart toxicity are summarized in Table 4.5. Briefly, Darby et al. and van den Bogaard et al. found that there is an increase in major coronary event for 1 Gy increase in mean heart dose, Nilsson et al. 2012 and Moignier et al. 2015 concluded that dose to coronary artery leads to stenosis, Marks et al. 2005 and Erven et al. 2011 found that irradiation of LV apical part effects myocardial function as noticed in cardiac imaging. Skytta et al. 2015 measured troponin levels during radiotherapy and found that different doses to

Table 4.5 Cardiac tissue dose constraints for conventional fractionated radiotherapy

Structure	Dose/fraction	Dose	Volume
Whole heart (Breast radiotherapy)	2 Gy	<2.5 Gy	Mean
Left ventricle (Breast radiotherapy)	2 Gy	<3 Gy V_5 V_{23}	Mean <17% <5%
LAD (Breast radiotherapy)	2 Gy	<10 Gy V_{30} V_{40}	Mean <2% <1%
Whole heart (Lung cancer)	1.8 Gy	60 Gy	33%
Whole heart (Lung cancer)	1.8 Gy	45 Gy	67%
Whole heart (Lung cancer)	1.8 Gy	40 Gy	100%
Whole heart (Lung cancer)	2 Gy	70 Gy	D_{max}
Whole heart (Lung cancer)	2 Gy	30 Gy	Mean
Whole heart (Lung cancer)	2 Gy	>30 Gy	50%
Whole heart (Lung cancer)	2 Gy	>40 Gy	35%
Whole heart (Lung cancer)	3 Gy	47 Gy	D_{max}
Whole heart (Lung cancer)	3 Gy	45 Gy	<30%

Left anterior descending artery (LAD), Dose maximum (D_{max})

heart, LV, LAD corelated with specific increase in troponin levels [94]. Use of hypofractionation does not show increase in cardiac toxicity [95, 96].

4.2.4.2 The Literature Review of SABR for Radiation Induced Cardiovascular Disease (RICVD)

Effect of SABR on heart is not well recognized; however, there is data regarding toxicity in some studies. Stam et al. 2017 after analyzing 803 patients with early NSCLC treated with SABR recognized that dose to 90% of superior vena cava (median 0.6 Gy) and maximum dose to left atrium (median 6.5 Gy) were associated with non-cancer death [97]. In two smaller cohorts, no specific dose to heart or its components could be correlated to mortality or toxicity [98, 99].

Cardiac tissue dose constraints for SBRT are summarized in Table 4.6.

4.2.5 Prevention

Limiting the dose and exposed volume of the heart as low as possible and respecting dose constraints is the main step in prevention. Use of advanced technology in diminishing margins (IGRT, inspiratory gating and deep inspirium breath

Table 4.6 Cardiac tissue dose constraints for SBRT

	Constraint	1 frx	3 frx -60Gy	4 frx	5 frx 50–55Gy	8 frx- 60Gy
Heart	D_{max}	22 Gy	30 Gy		35 or 105% PTV	50 Gy
Heart	15 cm^3	16 Gy	24 Gy		32 Gy	
Left atrium	D_{max}		6.5 Gy			

Fraction (frx), Dose maximum (D_{max})

hold-DIBHT in lung cancer and esophageal cancer), risk adopted dose de-escalation and field reduction (Hodgkin's disease and non-Hodgkin lymphoma), purposefully removing heart from RT field (DIBH in left breast irradiation), use of intensity modulated treatments to increase conformity (lung cancer), and proton therapy in pediatric tumors are necessary measures that a radiation oncologist should be aware of and implement in treatments involving thorax, when feasible. Consultation with a cardiologist before radiotherapy with the aim to distinguish additional risk factors in order to promptly and aggressively treating them (hyperlipidemia, hypertension, diabetes mellitus, smoking, obesity, sedentary lifestyle) in addition to a baseline echocardiography might be useful.

4.2.6 Follow-Up and Screening

Different guidelines proposed several types of screening for RICVD [100–104]. It can be summarized as:

1. Yearly physician visits and blood pressure control,
2. Twice a year lipid screening,
3. For patients with no additional risk factors: transthoracic echocardiography (TTE) 10 years after RT and repeat TTE every 5 years.
4. For patients with >1 additional risk factor: TTE 5 years after RT, repeat TTE every 5 years, noninvasive stress imaging every 5 years.
5. For patients with symptoms of chronic heart failure (CHF), angina, and new murmur: refer immediately for TTE and stress imaging.

Radioprotectants There is no drug to have been approved for use in mitigating or preventing RICVD. However, drugs which are used for other purposes are being tested. Statins, angiotensin converting enzyme inhibitors, amifostine and melatonin are some of the drugs which have shown good results in animal testing [74, 105–108].

4.2.7 Treatment

There is not much a radiation oncologist can do after symptoms related to RICVD emerge, beside referring the patient to a cardiologist. Treatments then vary according to the disease type:

- *Acute pericarditis:* Due to more stringent heart constraints, incidence of acute pericarditis is very low; however, it should be kept in mind when a patient who had being irradiated to high doses, or whose heavy burden tumor infiltrates pericardium or is positioned adjacent to it, develops symptoms of pericarditis such as pleuritic chest pain, fever, pericardial friction rub. These symptoms usually develop during or immediately after, in the weeks that follow RT. Even though the syndrome might be self-limiting it is prudent to refer the patient to cardiologist for advanced tests such as TTE or ECG which would show signs of pericardial effusion. It should be kept in mind that even though NSAIDS or colchicine might be sufficient as a treatment, there is the probability for the disease to progress to tamponade and an evaluation by the cardiologist is crucial [74].
- *Chronic pericarditis:* It usually presents itself as incidental pericardial effusion months or years after irradiation, but symptoms are similar to acute pericarditis. Due to its chronicity it rarely progresses to tamponade. TTE is the preferred imaging modality due to its feasibility; however, MRI might be useful in cases where differential diagnosis cannot be made since it can distinguish between constrictive pericarditis, transient constriction due to inflammation, and effusive constrictive pericarditis. If diagnosis of symptomatic constrictive pericarditis or recurrent symptomatic effusion develops, the treatment of choice is pericardiectomy [74]. Unfortunately, this procedure has high morbidity and mortality rate and prognosis is poor especially in irradiated patient either due to procedural difficulties or other RICDV [109–111]
- *Radiation induced cardiomyopathy (RICM):* It presents itself with typical heart failure symptoms such as exercise intolerance, volume overload, and shortness of breath. TTE or MRI is able to identify decrease in ejection fraction or fibrosis and inflammation in myocardium, respectively. Treatment is similar to heart failure due to other causes and depends on symptoms of the patient, starting with drugs such as ACE inhibitors, angiotensin receptor blocker, beta blocker, diuretics, isosorbide dinitrate, and digoxin. It should be kept in mind that these drugs are for symptomatic relief and do not cure the underlying disease. In more severe cases cardioverter-defibrillator (ICD) and heart transplant are needed. Again, the prognosis after surgery is not very good in patients undergoing transplant due to RICM, with 5 year survival rates after transplants as low as 47% [112, 113].
- *Valvular heart disease (VHD):* New murmur on physical examination together with symptoms of heart failure should be an alarm bell for VDH. Doppler TTE is the investigation of choice and TEE reserved for non-diagnostic TEE [100]. Incidence of VHD is higher in irradiated patients, with aortic valve being the most affected [114]. Repair of VHD in these patients has poor outcome, with one third of patients deteriorated after the procedure [114]. For this reason, valve replacement may be superior in RIVHD. Beside surgery, transfemoral transcatheter aortic valve replacement has gained popularity with proven equal results in intermediate and high-risk patients [115–117].
- *Coronary heart disease (CHD):* Angina pectoris in a patient irradiated to the chest requires attention and immediate coronary angiography is advised, since RT is an additional risk factor for CHD. As stenosis after RT occurs in the proximal coronary arteries it is difficult to be treated with transcatheter stent placement alone. In

older studies as much as 86% of patients showed restenosis after stent placement and 67% required balloon angioplasty after each angiography [118, 119]. Even surgical revascularization (by-pass surgery) is not without consequences. In retrospective data mortality and morbidity after surgery was found to be dose dependent and breast cancer patients show better outcome than HL patients [120, 121].

4.3 Chest Wall

Identifying toxicity of radiotherapy to chest wall (CW), such as chest wall pain and rib fractures, can be challenging due to many reasons. Firstly, rib fractions are, in many occasions, asymptomatic and might not be perceived or reported by the patient. As much as 61% and 65.9% of rib fractures were revealed only through imaging in two retrospective studies [122, 123]. Secondly, symptoms may develop several months after exposure to radiotherapy, making it difficult to identify radiation as the causing agent. Also, small changes in the bone structure can be easily overlooked when evaluating imaging studies.

Due to these reasons and its less frequent occurrence after conventional fractionation, chest wall toxicity has gained recognition after SBRT studies. With the widespread use of SBRT in thoracic tumors chest wall and ribs have emerged as "organ at risk" with higher rate of toxicity and constraints that need to be met.

4.3.1 Anatomy

By definition chest wall is the protective structure around vital structures in the thorax which helps support respiration and motion of upper extremities. It is composed of skin, fat, other connective tissue, muscles, and bones. Bones in the chest wall include ribs, sternum, and vertebra. However, conventionally skin, sternum, and vertebra are not identified as part of chest wall; they are not included in the contouring and these structures' toxicities are not considered as chest wall toxicity.

4.3.2 Contouring

Contouring of chest wall has been a reason for debate; in different studies different definitions of CW were used. Similarly, instead of a defining CW individual ribs were contoured for dosimetric purposes (Fig. 4.5) [122–126].

The contouring of CW accepted in RTOG studies is similar to that proposed by Mutter et al. and Kong et al. [3, 124].

- Chest wall can be auto-segmented from the ipsilateral lung with a 2-cm expansion in the lateral, anterior, and posterior directions within 3 cm range of PTV.
- It extends anteriorly and medially from the edge of the sternum and stops posteriorly and medially at the edge of the vertebral body with inclusion of the spinal nerve root exit site, excluding vertebrate bodies, sternum, and skin.

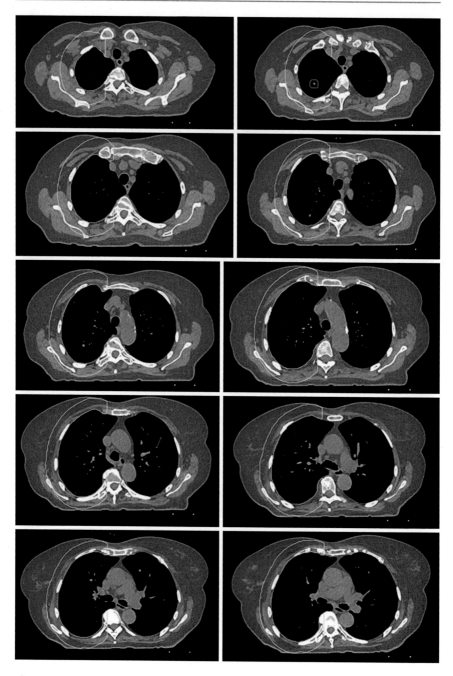

Fig. 4.5 Delineation of chest wall (yellow)

4.3.3 Pathophysiology

4.3.3.1 Pathophysiology of Rib Fracture (RF)

Effect of radiotherapy to bone in general is reviewed by Pacheco and Stock in 2013 [127]. Similar to the effect elsewhere, radiation to the bone causes increased endothelial cell permeability, edema, and migration of inflammatory cells [128]. Subsequent fibrosis, which in bone particularly, leads to vascular luminal narrowing and decrease in blood supply [129]. The fact that SBRT and hypofractionation in general, rather than conventional fractionation, are causing rib fracture may lead us to accept this hypothesis as the most plausible one. At the same time radiation causes an arrest in osteoblast cell cycle, leading to decrease in number [130]. Even in low doses, due to activation of inflammatory mediators and cytokines by radiation, simulation of osteoclasts occurs, resulting in imbalance between osteoblasts and osteoclasts number and function [130]. This translates into increased bone resorption, trabecular turnover which resembles osteoporosis. The radiation effects are more pronounced in actively dividing cells, like in trabecular bone which despite having a much higher rate of turnover and remodeling supports bone marrow, which is even more susceptible to radiation, resulting in marrow fibrosis. Especially in postmenopausal female patients these effects can be more evident since lack of estrogen causes overproduction of interleukin-6 by osteoblast, which in turn stimulates osteoclasts and bone resorption [131].

4.3.3.2 Pathophysiology of Chest Wall (CW) Pain

Bone pain after fracture might be the most straightforward explanation for chest wall pain; however, in literature roughly 60% of patients with fractures have no symptoms and many of patients with CW pain do not show overt fractures. Thus, it leads us to search for other explanations for pain, unrelated to fracture. One plausible cause might be injury to the nerves in the chest wall. Similar scenario is noticed after breast irradiation of supraclavicular fossa causing brachial plexopathy. In the study by Nambu et al. four patients without fracture but chest wall pain also showed edema at the nearest chest wall site with PTV which received the higher dose. Chronic inflammation or contraction due to underlying fibrosis was the explanation for the phenomenon [123]. The grading system for chest wall and rib toxicity according to CTCAE v5.0 (Common Terminology Criteria for adverse events) is shown in Table 4.7.

4.3.4 Dose Constraints

Although chest wall toxicity has gained recognition after high dose stereotactic treatments, chest wall pain and rib fracture have been noticed with less frequency after conventional fractionation. In early breast radiotherapy studies, incidence of

Table 4.7 Toxicity grading for chest wall and rib

	Grade 1	Grade 2	Grade 3	Grade 4	Grade 5
CTCAE v5.0 Chest wall pain	Mild pain	Moderate pain; limiting instrumental ADL	Severe pain; limiting self-care	–	–
CTCAE v5.0 Fracture	Asymptomatic; clinical or diagnostic observations only; intervention not indicated	Symptomatic but non-displaced; immobilization indicated	Severe symptoms; displaced or open wound with bone exposure; limiting self-care, operative intervention indicated	Life-threatening consequences; urgent intervention indicated	Death

CTCAE v5.0 (Common Terminology Criteria for adverse events)

rib fracture ranged from 0.4% in conventionally fractionated treatments with 6 MV to 19% in patients treated with hypofractionated regimens [132, 133]. The estimated alpha/beta ration was calculated to be between 1.8 and 2.8 [133]. Similar to the former study accelerated partial breast radiotherapy given with balloon catheter to the tumor site after surgery showed higher than anticipated incidence of CW toxicity [134]. They distinguished that postmenopausal status, use of chemotherapy, and osteoporosis were risk factors for CW toxicity.

4.3.4.1 The Literature Review of SABR for Chest Wall and Rib Toxicity

Studies related to chest wall toxicity, dosimetric predictors, and other risk factors are found in abundance in literature. One study by Ma et al. in 2018 summarizes 57 of these studied (5985 patients) [135].

Any grade CWP, grade >2, grade >3 was found to be 11%, 6.2%, and 1.2%, respectively. Distance from tumor to CW of less than 16–25 mm (risk of RF increases up to 36.7% in lesions abutting rib), BMI >29, maximum dose (D_{max}) of 0.5 cm^3 >60 Gy, 5 cm^3 >40 Gy, and the volume of CW or ribs receiving >30 Gy correlated with higher risk of CWP and RF. Rib fracture occurred in 6.3% of patients and female gender was an important risk factor for RF. The main dosimetric recommendation derived from studies summarized is found in Table 4.8.

All these recommendations are not mandatory since the rate and severity of chest wall toxicity do not justify withholding potentially curative treatment and decreasing dose to meet these constraints should not jeopardize local control. However, that should be taken in consideration and a less toxic schedule should be followed when feasible. In a recent study by Chipko et al. 2019 in the cohort of 100 patients it was noticed that 36% of the developed chest wall pain never resolved and more than 60% of fractures were accompanied by tissue fibrosis or heterotopic ossification.

Table 4.8 Chest wall toxicity dose constraints for SABR

	Constraint	3 frx	4 frx	5 frx	8 frx	Endpoint
Ribs	D_{max}	50–54 Gy				
CW	D0.5 cm³	60 Gy				50% RF
CW	D0.5 cm³			<39 Gy	<39 Gy	
CW	D2 cm³	21 Gy 27.3 Gy 50 Gy				0% RF 5% RF 50% RF
CW	D5 cm³	40 Gy				10% CWT
CW	D15 cm³	40 Gy				30% CWT
CW	V_{30}	>30 cm³	>35 Gy	13.3% Gr3 17.3% Gr2		
CW	V_{30}	>70 cm³		15.1% Gr3 27.8% Gr2		

Chest Wall (CW), Chest Wall Toxicity (CWT)

4.3.5 Treatment

Asymptomatic rib fracture that is not displaced does not require further treatment. Chest wall pain and pain due to fractures might require anti-inflammatory drugs according to the severity of symptoms. Over the counter drugs can be sufficient in grade 2; however, stronger drugs, such as opioids should be included in the treatment of grade 3 pain. Grade 4 rib fracture is deemed very rare, though the treatment in that case should be surgery.

4.3.6 Rx: Sample Prescriptions

- Mildly symptomatic: 2 × 1 tablet of ibuprofen or naproxen or diclofenac
- Moderately symptomatic: NSAID as above + fentanil patches or tramadol

4.4 Esophagus

4.4.1 Anatomy

Esophagus is the tubular part of the alimentary tract extending from the lower part of pharynx (inferior of cricoid cartilage at the C5-6 vertebra level) to the stomach (gastroesophageal junction at the T11 vertebra level). It is approximately 18–26 cm long in adults and consists of four layers; mucosa, submucosa, muscularis propria, and adventitia. Esophagus does not have a serosal covering, unlike other areas of gastrointestinal tract. While lack of serosa makes repair of luminal disruption more difficult, it also allows tumor to spread more easily and rendering it harder to treat surgically. Topographically, it consists of three regions: cervical (from pharyngo-esophageal junction to the suprasternal notch, approximately 4–5 cm), thoracic (from suprasternal notch to the diaphragmatic hiatus at T10 vertebral level), and the abdominal region (from diaphragmatic hiatus to the cardia of stomach, approximately 1 cm).

For most of its course esophagus runs anterior to the vertebral body and posterior to trachea. From the T8 vertebral level until the diaphragmatic hiatus it lies anterior to aorta [136].

4.4.2 Contouring

The RTOG 11-06 trial [137] defined contouring of esophagus as: 'The esophagus should be contoured from the beginning at the level just below the cricoid to its entrance to the stomach at GE junction, thus the entire length of the esophagus is identified, requiring that a portion of the neck and upper abdomen be included in the planning CT scan'. In some of the studies, where the upper (cervical) esophagus was not included the absolute esophageal volume was ~20% smaller than if it had been contoured entirely [138–140]. The esophagus will be contoured using mediastinal window/level on CT to correspond to the mucosal, submucosa, and all muscular layers out to the fatty adventitia.

When not contracting or when there is no food passing, esophagus lumen is closed, thus more difficult to be distinguished. Administration of small amount of diluted non-barium contrast liquid might improve visualization (Fig. 4.6).

Esophagus can move slightly even when not passing food. In a study it was found that during 4DCT, the upper, middle, and lower esophagus can move 5, 6–7, and 8–9 mm in medio-lateral and dorso-ventral directions, respectively [140].

4.4.3 Pathophysiology

4.4.3.1 Acute Esophagitis

Radiation induced acute esophagitis is a frequent toxicity of radiotherapy to the thorax or lower neck. By definition, acute refers to toxicity occurring <3 month after RT. It generally onsets 2–3 weeks after initiation of conventionally fractionated radiotherapy and may last up to 4 weeks after RT completion [141, 142].

It is usually self-limiting; however, according to its severity it may interfere with treatment course, leading to treatment delays, hospitalization, or interruption of RT. Grading of acute toxicity is shown in Table 4.9.

Esophagitis incidence depends of the timing and methods used to measure it, whether it is self-reported by the patients, quantified by quality of life questionnaires or reported by the physician [143, 144]. In studies regarding RIE after curative irradiation of lung cancers its incidences was grade 2 in 32.2%, grade 3 in 17.1%, and grade 4 in 0.9% of patients [145]. Its incidence was found to be even higher in the palliative setting of NSCLC. Mean rate of grade 3–4 esophagitis was 25.7% in higher fractionated regimens, ranging from 0 to 56% [143].

The mechanism of radiation induced esophagitis is not clear. Efforts to link genetic and transcription changes with RIE revealed a multistep and multifactorial

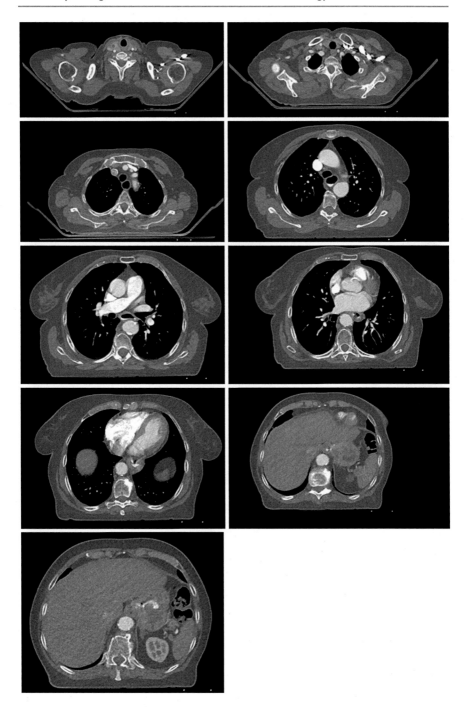

Fig. 4.6 Delineation of esophagus (light brown)

Table 4.9 Grading of acute toxicity according to CTCAE v5.0 (common terminology criteria for adverse events)

	Grade 1	Grade 2	Grade 3	Grade 4	Grade 5
CTCAE v5.0 Esophagitis	Asymptomatic; clinical or diagnostic observations only; intervention not indicated	Symptomatic; altered eating/ swallowing; oral supplements indicated	Severely altered eating/ swallowing; tube feeding, TPN, or hospitalization indicated	Life-threatening consequences; urgent operative intervention indicated	Death

process [146]. In study by Epperly MW reported that increased levels of proinflammatory cytokines such as TGF beta1, IL-1, TNF alpha, IL-18, and interferon gamma by ROS and SOD/liposome decrease it [147]. EGF on the other hand was shown to be decreased by RT and was proposed to be used as target for reduction of RİE in another study [148]. Irradiation of esophagus causes upregulation of 398 genes, including genes related to inflammation and immune response, cell growth, and proliferation and cell apoptosis, supporting the hypothesis that irradiation causes a heavy inflammatory response and slight oncogenicity. However, Fgfr3, Hgf, and Bcl2l14 among others are downregulated indicating that oncogenic genes might be more sensitive to irradiation. Similarly, up- or downregulation in long noncoding RNA and other epigenetic changes were noticed after irradiation [146].

Histopathologic findings include appearance of apoptotic bodies in the basal zone, sloughing of squamous epithelial layer, degeneration and decrease number of mucosal glands, submucosal endothelial swelling and capillary dilation, atypia of both epithelial and stromal cells [149]. Vascular bed also shows changes such as obliterative vasculitis, sclerosis, and intimal foam cell arteriopathy. Acute esophagitis and inflammatory changes that characterize it generally subside 3–4 weeks after RT.

Late toxicity: By definition, "late" refers to >3 months after the completion of RT; median time of onset of late esophageal injury is 6 months, with some instances diagnosed at 1 year or later [144].

Estimating incidence of late toxicity to the esophagus is even more challenging. Tumor recurrence whether patients are actively surveyed or self-reporting also effects incidence.

After acute esophagitis resolves or symptoms are alleviated, in some patients new changes occur. Submucosal thickening, edema, fibroblasts, and inflammatory cells infiltrate the muscle wall and mural fibrosis occurs, leading to stricture formation [144].

Esophageal wall necrosis, perforation, or fistulas may also develop as late toxicity; grading of late toxicity is shown in Table 4.10.

In one study the severity of acute esophagitis could be predictive of late toxicity [139]. This could be a plausible hypothesis since both toxicities have inflammatory background; however, many patients with more pronounced endoscopic findings do not show severe symptoms [150].

Table 4.10 Grading of late toxicity according to CTCAE (common terminology criteria for adverse events)

	Grade 1	Grade 2	Grade 3	Grade 4	Grade 5
RTOG/ EORTC Late esophagitis	Mild fibrosis; slight difficulty in swallowing solids; no pain on swallowing	Unable to take solid food normally; swallowing semisolid food; dilatation may be indicated	Severe fibrosis; able to swallow only liquids; may have pain on swallowing; dilatation required	Necrosis/perforation, fistula	Death
CTCAE v5.0 Esophageal stenosis	Asymptomatic; clinical ordiagnostic observations only; intervention not indicated	Symptomatic; altered GI function	Severely altered GI function; tube feeding or hospitalization indicated; elective operative intervention indicated	Life-threatening consequences; urgent operative interventionindicated	Death
CTCAE v5.0 Esophageal fistula Perforation Necrosis		Invasive intervention notindicated (not applicable for necrosis)	Invasive intervention indicated	Life-threateningconsequences; urgent operative interventionindicated	Death

This may lead to discordance between severity of symptoms and actual damage to the esophagus, which later translates to late toxicity. Likewise, severe symptoms in some patients (young, female) may be an indicator of altered pain perception rather than marker for toxicity.

4.4.4 Dose Constraints

4.4.4.1 The Literature Review of Conventional Fractionated Radiotherapy for Esophageal Toxicity

Non-small Cell Lung Cancer (NSCLC) Tolerance of esophagus to radiotherapy in the late phase, such as the maximum dose to specific volumes to esophagus were described by Emami et al. [151]. Toxicity end points area 5% complication rate at 5 years (TD5/5) and a 50% complication rate at 5 years (TD50/5); clinical stricture and perforation occurs in 5% of patient who have 60 Gy to one third of esophagus, 58 Gy to two thirds or 55 Gy to whole esophagus. TD50/5 is observed in patients irradiated 72 Gy to one third of esophagus, 70 Gy to two thirds, and 68 Gy to whole esophagus. Similarly, in older studies the tolerance of esophagus for late sequela was suggested to be 6000 rad given at 1000 rad per week [152].

However, the toxicity in the acute phase was not addressed in these studies.

With addition of chemotherapy higher toxicity was expected; Hirota et al. showed that 0% of patient given RT alone vs. 27% of patient given concomitant chemotherapy had endoscopic grade 3 esophagitis [150]. In another study by the same group the best predictor of esophagitis was found to be length of esophagus having circumferential doses of more than 40 or 45 Gy (V_{40} and V_{45}) [153]. In other early studies 46% of patient were reported to have grade 3–4 esophagitis after weekly paclitaxel-carboplatin [154]. Type of chemotherapy used also affect esophagitis with taxane and cisplatin combination more toxic than vinorelbine cisplatin [155]. In the same study V_{40} >23% increases Gr 2 esophagitis from 33% to 89% and V_{50} >26.5% increases Gr 3 esophagitis from 6.7% to 38.7% [155].

Hyperfractionation also was shown to increase toxicity; in one study where 57% of patients had hyperfractionated regimens more than 10% of patients suffered from acute or late esophagitis. Dosimetrical data showed that length of 100% circumference treated to greater than 50 Gy was the best predictor of toxicity [156]. Bradley et al. showed that length of esophagus receiving 60 Gy and surface area receiving 55 Gy correlates with development of acute esophagitis in both CRT and RT arms [157]. In the study by Werner–Wasik specific rates of grade 3 acute esophagitis by treatment groups were 6%, 0%, 18%, and 43% for RT alone, induction chemotherapy followed by radiation, concurrent chemotherapy with daily RT, and concurrent chemotherapy with twice-per-day RT, respectively [158]. Time to healing from esophagitis was also longer in the latter group: 14, 19, 29, and 87 days, respectively. No dosimetric data was found to effect esophagitis.

Similarly, in another study use of concurrent chemotherapy was found to be the most important factor increasing toxicity, together with V_{35}. In the non-concomitant group TD (50)=47 Gy (41–60 Gy) according to Lyman–Kutcher–Burman normal tissue complication probability model [159]. While using the same model Chapet et al. found that TD_{50} was 51 Gy and that significant association is found between esophagitis and dose/volume parameters V_{40} ($P = 0.001$) to V_{70} ($P = 0.024$) [138].

In the study by Wang et al. low levels of IL-8, age younger than 70 years, and equivalent uniform dose of 41.4 Gy were associated with higher risk of Gr >2 esophagitis [160].

In a large review of literature by Werner and Wasik et al. concluded that it is not possible to identify a cut-off for volumetric parameters. However, they suggest that esophagus does not receive doses higher than the prescription dose (i.e., 60 Gy) and that mean dose to esophagus be kept below 34 Gy, as suggested in the RTOG 0617 trial. They also stressed the fact that according to the studies reviewed the toxicity correlated with volume receiving doses larger than 40–50 Gy. They encourage institutions to analyze and determine their own constraints, since esophagitis may change according to the type of chemotherapy, radiotherapy protocol and schedule, as well as the population studied [161].

In an individual based meta-analysis of NSCLC patients treated with CRT best predictor of esophagitis was found to be V_{60}. In that study recursive partitioning identified 3 risk groups for developing grade >2 and >3 esophagitis: low ($V_{60} < 0.07\%$), intermediate (V_{60} 0.07% to 16.99%), and high (V_{60} 17%) [145]. Similarly, in another study a V_{60} of ≥15% had a 37.8% risk of grade 3 RE compared to a 6.1% risk among those with a V_{60} of <15% in NSCLC patients treated with hyperfracionated regimen (64 Gy in 40 fractions twice daily) [162]. In a study in which hyperfractionated therapy (73.8–90 Gy, median 79.2 Gy in twice daily fractions of 1.8 Gy) was given after induction chemotherapy it was noticed that >2 grade esophagitis occurs in 35% of patients and V_{38} was the best predictor, where ≥ grade 2 is 30% or less if V_{38} does not exceed 34% [163].

In the era of intensity modulated radiotherapy (IMRT) esophagitis remains of concern. In the study by Uyterlinde et al. where 153 NSCLC were given low dose daily cisplatin concurrent with 66 Gy in 24 fractions, 37% experienced Gr 2, and 20% gr 3 esophagitis. Esophagus V_{50}, non-Caucasian ethnic background, and the number of cisplatin administrations higher than 20 significantly correlated with grade 3 toxicity [164]. In another study, where IMRT was used exclusively (IMRT or VMAT) to treat 193 NSCLC patients in 30 fractions to 60 Gy, the rate of grade 2 and grade 3 esophagitis was 23.7% and 5.1%, respevtively. Female gender, concurrent versus sequential chemotherapy, mean dose, and upper esophageal position were found to be risk factors for grade >2 esophagitis [165].

According to one study protecting the contralateral side ($V_{45} < 2.5$ cc, $V_{55} < 0.5$) helps in preventing gr >3 esophagitis (no patient had severe esophagitis in the experimental arm) [166]. Likewise, in the study by Kao J 2015, protecting the contralateral lung and esophagus resulted in lower gr >3 esophagitis [167]. In another study whole esophagus was protected (max <65 Gy, $V_{50} < 30\%$) which resulted in better nutritional status and lower gr >3 esophagitis, as compared to patients in which constraints suggested in the NCCN guideline were respected (4.5% vs. 30.2%) [168].

SCLC: In a study where limited stage SCLC patients were given hyperfractionated chemoradiotherapy of 45 Gy in twice daily fractions of 1.5 Gy 26% of 3-D conformal RT patients and 11.5% of the IMRT patients developed grade 3 esophagitis [169]. Besides confirming the protectant effect of IMRT to esophagus, it was also noticed that 26% of patients having grade 3 acute esophagitis developed late toxicity (strictures) as compared to only 2% in patients with less severe acute injury. Mean esophagus dose and V_{45} were the best predictor of late toxicity, with 13.7% of patients developing esophagus strictures if V_{45} exceeded 37.5%. Acute esophagitis correlated more with volume receiving low-mid doses between V_5 and V_{40}. Patients with V_5 higher than 74% had a 44.4% risk of acute esophagitis. In the study by Guliani et al. where two different radiotherapy schedules were used (40 Gy in 15 fractions or 45 Gy in 30 fractions, twice daily) the best predictor for grade >3 esophagitis were mean esophageal dose and dose to the hottest part of esophagus (D_{45}) [170].

Esophageal cancer: After implementation of new neoadjuvant chemoradiotherapy protocols, use of high doses that may cause acute or late toxicity in the mid and lower esophagus is limited, since the dose used is low (41.4 Gy). In the cervical esophagus surgery is associated with high morbidity and decreased quality of life and definitive chemoradiotherapy is the best alternative. However, high doses given to large portion of esophagus and unavoidably to its whole circumference lead to acute and late toxicity. In the studies by Kim et al. and Atsumi et al. rather than dosimetric parameters, extent of circumferential involvement (in both studies complete involvement) and tumor regression, T stage, wall thickness of the tumor region in the later study were associated with stenosis [171, 172].

Palliative radiotherapy: As mentioned early, risk of esophagitis after palliative treatments is unacceptably high, as noticed in a large review by Stevens et al., with as much as 56% of patients suffering from esophagitis [143]. In a multicenter trial, Cancer Trials Ireland (ICORG) 06–34, 3-D conformal radiotherapy with dose regimens of 39 Gy in 13 fractions, 20 Gy in 5 fractions or 17 Gy in 2 fractions is used for palliative purpose [173]. Although number of patients was small, an incidence of grade 2 acute toxicity of 14% was recorded, mean D_{max} and mean D_{mean} for 5 fraction and 13 fraction schedules were 18.3 Gy, 12.9 Gy and 38.2 Gy, 23.3 Gy, respectively. Esophagus sparing IMRT is a proposed method to decrease esophagus toxicity from 13% to 2% by limiting the maximum dose to esophagus to 24 Gy (80% of the prescribed dose of 30 Gy in 10 fractions) [174]. This data led to the randomized phase III study of palliative radiation of advanced central lung tumors with intentional avoidance of the esophagus (PROACTIVE) with the goal of assessing the clinical benefit of ES-IMRT in 30 Gy in 10 fractions and 20 Gy in 5 fractions.

Normal esophageal tissue dose constraints for conventional fractionated radiotherapy are summarized in Table 4.11.

4.4.4.2 The Literature Review of SABR for Esophageal Toxicity

Stereotactic treatments to the mediastinum have resulted in esophageal toxicity as well. The Grimm et al. study [44] provides us with a basal review of constraints from RTOG and other studies. With increased experience and knowledge on

Table 4.11 Normal esophageal tissue dose constraints for Conventional Fractionated Radiotherapy

Structure	Dose/fraction	Dose	Volume
Esophagus whole	1.8 Gy	34 Gy	Mean
Esophagus whole	1.8 Gy	60 Gy	10 cm
Esophagus, cervical	2 Gy	30 Gy	Mean
Esophagus (irradiated part)	3 Gy	23.3 Gy	Mean
Esophagus (palliative 10 frx)	3 Gy	24 Gy	Max
Esophagus (irradiated part)	4 Gy	18.3 Gy	Mean
Esophagus	4 Gy	12.9 Gy	Max
Esophagus	1.8–2 Gy	60 Gy	17%

stereotactic treatments more conservative constraints were reviewed [175]. According to the later study, D_{1cc} at a dose of 32.9 Gy and D_{max} dose of 43.4 Gy led to a complication probability of 50% for grade 2 toxicity, where analysis was performed in terms of 5 fraction equivalent dosing. One of the latest studies by Yao et al. argues that constraints to esophagus might be too conservative since in their large cohort of patients only 1 patient out of 632 experienced grade 3 esophagitis and 21 patients had grade 2 or less toxicity. Of notice is the use of 60 Gy in 8 fractions for central lesions and alternate day schedule. They found that a 15% risk of esophageal toxicity was associated with EQD_2 of D_{max} 141.6 Gy, D_{1cc} 123.61, and D_{2cc} 117.6 Gy which correspond to 48, 44, and 42.8 Gy for 4 fraction and 64, 59, and 57.6 Gy for 8 fraction treatment [176]. In another study with a large cohort of patients, no grade 3–5 esophageal toxicity was observed and a D_{max} of 56 Gy EQD^{10}_2 and a D_{5cc} of 35.5 Gy EQD_2 could be delivered with 17% risk of grade 2 esophagitis. Grade 1–2 esophagitis was significantly associated with D_{5cc} and female gender [177].

In the study by Wu et al. D_{5cc} to the esophagus should be kept less than 16.8, 18.1, and 19.0 Gy for 3, 4, and 5 fractions, respectively, to keep the acute toxicity rate <20%, which corresponds to $D_{5cc} \leq 26.3$ BED_{10} [178].

Late toxicity in the form of fistula was related to D_{max} higher than 51 Gy and D_{1cc} greater than 48 Gy and correlated with use of anti VEGF agents [179].

Normal esophageal tissue dose constraints for SABR are summarized in Table 4.12.

4.4.5 Treatment

4.4.5.1 Prevention

Amifostine: One of the most studied substance used for prevention of radiation side effects is indisputably amifostine. Studies to prevent esophagitis after radiotherapy for SCLC and NSCLC include three phase 2 and five phase 3 trials [59, 180–186]. Beside three studies [59, 183, 185], all others reported no difference in esophagitis between patients given amifostine and the others. The largest and latest study by Movsas et al., the RTOG 98-01 study, included 243 NSCLC patients receiving

Table 4.12 Normal esophageal tissue dose constraints for SABR

	Constraint	1 frx	3 frx	4 frx-	5 frx	6 frx	8 frx	EQD2 ($\alpha/\beta = 10$)
Esophagus	Max	14 Gy	20 Gy	20.8 Gy	29 Gy		64 Gy	56 Gy
Esophagus	0.5 cc					30 Gy		
Esophagus	1 cc				25 Gy		59 Gy	
Esophagus	2 cc						57.6 Gy	
Esophagus	5 cc	11.9 Gy	16.8 Gy	18.1 Gy	19 Gy			35.5 Gy
Esophagus	10 cc		16.2 Gy		19.5 Gy			

induction chemotherapy followed by concurrent hyperfractionated radiotherapy (69.6 Gy at 1.2 Gy twice daily) and chemotherapy with or without amifostine. Beside not being able to reduce grade 3 esophagitis amifostine was associated with significantly higher rates of nausea, vomiting, cardiovascular toxicity and infection or febrile neutropenia [182]. Another analysis of a smaller number of patients from the same study suggested that amifostine might be able to decrease pain and weight loss [187]. In spite of some benefits from amifostine, its use in prevention of esophagitis in NSCLC chemoradiotherapy setting is not justified, and one guideline recommended against its use [188].

Manuka honey: According to one study, Manuka honey does not prevent esophagitis in lung cancer treated with CRT; however, it may decrease use of opioids at 4th week [189].

Glutamine: The role of glutamine in prevention of stomatitis and esophagitis in head and neck and thoracis malignancies were reviewed [190]. Ten grams given 3 times a day reduced esophagitis or depletion of lymphocytes in NSCLC or esophageal cancer patients on chemoradiotherapy in five randomized controlled trials [191–195].

Soy flavonoids: Soy isoflavones are known to act as radiosensitizers and radioprotectants in many cancer models in preclinical studies [196]. In an animal study by Fountain et al., tissue damage induced by radiation both at 10 and 25 Gy given in single fraction was reduced [197].

4.4.5.2 Treatment/Prevention Recommendations

1. Avoid irritant food and consider behavioral changes (stop cigarette use, avoid alcohol, coffee, acidic and spicy food) [144, 198–200]:
2. Consider dietician referral, encourage use of small, frequent meals, soft diet
3. Start glutamine 30 g per day
4. Consider antacid to decrease acid reflux and PPI at first symptoms of esophagitis.
5. Nystatin solutions may be considered as prophylaxis. Oral antifungals may be required for refractory cases
6. After establishment of esophagitis support nutrition with oral supplements, i.v. hydration
7. Combination of antacid (sucralfate may be prioritized in patients with no nausea and vomiting) with topical analgesics (viscous lidocaine)
8. Opioid analgesics (tramadol, phentanyl, liquid morphine)
9. For prolonged symptoms enteral tube feeding or total parenteral nutrition may be required

4.4.6 Rx: Prescription Samples

- Asymptomatic:
  Glutamine 3 × 10 g
  Antacid 2 times per day
  Consider nystatin

- Mildly symptomatic:
  Glutamine 3 × 10 g
  PPI once daily (e.g., Lansoprazole 30 mg)
  Mixtures containing nystatin and equal parts of viscous xylocaine 2%, aluminum hydroxide-magnesium carbonate, and diphenhydramine
- Moderately symptomatic, >5% weight loss:
  Glutamine 3 × 10 g
  PPI once daily (e.g., Lansoprazol 30 mg)
  Mixtures containing nystatin and equal parts of viscous xylocaine 2%, aluminum hydroxide-magnesium carbonate, and diphenhydramine
  Three times 10 drops of oral tramadol
  Phentanyl patches starting with lowest dose (12 µg/h)
  Oral enteral nutrition support
- Severely symptomatic, no oral intake:
  Phentanyl patches
  Gastrostomy or TPN
- Stricture:
  Refer to gastroenterologist for dilation to achieve 13 mm opening
  Continue PPI
  If several attempted dilatations are unsuccessful consider gastrostomy
- Perforation/fistula/necrosis:
  Refer to surgery

4.5 Major Vessels

4.5.1 Anatomy

Circulatory system is composed of the heart and vessels. Due to their position, size, structure, and function, some of these vessels require special consideration. The great vessels are arteries and veins that transport blood from or to the heart, namely, aorta, pulmonary artery (PA), pulmonary veins (PV), inferior vena cava (IVC), and superior vena cava (SVC).

Aorta: It originates from the left ventricle, between which lays the aortic semi-lunar valve. According to its position, aorta is named as thoracic (from origin until it passes the diaphragm at T12 vertebral level) and abdominal (from T12 to L4 vertebral level where it bifurcates into right and left common iliac artery). The thoracic aorta can be divided into ascending, aortic arch and descending aorta. The ascending aorta is the first part, from which right and left coronary artery originates and extends until the level of T4 vertebra. Then, it arches posteriorly and to the left to from the aortic arch from which brachiocephalic artery, left common carotid, and subclavian artery originate. Thereafter it is considered as descending aorta, which gives off superior phrenic arteries, posterior intercostal arteries, subcostal arteries, and arteries to supply the pericardium, bronchi, mediastinum, and esophagus.

Structurally, from inside out it is composed of three layers; Tunica intima: The innermost layer of simple squamous epithelium, Tunica media: The middle layer of connective tissue made up of elastin and smooth muscles, Tunica adventitia: The outermost layer of thick collagenous tissue. Additionally, different from other arteries, it contains smooth muscle, collagen, and elastin within both the tunica media and tunica adventitia, making it the thickest artery in the body. This robust structure needs a good blood supply, since simple diffusion could not be sufficient. Blood vessels that supply aorta form two networks, the vasa vasorum interna supplied by the lumen and externa found in the tunica adventitia. Veins, known as venous vasa vasorae are mostly found in the tunica adventitia. It is innervated by sympathetic and parasympathetic fibers which cause vasoconstriction and dilatation, respectively [201, 202].

Pulmonary artery: It originates from the right ventricle and divides into right (RPA) and left pulmonary artery (LPA). It has a diameter of 2–3 cm and approximately 5 cm long, lies to the left of ascending aorta and its bifurcation is at the level of carina at T4 where RPA and LPA divide at a right angle. RPA courses between ascending and descending aorta, anterior to right main bronchus, LPA lies anterior to descending aorta and superior to left main bronchus. Its structure, vascular supply is similar to aorta, but without smooth muscle in the tunica adventitia [203].

Superior vena cava: It drains venous blood from the thorax, upper extremities, head, and neck region. Two brachiocephalic veins (left and right) join to form SVC at the posterior and inferior level of the first right costal cartilage. Azigos is another vein that drains to the 7 cm long SVA before it enters the right atrium at the third right costal cartilage level. Similar to IVC, but different from other veins, it has no valves. Structurally it is similar to great arteries, but with much less muscular tissue [204].

Inferior vena cava: It drains blood from the abdomen and lower extremities, it has a very small intrathoracic part and most of it lies in the retroperitoneal area. For this reason, it is not usually considered as an organ at risk during thoracic radiotherapy.

Pulmonary veins: PV are the only veins in the body that carry more oxygenated blood than their counterpart arteries, the PA. There are two PV carrying blood from each lung, to a total of four [205]. To our knowledge IVC and PV injury has not been recognized from thoracic irradiation.

4.5.2 Contouring

There is not much consensus even in RTOG studies on how and which great vessels to include in contouring. According to a study protocol where conventional fractionation is used, the RTOG 1106, all great vessels should be contoured, while on a SABR related study protocol, the RTOG 0813, only aorta and vena cava should be included. Considering that only few cases in literature report of RT induced injury to the vena cava and more reports could be found in relation to PA toxicity we suggest that PA contouring should be added in SABR planning too [206–209]. According to RTOG 1106, vessels should be contoured in mediastinal windowing.

It should include the vascular wall and all muscular layers out to the fatty adventitia (5 mm from the contrast enhanced vascular wall). For right sided tumors, SVC will be contoured, and for left sided tumors, the aorta will be contoured. The ipsilateral PA will be delineated for tumor of either side. The great vessel should be contoured starting at least 3 cm above the superior extent of the PTV and continuing on every CT slice to at least 3 cm below the inferior extent of the PTV. On the other hand, according to RTOG 0813 study protocol the great vessel should be contoured starting 10 cm above the superior extent of the PTV and continuing to 10 cm below the inferior extent of the PTV. Additionally, the nonadjacent wall corresponding to the half circumference of the tubular structure not immediately touching the GTV or PTV should be contoured in SABR. Given the literature above, contouring of great vessels are shown in Figs. 4.7 and 4.8.

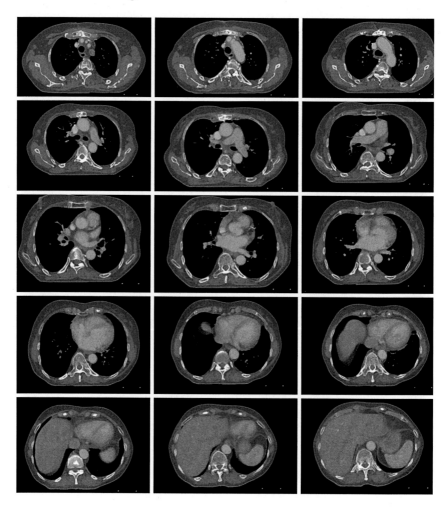

Fig. 4.7 Delineation of Aorta (green)

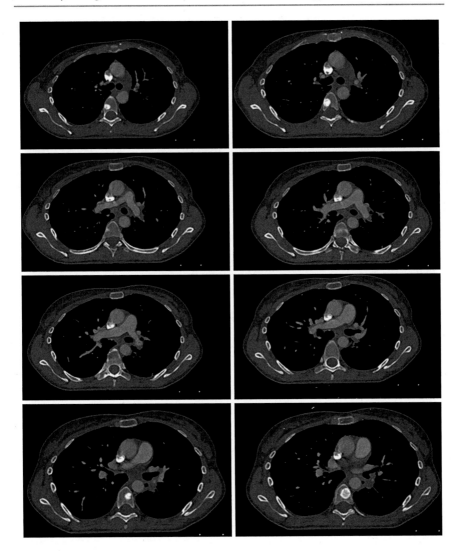

Fig. 4.8 Delineation of Pulmonary Artery (pink)

4.5.3   Pathophysiology

Radiation injury in normal tissues is studied thoroughly and summarized in many reviews. Beside small differences, mechanism of radiation induced injury is generally explained as combination of progenitor cell loss, oxidative stress, vascular endothelial dysfunction, increased and uncontrolled inflammation ultimately leading to fibrosis [210]. Vessels, especially the arteries, have a structure very similar to heart; highly perfused organ, made mostly of muscular tissue and endothelium. The

Table 4.13 Grading of great vessel toxicity according to CTCAE version 5

	Grade 1[a]	Grade 2	Grade 3	Grade 4	Grade 5
CTCAE v5.0 Vascular injury	Asymptomatic diagnostic finding; intervention not indicated	Symptomatic; repair or revision not indicated	Severe symptoms; limiting self-care ADL; repair or revision indicated	Life-threatening consequences; evidence of end organ damage; urgent operative intervention indicated	Death

[a]There is no grade 1 grading for Aortic injury

mechanism used to explain injury to the heart might be suitable for arterial injury and venous injury as well. Grading of great vessel toxicity according to CTCAE version 5 is shown in Table 4.13.

4.5.4 Dose Constraints

4.5.4.1 The Literature Review of Conventional Fractionated Radiotherapy for Great Vessel Toxicity

Lung Cancer

Few early reports regarding injury to great arteries could be found in the pre SABR era [207, 208]. Due to lower doses and poor survival of patients no dose toxicity relation could be drawn. In later studies the effect of conventional fractionation on vessels could be noticed. In one study where late toxicity of patients recruited in prospective high dose chemoradiation trials were investigated it was noticed that most of grade 5 toxicities were due to causes unrelated to vascular toxicity, with one hemoptysis due to bronchial injury [211]. In a single arm phase two study where mid-treatment PET-CT is performed in order to escalate radiation dose accordingly, it was noticed that out of 42 patients, four had fatal hemoptysis due to known causes; however, all of them had T4 tumors invading PA [79]. This explanation, though plausible, cannot be definitive, since according to another study where patients with great vessel invasion (mostly PA) were retrospectively investigated for toxicity showed that fatal hemoptysis does not correlate with invasion to vessels [212]. In the study two of the 37 patients studied showed hemoptysis unrelated to their invasion. In the studies by Han et al. 2014 and Ma et al. 2017, 100 and 141 patients were retrospectively investigated and invasion grade to PA and $V_{40}-V_{60}$ correlated with overall survival [213, 214]. In the later study PA V40 > 80%, V45 > 68%, V50 > 45%, and V55 > 32% were independent predictors for OS and OS according to PA invasion was; Gr 0-41.8 months, Gr1 27.8 months, Gr2 12.7 months, and Gr3 7.5 month. Grading of invasion according to these studies were: Grade 0 (no invasion); No evidence of vessel invasion, ≥1 mm from the closest pulmonary vessel wall (presence of a fat plane between tumor and vessel wall), grade 1 (minimal invasion); Tumor invasion with 0 mm to the closest pulmonary vessel wall, no fat plane, without presence of narrowing or truncation of vessels, nor signs of vessel wall damage (irregularity, discontinuity, or intra-luminal mass formation), grade 2 (moderate invasion); Circumferential involvement with narrowing or truncation, grade 3 (extensive invasion); Tumor invading pulmonary vessel extensively with any sign of vessel wall damage: irregularity, discontinuity or intra-luminal mass formation or massive hemorrhage due to the tumor invading pulmonary artery.

Reirradiation: Reirradiation of centrally located tumors, even if not treated with SABR, is not without consequences. In retrospective studies it is noticed that aorta can withstand composite doses as high as 120 Gy, and most of patients who exceed this dose might be free of toxicity but due to irreversible fatal damage most authors advice keeping aortic doses less than 120 Gy, since higher doses might result in 25% risk of severe aortic toxicity [215–217].

4.5.4.2 The Literature Review of Sterotactic Ablative Radiotherapy (SABR) for Great Vessel Toxicity

SABR

In 2006 Timmerman et al. published the high impact study that determined the central location as a main factor for fatal toxicity in SABR [218]. In the following decade more data emerged regarding the effect of central location, i.e., high dose to tracheobronchial tree. Most of these studies are elegantly reviewed by Bang and Bezjak in 2019 [219]. In the prospective and retrospective studies reviewed hemoptysis appears to be one of the most common cause of grade 5 toxicity. Endobronchial lesions (ultracentral), anti-VEGF use, and iatrogenic manipulation of irradiated bronchus were found to be the most important risk factors, in addition to dose per fraction. Major airways rather than vascular toxicity were the cause of toxicity. In the study by Nishimura et al. 2014, 398 OAR/133 patients with centrally located lesions treated with SABR in five fractions to doses up to 60 Gy were analyzed [206]. They did not find any toxicity related to aorta, vena cava, or PV; however, 2 patients with grade 5 hemoptysis received high doses to the PA and bronchus ((59.2 and 54.4 Gy, and 61.3 and 59.6 Gy, respectively).

In 2016 Xue et al. made a validation of SABR constraints for aorta and great vessels [220]. They concluded that constraints used in clinical trials would result in low risk of aortic or great vessel injury, even in 3 fraction schemes the risk would be less than 3%.

In the largest prospective trial regarding 5 fraction SABR to centrally located NSCLC lesions, the RTOG 0813 trial published in 2019, a total of 6 patients had grade 5 toxicity, mostly bronchopulmonary hemorrhage, no toxicity related to great vessels was noticed [221].

Summary of dose constraints used is shown in Table 4.14.

4.5.5   Treatment

Major vessel injury should be considered in cases of patients previously irradiated to high doses to the chest who present with hemodynamic instability or hemoptysis. It is an emergency that should be promptly investigated.

Table 4.14 Great vessels dose constraints for Conventional Fractionated Radiotherapy and SABR

	Constraint	1 frx - 3 frx - 4 frx	5 frx	8 frx	10 frx	Conventional fractionation
Great vessels, nonadjacent wall	D_{max}	Not recommended in central lesions	105% of PTV		75 Gy	120 Gy
Great vessels, nonadjacent wall	1 cc				50 Gy	
Great vessels, nonadjacent wall	10 cc		47 Gy	47 y		

4.6 Major Airways

4.6.1 Anatomy

Airways are part of respiratory system that allows passage of air during ventilation. The upper airway is found in the head and neck region and is not included in the major airways of the thoracic region. The lower airway is composed of trachea, main bronchi (right and left), lobar bronchi (3 on the right and 2 on the left), segmental bronchi, conducting bronchioles, terminal bronchioles, respiratory bronchioles, and alveoli. Even though segmental bronchi to alveoli are part of respiratory tract, they are described as the lung parenchyma. That leaves trachea, main bronchi, and lobar bronchi as major airway components [222]. Trachea and bronchi form the tracheobronchial tree. Structurally they are composed of cartilage to prevent collapse due to pressure change during respiration, smooth muscles and mucosal lining; the ciliated pseudostratified columnar epithelium. Bronchial arteries (BA) supply oxygenated blood to the airway; the left BA arises from aorta and right may arise from superior posterior intercostal arteries or a common trunk with the left superior bronchial artery.

4.6.2 Contouring

Major airways have been afflicted with radiotherapy induced injury after both conventional fractionation and SABR; however, it is the later technique that has caused much more damage and needs special attention. Even though contouring of airways is important in both cases, it is from the SABR trials that we have the most accurate description of airway delineation. In the latest of RTOG studies related to central SABR, the RTOG 0813 trial, it is required that [221]:

- The trachea and proximal bronchial tree will be contoured as two separate structures using mediastinal windows on CT to correspond to the mucosal, submucosa and cartilage rings and airway channels associated with these structures.

- Trachea will be divided into two sections: the proximal trachea and the distal 2 cm of trachea.
- Proximal Trachea: Contouring of the proximal trachea should begin at least 10 cm superior to the extent of the PTV or 5 cm superior to the carina (whichever is more superior) and continue inferiorly to the superior aspect of the proximal bronchial tree.
- Proximal Bronchial Tree: The proximal bronchial tree will include the most inferior 2 cm of distal trachea and the proximal airways on both sides.
- The following airways will be included according to standard anatomic relationships: the distal 2 cm of trachea, the carina, the right and left mainstem bronchi, the right and left upper lobe bronchi, the intermedius bronchus, the right middle lobe bronchus, the lingular bronchus, and the right and left lower lobe bronchi.
- Contouring of the lobar bronchi will end immediately at the site of a segmental bifurcation.
- If there are parts of the proximal bronchial tree that are within GTV, they should be contoured separately, as "proximal bronchial tree GTV," not as part of the "proximal bronchial tree."

The contouring, the trachea, and proximal bronchial tree in the light of these description are shown in Figs. 4.9 and 4.10.

4.6.3 Pathophysiology

Pathophysiology of radiation induced normal-tissue inflammation, endothelial damage, necrosis, and fibrosis has been explained in detail in other chapters.

The result of fibrosis and necrosis in trachea and bronchi is hemoptysis, strictures, fistulas, perforation, and increased risk of infection. Grading according to common terminology criteria for adverse events (CTCAE) version 5 is shown in Table 4.15.

4.6.4 Dose Constraints

4.6.4.1 The Literature Review of Endobronchial Brachytherapy for Major Airways

We will not go into an in-depth literature review but as a possible option for treatment in extreme cases this type of increasingly abandoned modality is worth mentioning.

In one large retrospective study where 189 patients were given brachytherapy weekly in 3 to 4, 8 to 10 Gy fractions at a radius of 10 mm from the center of the source, the rate of >3 grade toxicity such as massive hemoptysis ($n = 13$), bronchial stenosis ($n = 12$), soft tissue necrosis ($n = 8$), and bronchial fistula ($n = 3$) occurred at a rate of 17% [223].

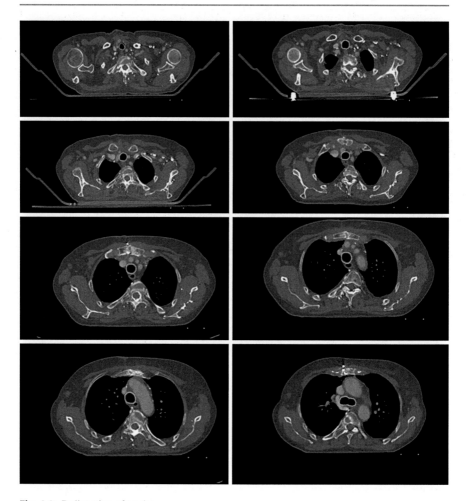

Fig. 4.9 Delineation of trachea

In order to decrease this high rate of toxicity newer techniques are being investigated and in a later study by Nomoto et al. in 2017 no chronic bronchitis or hemoptysis was noticed after a median follow-up of 36 months [224]. They treated 15 patients with combined external RT of 40 Gy in 20 fraction and brachytherapy of 18 Gy in 3 fractions with curative intent. They had excellent local control (100%) and 79% 3-year overall survival. They used a source centralizing applicator that held the source in the middle of the bronchus and prescribed the dose according to bronchus diameter (5–7 mm).

Palliative endobronchial brachytherapy was analyzed in a systematic review and it was concluded that external RT alone is superior to brachytherapy alone and there is no data in support of their combination; however, brachytherapy may be considered in selective cases when symptomatic patients present after previous external RT [225].

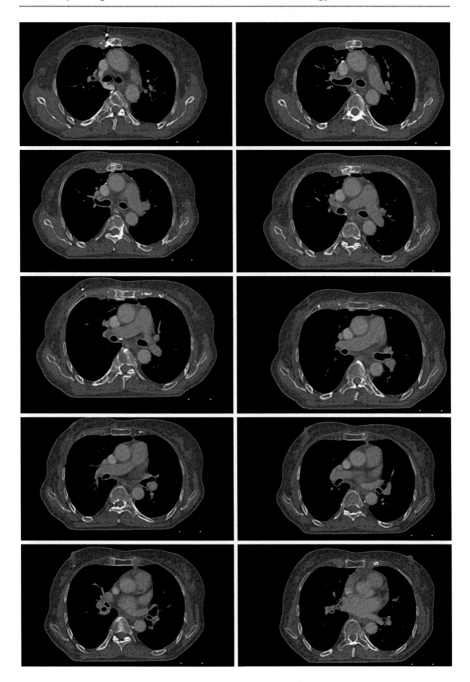

Fig. 4.10 Delineation of proximal bronchial tree

Table 4.15 Grading according to common terminology criteria for adverse events (CTCAE) version 5

	Grade 1	Grade 2	Grade 3	Grade 4	Grade 5
CTCAE v5.0 Bronchial stricture	Asymptomatic diagnostic finding; intervention not indicated	Symptomatic (e.g., rhonchi or wheezing) but without respiratory distress; medical intervention indicated (e.g., steroids, bronchodilators)	Shortness of breath with stridor; endoscopic intervention indicated (e.g., laser, stent placement)	Life-threatening respiratory or hemodynamic compromise; intubation or urgent intervention indicated	Death
Bronchial fistula	Asymptomatic	Symptomatic invasive intervention not indicated	intervention indicated; hospitalization	Life-threatening consequences; urgent intervention indicated	Death
Broncho-pulmonary hemorrhage	Mild symptoms, intervention not indicated	Moderate symptoms, invasive intervention not indicated	Transfusion indicated; invasive intervention indicated; hospitalization	Life-threatening consequences; intubation or urgent intervention indicated	Death

4.6.4.2 The Literature Review of Conventional fractionation for Major Airways

Poor survival in lung and esophageal cancer and use of lower doses have made toxicity to the airways to go unnoticed for a long time.

In 1995 Mehta and Dweik reported of 4 cases of bronchial necrosis resulting in fatal hemoptysis or pneumonia after 50–64 Gy for squamous cell carcinoma [226]. After use of dose escalation in lung cancer trials reporting of toxicity started to increase and more cases and studies emerged. In the study by Miller et al. the risk of bronchial stenosis was 4% after 74 Gy and 25% after 86 Gy [227]. In a similar study, radiation induced narrowing was found to increase with increased dose and use of chemotherapy, time elapsed and be more pronounced in bronchi than in trachea in patients treated with >73.6 Gy [228]. In a pooled analysis of 88 patients who were given >66 Gy doses for NSCLC in prospective trials late toxicity was investigated [211]. Among the 28 late complications occurring in 21 (24%) of patients, fatal hemoptysis (2 patients) and bronchial stenosis (3 patients) could be considered as airway toxicity. Late toxicity occurred in patients receiving from 66 Gy to 90 Gy; however, more patients who received 82, 86, and 90 Gy dose levels were in the toxicity group.

4.6.4.3 The Literature Review of SABR for Major Airways

As mentioned in the "Lung" section, lesions are described according to their position in relation to airways, central; if within 2 cm of tracheobronchial tree or peripheral. Definition of central has evolved and proximity to other mediastinal structures is defined as central in the International Association for the Study of Lung Cancer (IASLC) prescription [2]. Whatever the definition, studies reporting toxicities related to central position mostly describe airway related side effects such hemorrhage, pneumonitis, bronchial stenosis among the most common grade 3–5 adverse effects [229–232]. After recognition of central location as one important toxicity predisposing factor in SABR by Timmerman et al. in 2006 many other prospective and retrospective studies have found similar results [218, 221, 233–238].

Collectively, these studies showed that grade >3 toxicity is higher for patients with central lesions as compared to peripheral and 3 fraction regimen is more toxic than more fractionated regimens.

In order to achieve a good local control and increased survival, BED10 should be higher than 100 Gy. While peripheral lesions could be successfully treated with high ablative dose without significant side effect, a more protracted treatment protocol is needed for lesions near the central airway. Many groups tried different schedules and 70 Gy in 10 fractions, 60 Gy in 8 fractions, 50–60 Gy in 5 fractions, 50 Gy in 4 fractions have all been used and achieved similar local control to peripheral lesions [229, 231, 237, 239].

Taking in account these and many other published trials, in 2017 an evidence-based ASTRO guideline for SABR to early- stage non-small cell lung cancer concluded that [240]:

- The use of 3-fraction regimens should be avoided in centrally located early stage lung tumors.
- SABR directed at central lung tumors should be delivered in 4 or 5 fractions.
- For central tumors for which SABR is deemed too high risk, hypofractionated radiation therapy utilizing 6 to 15 fractions can be considered.

In the guideline, beside other factors regarded as high risk, proximity or involvement of mediastinal structures and chest wall was mentioned. The most important is proximity or involvement of bronchial tree, sometimes referred to as "ultracentral." Similar to the definition of central location, ultracentral notification is also arbitrary and vary between studies, it can be either GTV or PTV intersecting with bronchial tree. In most studies, toxicity of SABR to ultracentral lesions surpasses that of general central lesions, with grade >3 toxicity as high as 38%, when compared to roughly10–20% in general central lesions [241–244]. In an early report of Nordic HILUS-Trial it was noticed that main bronchi position is more prone to high toxicity as compared to lobar bronchi [245]. Of note is the fact that this increase in toxicity in ultracentral SABR occurs despite the use of 5–8 fraction regimens. In order to identify the least toxic regimen for ultracentral lesions the results of the SUNSET trial is awaited [246]. Beside defining the best dose for lesions overlapping with bronchial tree the study will investigate also lesions whose PTV is overlapping with pulmonary artery, veins, and esophagus.

The latest prospective trial regarding SABR to central lesions recently reported its results [221]. In the study central lesions were treated in 5 fractions of 10, 10.5, 11, 11.5 or 12 Gy delivered in 1.5–2 weeks. The maximum tolerated dose was found to be 12 Gy/fraction and grade >3 toxicity in the first year was 7.2% for this group.

Table 4.16 Major Airways dose constraints for toxicity

	Constraint	1 frx - 3 frx	4 frx	5 frx	8 frx	10 frx	Conventional fractionation
Trachea and ipsilateral bronchus, nonadjacent wall	D_{max}	Not recommended in central lesions	15.6 Gy	105% of PTV			74 Gy
Trachea and ipsilateral bronchus, nonadjacent wall	4 cc	Not recommended in central lesions		18 Gy	18 Gy		
Central airways	0.5 cc	Not recommended in central lesions		21 Gy			
Central airways	1 cc	Not recommended in central lesions	35 Gy			50 Gy	

After a median follow-up of 37.9 months, 2-year local control in the remaining 71 patients in the 11.5 and 12 Gy/fraction groups was 89.4% and 87.9%, overall survival was 67.9% and 72.7%, respectively, which was commented to be similar to that achieved in peripheral lesions. In the study, dose limiting toxicity was defined as '*any treatment-related grade 3 or worse predefined toxicity that occurred within the first year*'. Only 4 patients (12.1%) given 11.5 and 12 Gy/fraction had grade >3 toxicity in the first year and no patient showed predefined grade 5 toxicity. However, beyond the first year, 4 patients in the 11.5 Gy/frx and 12 Gy/frx groups had grade 5 toxicity; 3 hemorrhages and one "non otherwise identified death". Dose constraints used in the protocol are shown in Table 4.16.

4.6.5 Treatment

There is no known mitigating, preventive measures to decrease major airway toxicity, beside modulation of dose and fractionation, respecting dose constraints, and recognizing risk factors that lead to toxicity.

High dose per fraction, total circumferential irradiation and total dose, invasion of bronchi, use of VEGF inhibitors (Bevacizumab), squamous cell histology, presence of cavities in the lesion are known factors for hemorrhages in conventional fractionation RT or SABR [247–250]. Additionally, instrumentation, invasive procedures in the irradiated bronchus may result in high grade 5 toxicity [231].

To our knowledge there is no guideline that suggest active surveillance of RT induced toxicity in high-risk patients. Patients should be followed and informed about high risks of RT and they should recognize and promptly seek medical attention when they occur. Hemoptysis, increasing difficulty in breathing, coughing, wheezing, frequent infections should not be left without investigation. After the patient is suspected of having RT related toxicity referral to a specialized pneumology and thoracic surgeon should be made. Once toxicity occurs it is managed according to its severity. Preferably discussion in a multidisciplinary meeting could be of use. However, most of symptomatic patients require surgical intervention, some of them urgent.

Surgical Treatment
In a study by Dickoff et al., where 15 patients were operated due to different types of toxicity after 66 Gy RT, they reported of a 90-day 27% mortality rate and 19 month median survival [251]. They concluded that operating in post radiotherapy setting is technically challenging and should be done in specialized experienced tertiary centers, since rate of complications and mortality is high.

Non-surgical Treatments

- Stenting: In a review of stent placement in stenotic bronchi due to malignant or benign reasons, complications rate as high as 34% was noticed [252].
- Balloon dilation: In a small retrospective series of 10 patients, 6 (60%) achieved full recovery without any other treatment, 2 had repeated balloon dilation and others had stent or cutting balloon dilation [253].

Hemoptysis: Abundant hemoptysis is an emergency in a cancer patient, even without history of irradiation since it carries a mortality rate of 80% [254]. Airway must be kept open since death results from asphyxiation as well as exsanguination. A detailed algorithm of treatment of hemoptysis is given by Khalil et al. [255]. Hospitalization, preferably in the intensity care unit, consultation with pulmonologist and thoracic surgeon, keeping the airway opened, replacing of fluid loss and immediate measures to identify the bleeding site with multidetector CT angiography and bronchoscopy should be made. Arterial embolization, as the first line therapy, and surgical intervention (when embolization fails or is not feasible) are the possible life saving treatments [256].

References

1. Chaudhry R, Bordoni B. Anatomy, thorax, lungs. Treasure Island (FL): StatPearls; 2019.
2. Chang JY, Bezjak A, Mornex F, Committee IART. Stereotactic ablative radiotherapy for centrally located early stage non-small-cell lung cancer: what we have learned. J Thorac Oncol. 2015;10(4):577–85.
3. Kong FM, Ritter T, Quint DJ, Senan S, Gaspar LE, Komaki RU, et al. Consideration of dose limits for organs at risk of thoracic radiotherapy: atlas for lung, proximal bronchial tree, esophagus, spinal cord, ribs, and brachial plexus. Int J Radiat Oncol Biol Phys. 2011;81(5):1442–57.
4. Uchida Y, Tsugawa T, Tanaka-Mizuno S, Noma K, Aoki K, Shigemori W, et al. Exclusion of emphysematous lung from dose-volume estimates of risk improves prediction of radiation pneumonitis. Radiat Oncol. 2017;12(1):160.

5. Wang W, Xu Y, Schipper M, Matuszak MM, Ritter T, Cao Y, et al. Effect of normal lung definition on lung dosimetry and lung toxicity prediction in radiation therapy treatment planning. Int J Radiat Oncol Biol Phys. 2013;86(5):956–63.
6. Meng Y, Yang H, Wang W, Tang X, Jiang C, Shen Y, et al. Excluding PTV from lung volume may better predict radiation pneumonitis for intensity modulated radiation therapy in lung cancer patients. Radiat Oncol. 2019;14(1):7.
7. Evans WALT. Intrathoracic changes induced by heavy radiation. Am J Roentgenol. 1925;13:203–20.
8. Graves PR, Siddiqui F, Anscher MS, Movsas B. Radiation pulmonary toxicity: from mechanisms to management. Semin Radiat Oncol. 2010;20(3):201–7.
9. Choi YW, Munden RF, Erasmus JJ, Park KJ, Chung WK, Jeon SC, et al. Effects of radiation therapy on the lung: radiologic appearances and differential diagnosis. Radiographics. 2004;24(4):985–97; discussion 98
10. Hanania AN, Mainwaring W, Ghebre YT, Hanania NA, Ludwig M. Radiation-induced lung injury: assessment and management. Chest. 2019;156(1):150–62.
11. Tsoutsou PG, Koukourakis MI. Radiation pneumonitis and fibrosis: mechanisms underlying its pathogenesis and implications for future research. Int J Radiat Oncol Biol Phys. 2006;66(5):1281–93.
12. Huang Y, Zhang W, Yu F, Gao F. The cellular and molecular mechanism of radiation-induced lung injury. Med Sci Monit. 2017;23:3446–50.
13. Palma DA, Senan S, Tsujino K, Barriger RB, Rengan R, Moreno M, et al. Predicting radiation pneumonitis after chemoradiation therapy for lung cancer: an international individual patient data meta-analysis. Int J Radiat Oncol Biol Phys. 2013;85(2):444–50.
14. Onishi H, Yamashita H, Shioyama Y, Matsumoto Y, Takayama K, Matsuo Y, et al. Stereotactic body radiation therapy for patients with pulmonary interstitial change: high incidence of fatal radiation pneumonitis in a retrospective multi-institutional study. Cancers (Basel). 2018;10(8)
15. Chen H, Senan S, Nossent EJ, Boldt RG, Warner A, Palma DA, et al. Treatment-related toxicity in patients with early-stage non-small cell lung cancer and coexisting interstitial lung disease: a systematic review. Int J Radiat Oncol Biol Phys. 2017;98(3):622–31.
16. Yamaguchi S, Ohguri T, Matsuki Y, Yahara K, Oki H, Imada H, et al. Radiotherapy for thoracic tumors: association between subclinical interstitial lung disease and fatal radiation pneumonitis. Int J Clin Oncol. 2015;20(1):45–52.
17. Glick D, Lyen S, Kandel S, Shapera S, Le LW, Lindsay P, et al. Impact of pretreatment interstitial lung disease on radiation pneumonitis and survival in patients treated with lung stereotactic body radiation therapy (SBRT). Clin Lung Cancer. 2018;19(2):e219–e26.
18. Kreuter M, Ehlers-Tenenbaum S, Schaaf M, Oltmanns U, Palmowski K, Hoffmann H, et al. Treatment and outcome of lung cancer in idiopathic interstitial pneumonias. Sarcoidosis Vasc Diffuse Lung Dis. 2015;31(4):266–74.
19. Onishi H, Marino K, Yamashita H, Terahara A, Onimaru R, Kokubo M, et al. Case series of 23 patients who developed fatal radiation pneumonitis after stereotactic body radiotherapy for lung cancer. Technol Cancer Res Treat. 2018;17:1533033818801323.
20. Fujita J, Bandoh S, Ohtsuki Y, Dobashi N, Hiroi M, Takeuchi T, et al. The role of anti-epithelial cell antibodies in the pathogenesis of bilateral radiation pneumonitis caused by unilateral thoracic irradiation. Respir Med. 2000;94(9):875–80.
21. Pang Q, Wei Q, Xu T, Yuan X, Lopez Guerra JL, Levy LB, et al. Functional promoter variant rs2868371 of HSPB1 is associated with risk of radiation pneumonitis after chemoradiation for non-small cell lung cancer. Int J Radiat Oncol Biol Phys. 2013;85(5):1332–9.
22. Mehta V. Radiation pneumonitis and pulmonary fibrosis in non-small-cell lung cancer: pulmonary function, prediction, and prevention. Int J Radiat Oncol Biol Phys. 2005;63(1):5–24.
23. Tonison JJ, Fischer SG, Viehrig M, Welz S, Boeke S, Zwirner K, et al. Radiation pneumonitis after intensity-modulated radiotherapy for esophageal cancer: institutional data and a systematic review. Sci Rep. 2019;9(1):2255.

24. Zhang XJ, Sun JG, Sun J, Ming H, Wang XX, Wu L, et al. Prediction of radiation pneumonitis in lung cancer patients: a systematic review. J Cancer Res Clin Oncol. 2012;138(12):2103–16.
25. Rodrigues G, Lock M, D'Souza D, Yu E, Van Dyk J. Prediction of radiation pneumonitis by dose - volume histogram parameters in lung cancer--a systematic review. Radiother Oncol. 2004;71(2):127–38.
26. Bradley JD, Hope A, El Naqa I, Apte A, Lindsay PE, Bosch W, et al. A nomogram to predict radiation pneumonitis, derived from a combined analysis of RTOG 9311 and institutional data. Int J Radiat Oncol Biol Phys. 2007;69(4):985–92.
27. Marks LB, Bentzen SM, Deasy JO, Kong FM, Bradley JD, Vogelius IS, et al. Radiation dose-volume effects in the lung. Int J Radiat Oncol Biol Phys. 2010;76(3 Suppl):S70–6.
28. Wu K, Xu X, Li X, Wang J, Zhu L, Chen X, et al. Radiation pneumonitis in lung cancer treated with volumetric modulated arc therapy. J Thorac Dis. 2018;10(12):6531–9.
29. Miles EF, Larrier NA, Kelsey CR, Hubbs JL, Ma J, Yoo S, et al. Intensity-modulated radiotherapy for resected mesothelioma: the Duke experience. Int J Radiat Oncol Biol Phys. 2008;71(4):1143–50.
30. Blom-Goldman U, Svane G, Wennberg B, Lidestahl A, Lind PA. Quantitative assessment of lung density changes after 3-D radiotherapy for breast cancer. Acta Oncol. 2007;46(2):187–93.
31. Blom Goldman U, Wennberg B, Svane G, Bylund H, Lind P. Reduction of radiation pneumonitis by V20-constraints in breast cancer. Radiat Oncol. 2010;5:99.
32. Gokula K, Earnest A, Wong LC. Meta-analysis of incidence of early lung toxicity in 3-dimensional conformal irradiation of breast carcinomas. Radiat Oncol. 2013;8:268.
33. Lee TF, Chao PJ, Chang L, Ting HM, Huang YJ. Developing multivariable normal tissue complication probability model to predict the incidence of symptomatic radiation pneumonitis among breast cancer patients. PLoS One. 2015;10(7):e0131736.
34. Vogelius IR, Bentzen SM. A literature-based meta-analysis of clinical risk factors for development of radiation induced pneumonitis. Acta Oncol. 2012;51(8):975–83.
35. Zhou ZR, Han Q, Liang SX, He XD, Cao NY, Zi YJ. Dosimetric factors and Lyman normal-tissue complication modelling analysis for predicting radiation-induced lung injury in postoperative breast cancer radiotherapy: a prospective study. Oncotarget. 2017;8(20):33855–63.
36. Lind PA, Marks LB, Hardenbergh PH, Clough R, Fan M, Hollis D, et al. Technical factors associated with radiation pneumonitis after local +/− regional radiation therapy for breast cancer. Int J Radiat Oncol Biol Phys. 2002;52(1):137–43.
37. Lind PA, Wennberg B, Gagliardi G, Fornander T. Pulmonary complications following different radiotherapy techniques for breast cancer, and the association to irradiated lung volume and dose. Breast Cancer Res Treat. 2001;68(3):199–210.
38. Ho AY, Ballangrud A, Li G, Gupta GP, McCormick B, Gewanter R, et al. Long-term pulmonary outcomes of a feasibility study of inverse-planned, multibeam intensity modulated radiation therapy in node-positive breast cancer patients receiving regional nodal irradiation. Int J Radiat Oncol Biol Phys. 2019;103(5):1100–8.
39. Haviland JS, Owen JR, Dewar JA, Agrawal RK, Barrett J, Barrett-Lee PJ, et al. The UK standardisation of breast radiotherapy (START) trials of radiotherapy hypofractionation for treatment of early breast cancer: 10-year follow-up results of two randomised controlled trials. Lancet Oncol. 2013;14(11):1086–94.
40. Baumann P, Nyman J, Hoyer M, Wennberg B, Gagliardi G, Lax I, et al. Outcome in a prospective phase II trial of medically inoperable stage I non-small-cell lung cancer patients treated with stereotactic body radiotherapy. J Clin Oncol. 2009;27(20):3290–6.
41. Zheng X, Schipper M, Kidwell K, Lin J, Reddy R, Ren Y, et al. Survival outcome after stereotactic body radiation therapy and surgery for stage I non-small cell lung cancer: a meta-analysis. Int J Radiat Oncol Biol Phys. 2014;90(3):603–11.
42. Palma DA, Olson R, Harrow S, Gaede S, Louie AV, Haasbeek C, et al. Stereotactic ablative radiotherapy versus standard of care palliative treatment in patients with oligometastatic cancers (SABR-COMET): a randomised, phase 2, open-label trial. Lancet. 2019;393(10185):2051–8.

43. Zhao J, Yorke ED, Li L, Kavanagh BD, Li XA, Das S, et al. Simple factors associated with radiation-induced lung toxicity after stereotactic body radiation therapy of the thorax: a pooled analysis of 88 studies. Int J Radiat Oncol Biol Phys. 2016;95(5):1357–66.
44. Grimm J, LaCouture T, Croce R, Yeo I, Zhu Y, Xue J. Dose tolerance limits and dose volume histogram evaluation for stereotactic body radiotherapy. J Appl Clin Med Phys. 2011;12(2):3368.
45. Pollom EL, Chin AL, Diehn M, Loo BW, Chang DT. Normal tissue constraints for abdominal and thoracic stereotactic body radiotherapy. Semin Radiat Oncol. 2017;27(3):197–208.
46. Hanna GG, Murray L, Patel R, Jain S, Aitken KL, Franks KN, et al. UK consensus on normal tissue dose constraints for stereotactic radiotherapy. Clin Oncol (R Coll Radiol). 2018;30(1):5–14.
47. Chun SG, Hu C, Choy H, Komaki RU, Timmerman RD, Schild SE, et al. Impact of intensity-modulated radiation therapy technique for locally advanced non-small-cell lung cancer: a secondary analysis of the NRG oncology RTOG 0617 randomized clinical trial. J Clin Oncol. 2017;35(1):56–62.
48. Boda-Heggemann J, Knopf AC, Simeonova-Chergou A, Wertz H, Stieler F, Jahnke A, et al. Deep inspiration breath hold-based radiation therapy: a clinical review. Int J Radiat Oncol Biol Phys. 2016;94(3):478–92.
49. Cole AJ, Hanna GG, Jain S, O'Sullivan JM. Motion management for radical radiotherapy in non-small cell lung cancer. Clin Oncol (R Coll Radiol). 2014;26(2):67–80.
50. Sonke JJ, Belderbos J. Adaptive radiotherapy for lung cancer. Semin Radiat Oncol. 2010;20(2):94–106.
51. De Ruysscher D, Faivre-Finn C, Moeller D, Nestle U, Hurkmans CW, Le Pechoux C, et al. European organization for research and treatment of cancer (EORTC) recommendations for planning and delivery of high-dose, high precision radiotherapy for lung cancer. Radiother Oncol. 2017;124(1):1–10.
52. Kim H, Pyo H, Noh JM, Lee W, Park B, Park HY, et al. Preliminary result of definitive radiotherapy in patients with non-small cell lung cancer who have underlying idiopathic pulmonary fibrosis: comparison between X-ray and proton therapy. Radiat Oncol. 2019;14(1):19.
53. McGovern K, Ghaly M, Esposito M, Barnaby K, Seetharamu N. Radiation recall pneumonitis in the setting of immunotherapy and radiation: a focused review. Future Sci OA. 2019;5(5):FSO378.
54. Ding X, Ji W, Li J, Zhang X, Wang L. Radiation recall pneumonitis induced by chemotherapy after thoracic radiotherapy for lung cancer. Radiat Oncol. 2011;6:24.
55. Awad R, Nott L. Radiation recall pneumonitis induced by erlotinib after palliative thoracic radiotherapy for lung cancer: Case report and literature review. Asia Pac J Clin Oncol. 2016;12(1):91–5.
56. Sanchis-Borja M, Parrot A, Sroussi D, Rivin Del Campo E, Fallet V, Cadranel J. Dramatic radiation recall pneumonitis induced by osimertinib after palliative thoracic radiotherapy for lung cancer. J Thorac Oncol. 2019;14(10):e224–e6.
57. Bourgier C, Massard C, Moldovan C, Soria JC, Deutsch E. Total recall of radiotherapy with mTOR inhibitors: a novel and potentially frequent side-effect? Ann Oncol. 2011;22(2):485–6.
58. Schwarte S, Wagner K, Karstens JH, Bremer M. Radiation recall pneumonitis induced by gemcitabine. Strahlenther Onkol. 2007;183(4):215–7.
59. Antonadou D, Coliarakis N, Synodinou M, Athanassiou H, Kouveli A, Verigos C, et al. Randomized phase III trial of radiation treatment +/− amifostine in patients with advanced-stage lung cancer. Int J Radiat Oncol Biol Phys. 2001;51(4):915–22.
60. Ozturk B, Egehan I, Atavci S, Kitapci M. Pentoxifylline in prevention of radiation-induced lung toxicity in patients with breast and lung cancer: a double-blind randomized trial. Int J Radiat Oncol Biol Phys. 2004;58(1):213–9.
61. Kwok E, Chan CK. Corticosteroids and azathioprine do not prevent radiation-induced lung injury. Can Respir J. 1998;5(3):211–4.
62. Kim KI, Jun JH, Baek H, Kim JH, Lee BJ, Jung HJ. Oral administration of herbal medicines for radiation pneumonitis in lung cancer patients: a systematic review and meta-analysis. PLoS One. 2018;13(5):e0198015.

63. Wang LW, Fu XL, Clough R, Sibley G, Fan M, Bentel GC, et al. Can angiotensin-converting enzyme inhibitors protect against symptomatic radiation pneumonitis? Radiat Res. 2000;153(4):405–10.
64. Williams JP, Johnston CJ, Finkelstein JN. Treatment for radiation-induced pulmonary late effects: spoiled for choice or looking in the wrong direction? Curr Drug Targets. 2010;11(11):1386–94.
65. Jain V, Berman AT. Radiation pneumonitis: old problem, new tricks. Cancers (Basel). 2018;10(7):222.
66. De Ruysscher D, Granton PV, Lieuwes NG, van Hoof S, Wollin L, Weynand B, et al. Nintedanib reduces radiation-induced microscopic lung fibrosis but this cannot be monitored by CT imaging: a preclinical study with a high precision image-guided irradiator. Radiother Oncol. 2017;124(3):482–7.
67. Wollin L, Distler JHW, Redente EF, Riches DWH, Stowasser S, Schlenker-Herceg R, et al. Potential of nintedanib in treatment of progressive fibrosing interstitial lung diseases. Eur Respir J. 2019;54(3)
68. Simone NL, Soule BP, Gerber L, Augustine E, Smith S, Altemus RM, et al. Oral pirfenidone in patients with chronic fibrosis resulting from radiotherapy: a pilot study. Radiat Oncol. 2007;2:19.
69. Knuppel L, Ishikawa Y, Aichler M, Heinzelmann K, Hatz R, Behr J, et al. A novel antifibrotic mechanism of nintedanib and pirfenidone. Inhibition of collagen fibril assembly. Am J Respir Cell Mol Biol. 2017;57(1):77–90.
70. Cerqueira MD, Weissman NJ, Dilsizian V, Jacobs AK, Kaul S, Laskey WK, et al. Standardized myocardial segmentation and nomenclature for tomographic imaging of the heart. A statement for healthcare professionals from the Cardiac Imaging Committee of the Council on Clinical Cardiology of the American Heart Association. Circulation. 2002;105(4):539–42.
71. Feng M, Moran JM, Koelling T, Chughtai A, Chan JL, Freedman L, et al. Development and validation of a heart atlas to study cardiac exposure to radiation following treatment for breast cancer. Int J Radiat Oncol Biol Phys. 2011;79(1):10–8.
72. Duane F, Aznar MC, Bartlett F, Cutter DJ, Darby SC, Jagsi R, et al. A cardiac contouring atlas for radiotherapy. Radiother Oncol. 2017;122(3):416–22.
73. Wynn TA. Cellular and molecular mechanisms of fibrosis. J Pathol. 2008;214(2):199–210.
74. Cuomo JR, Sharma GK, Conger PD, Weintraub NL. Novel concepts in radiation-induced cardiovascular disease. World J Cardiol. 2016;8(9):504–19.
75. Haydont V, Mathe D, Bourgier C, Abdelali J, Aigueperse J, Bourhis J, et al. Induction of CTGF by TGF-beta1 in normal and radiation enteritis human smooth muscle cells: Smad/Rho balance and therapeutic perspectives. Radiother Oncol. 2005;76(2):219–25.
76. Lee CH, Shah B, Moioli EK, Mao JJ. CTGF directs fibroblast differentiation from human mesenchymal stem/stromal cells and defines connective tissue healing in a rodent injury model. J Clin Invest. 2010;120(9):3340–9.
77. Weigel C, Schmezer P, Plass C, Popanda O. Epigenetics in radiation-induced fibrosis. Oncogene. 2015;34(17):2145–55.
78. Bradley JD, Paulus R, Komaki R, Masters G, Blumenschein G, Schild S, et al. Standard-dose versus high-dose conformal radiotherapy with concurrent and consolidation carboplatin plus paclitaxel with or without cetuximab for patients with stage IIIA or IIIB non-small-cell lung cancer (RTOG 0617): a randomised, two-by-two factorial phase 3 study. Lancet Oncol. 2015;16(2):187–99.
79. Kong FM, Ten Haken RK, Schipper M, Frey KA, Hayman J, Gross M, et al. Effect of midtreatment PET/CT-adapted radiation therapy with concurrent chemotherapy in patients with locally advanced non-small-cell lung cancer: a phase 2 clinical trial. JAMA Oncol. 2017;3(10):1358–65.
80. Speirs CK, DeWees TA, Rehman S, Molotievschi A, Velez MA, Mullen D, et al. Heart dose is an independent dosimetric predictor of overall survival in locally advanced non-small cell lung cancer. J Thorac Oncol. 2017;12(2):293–301.

81. Dess RT, Sun Y, Matuszak MM, Sun G, Soni PD, Bazzi L, et al. Cardiac events after radiation therapy: combined analysis of prospective multicenter trials for locally advanced non-small-cell lung cancer. J Clin Oncol. 2017;35(13):1395–402.
82. Wang K, Pearlstein KA, Patchett ND, Deal AM, Mavroidis P, Jensen BC, et al. Heart dosimetric analysis of three types of cardiac toxicity in patients treated on dose-escalation trials for Stage III non-small-cell lung cancer. Radiother Oncol. 2017;125(2):293–300.
83. Vivekanandan S, Landau DB, Counsell N, Warren DR, Khwanda A, Rosen SD, et al. The impact of cardiac radiation dosimetry on survival after radiation therapy for non-small cell lung cancer. Int J Radiat Oncol Biol Phys. 2017;99(1):51–60.
84. Cuzick J, Stewart H, Rutqvist L, Houghton J, Edwards R, Redmond C, et al. Cause-specific mortality in long-term survivors of breast cancer who participated in trials of radiotherapy. J Clin Oncol. 1994;12(3):447–53.
85. Darby S, McGale P, Peto R, Granath F, Hall P, Ekbom A. Mortality from cardiovascular disease more than 10 years after radiotherapy for breast cancer: nationwide cohort study of 90 000 Swedish women. BMJ. 2003;326(7383):256–7.
86. Darby SC, McGale P, Taylor CW, Peto R. Long-term mortality from heart disease and lung cancer after radiotherapy for early breast cancer: prospective cohort study of about 300,000 women in US SEER cancer registries. Lancet Oncol. 2005;6(8):557–65.
87. Roychoudhuri R, Robinson D, Putcha V, Cuzick J, Darby S, Moller H. Increased cardiovascular mortality more than fifteen years after radiotherapy for breast cancer: a population-based study. BMC Cancer. 2007;7:9.
88. Piroth MD, Baumann R, Budach W, Dunst J, Feyer P, Fietkau R, et al. Heart toxicity from breast cancer radiotherapy: Current findings, assessment, and prevention. Strahlenther Onkol. 2019;195(1):1–12.
89. Darby SC, Ewertz M, McGale P, Bennet AM, Blom-Goldman U, Bronnum D, et al. Risk of ischemic heart disease in women after radiotherapy for breast cancer. N Engl J Med. 2013;368(11):987–98.
90. van den Bogaard VA, Ta BD, van der Schaaf A, Bouma AB, Middag AM, Bantema-Joppe EJ, et al. Validation and modification of a prediction model for acute cardiac events in patients with breast cancer treated with radiotherapy based on three-dimensional dose distributions to cardiac substructures. J Clin Oncol. 2017;35(11):1171–8.
91. Marks LB, Yu X, Prosnitz RG, Zhou SM, Hardenbergh PH, Blazing M, et al. The incidence and functional consequences of RT-associated cardiac perfusion defects. Int J Radiat Oncol Biol Phys. 2005;63(1):214–23.
92. Erven K, Jurcut R, Weltens C, Giusca S, Ector J, Wildiers H, et al. Acute radiation effects on cardiac function detected by strain rate imaging in breast cancer patients. Int J Radiat Oncol Biol Phys. 2011;79(5):1444–51.
93. Moignier A, Broggio D, Derreumaux S, Beaudre A, Girinsky T, Paul JF, et al. Coronary stenosis risk analysis following Hodgkin lymphoma radiotherapy: a study based on patient specific artery segments dose calculation. Radiother Oncol. 2015;117(3):467–72.
94. Skytta T, Tuohinen S, Boman E, Virtanen V, Raatikainen P, Kellokumpu-Lehtinen PL. Troponin T-release associates with cardiac radiation doses during adjuvant left-sided breast cancer radiotherapy. Radiat Oncol. 2015;10:141.
95. Whelan TJ, Pignol JP, Levine MN, Julian JA, MacKenzie R, Parpia S, et al. Long-term results of hypofractionated radiation therapy for breast cancer. N Engl J Med. 2010;362(6):513–20.
96. James M, Swadi S, Yi M, Johansson L, Robinson B, Dixit A. Ischaemic heart disease following conventional and hypofractionated radiation treatment in a contemporary breast cancer series. J Med Imaging Radiat Oncol. 2018;62(3):425–31.
97. Stam B, Peulen H, Guckenberger M, Mantel F, Hope A, Werner-Wasik M, et al. Dose to heart substructures is associated with non-cancer death after SBRT in stage I-II NSCLC patients. Radiother Oncol. 2017;123(3):370–5.
98. Reshko LB, Kalman NS, Hugo GD, Weiss E. Cardiac radiation dose distribution, cardiac events and mortality in early-stage lung cancer treated with stereotactic body radiation therapy (SBRT). J Thorac Dis. 2018;10(4):2346–56.

99. Tembhekar AR, Wright CL, Daly ME. Cardiac dose and survival after stereotactic body radiotherapy for early-stage non-small-cell lung cancer. Clin Lung Cancer. 2017;18(3):293–8.
100. Lancellotti P, Nkomo VT, Badano LP, Bergler-Klein J, Bogaert J, Davin L, et al. Expert consensus for multi-modality imaging evaluation of cardiovascular complications of radiotherapy in adults: a report from the European Association of Cardiovascular Imaging and the American Society of Echocardiography. Eur Heart J Cardiovasc Imaging. 2013;14(8):721–40.
101. Ha CS, Hodgson DC, Advani R, Dabaja BS, Dhakal S, Flowers CR, et al. ACR appropriateness criteria follow-up of Hodgkin lymphoma. J Am Coll Radiol. 2014;11(11):1026-33 e3.
102. van Leeuwen-Segarceanu EM, Bos WJ, Dorresteijn LD, Rensing BJ, der Heyden JA, Vogels OJ, et al. Screening Hodgkin lymphoma survivors for radiotherapy induced cardiovascular disease. Cancer Treat Rev. 2011;37(5):391–403.
103. Chen AB, Punglia RS, Kuntz KM, Mauch PM, Ng AK. Cost effectiveness and screening interval of lipid screening in Hodgkin's lymphoma survivors. J Clin Oncol. 2009;27(32):5383–9.
104. Armstrong GT, Plana JC, Zhang N, Srivastava D, Green DM, Ness KK, et al. Screening adult survivors of childhood cancer for cardiomyopathy: comparison of echocardiography and cardiac magnetic resonance imaging. J Clin Oncol. 2012;30(23):2876–84.
105. Kruse JJ, Strootman EG, Wondergem J. Effects of amifostine on radiation-induced cardiac damage. Acta Oncol. 2003;42(1):4–9.
106. Ran XZ, Ran X, Zong ZW, Liu DQ, Xiang GM, Su YP, et al. Protective effect of atorvastatin on radiation-induced vascular endothelial cell injury in vitro. J Radiat Res. 2010;51(5):527–33.
107. van der Veen SJ, Ghobadi G, de Boer RA, Faber H, Cannon MV, Nagle PW, et al. ACE inhibition attenuates radiation-induced cardiopulmonary damage. Radiother Oncol. 2015;114(1):96–103.
108. Gurses I, Ozeren M, Serin M, Yucel N, Erkal HS. Histopathological evaluation of melatonin as a protective agent in heart injury induced by radiation in a rat model. Pathol Res Pract. 2014;210(12):863–71.
109. Bertog SC, Thambidorai SK, Parakh K, Schoenhagen P, Ozduran V, Houghtaling PL, et al. Constrictive pericarditis: etiology and cause-specific survival after pericardiectomy. J Am Coll Cardiol. 2004;43(8):1445–52.
110. Avgerinos D, Rabitnokov Y, Worku B, Neragi-Miandoab S, Girardi LN. Fifteen-year experience and outcomes of pericardiectomy for constrictive pericarditis. J Card Surg. 2014;29(4):434–8.
111. Szabo G, Schmack B, Bulut C, Soos P, Weymann A, Stadtfeld S, et al. Constrictive pericarditis: risks, aetiologies and outcomes after total pericardiectomy: 24 years of experience. Eur J Cardiothorac Surg. 2013;44(6):1023–8; discussion 8
112. DePasquale EC, Nasir K, Jacoby DL. Outcomes of adults with restrictive cardiomyopathy after heart transplantation. J Heart Lung Transplant. 2012;31(12):1269–75.
113. Saxena P, Joyce LD, Daly RC, Kushwaha SS, Schirger JA, Rosedahl J, et al. Cardiac transplantation for radiation-induced cardiomyopathy: the Mayo Clinic experience. Ann Thorac Surg. 2014;98(6):2115–21.
114. Galper SL, Yu JB, Mauch PM, Strasser JF, Silver B, Lacasce A, et al. Clinically significant cardiac disease in patients with Hodgkin lymphoma treated with mediastinal irradiation. Blood. 2011;117(2):412–8.
115. Mollmann H, Bestehorn K, Bestehorn M, Papoutsis K, Fleck E, Ertl G, et al. In-hospital outcome of transcatheter vs. surgical aortic valve replacement in patients with aortic valve stenosis: complete dataset of patients treated in 2013 in Germany. Clin Res Cardiol. 2016;105(6):553–9.
116. Adams DH, Popma JJ, Reardon MJ, Yakubov SJ, Coselli JS, Deeb GM, et al. Transcatheter aortic-valve replacement with a self-expanding prosthesis. N Engl J Med. 2014;370(19):1790–8.
117. Beohar N, Kirtane AJ, Blackstone E, Waksman R, Holmes D Jr, Minha S, et al. Trends in complications and outcomes of patients undergoing transfemoral transcatheter aortic valve replacement: experience from the PARTNER continued access registry. JACC Cardiovasc Interv. 2016;9(4):355–63.

118. Schomig K, Ndrepepa G, Mehilli J, Pache J, Kastrati A, Schomig A. Thoracic radiotherapy in patients with lymphoma and restenosis after coronary stent placement. Catheter Cardiovasc Interv. 2007;70(3):359–65.
119. Liang JJ, Sio TT, Slusser JP, Lennon RJ, Miller RC, Sandhu G, et al. Outcomes after percutaneous coronary intervention with stents in patients treated with thoracic external beam radiation for cancer. JACC Cardiovasc Interv. 2014;7(12):1412–20.
120. Handa N, McGregor CG, Danielson GK, Orszulak TA, Mullany CJ, Daly RC, et al. Coronary artery bypass grafting in patients with previous mediastinal radiation therapy. J Thorac Cardiovasc Surg. 1999;117(6):1136–42.
121. Chang AS, Smedira NG, Chang CL, Benavides MM, Myhre U, Feng J, et al. Cardiac surgery after mediastinal radiation: extent of exposure influences outcome. J Thorac Cardiovasc Surg. 2007;133(2):404–13.
122. Andolino DL, Forquer JA, Henderson MA, Barriger RB, Shapiro RH, Brabham JG, et al. Chest wall toxicity after stereotactic body radiotherapy for malignant lesions of the lung and liver. Int J Radiat Oncol Biol Phys. 2011;80(3):692–7.
123. Nambu A, Onishi H, Aoki S, Tominaga L, Kuriyama K, Araya M, et al. Rib fracture after stereotactic radiotherapy for primary lung cancer: prevalence, degree of clinical symptoms, and risk factors. BMC Cancer. 2013;13:68.
124. Mutter RW, Liu F, Abreu A, Yorke E, Jackson A, Rosenzweig KE. Dose-volume parameters predict for the development of chest wall pain after stereotactic body radiation for lung cancer. Int J Radiat Oncol Biol Phys. 2012;82(5):1783–90.
125. Woody NM, Videtic GM, Stephans KL, Djemil T, Kim Y, Xia P. Predicting chest wall pain from lung stereotactic body radiotherapy for different fractionation schemes. Int J Radiat Oncol Biol Phys. 2012;83(1):427–34.
126. Bongers EM, Haasbeek CJ, Lagerwaard FJ, Slotman BJ, Senan S. Incidence and risk factors for chest wall toxicity after risk-adapted stereotactic radiotherapy for early-stage lung cancer. J Thorac Oncol. 2011;6(12):2052–7.
127. Pacheco R, Stock H. Effects of radiation on bone. Curr Osteoporos Rep. 2013;11(4):299–304.
128. Knospe WHBJ, Crosby WH. Regeneration of locally irradiated bone marrow. I. Dose dependent, long-term changes in the rat, with particular emphasis upon vascular and stromal reaction. Blood. 1966;28(3):398–415.
129. Pitkanen MA, Hopewell JW. Functional changes in the vascularity of the irradiated rat femur. Implications for late effects. Acta Radiol Oncol. 1983;22(3):253–6.
130. Hui SK, Sharkey L, Kidder LS, Zhang Y, Fairchild G, Coghill K, et al. The influence of therapeutic radiation on the patterns of bone marrow in ovary-intact and ovariectomized mice. PLoS One. 2012;7(8):e42668.
131. Masiukiewicz US, Mitnick M, Grey AB, Insogna KL. Estrogen modulates parathyroid hormone-induced interleukin-6 production in vivo and in vitro. Endocrinology. 2000;141(7):2526–31.
132. Pierce SM, Recht A, Lingos TI, Abner A, Vicini F, Silver B, et al. Long-term radiation complications following conservative surgery (CS) and radiation therapy (RT) in patients with early stage breast cancer. Int J Radiat Oncol Biol Phys. 1992;23(5):915–23.
133. Overgaard M. Spontaneous radiation-induced rib fractures in breast cancer patients treated with postmastectomy irradiation. A clinical radiobiological analysis of the influence of fraction size and dose-response relationships on late bone damage. Acta Oncol. 1988;27(2):117–22.
134. Brashears JH, Dragun AE, Jenrette JM. Late chest wall toxicity after MammoSite breast brachytherapy. Brachytherapy. 2009;8(1):19–25.
135. Ma JT, Liu Y, Sun L, Milano MT, Zhang SL, Huang LT, et al. Chest wall toxicity after stereotactic body radiation therapy: a pooled analysis of 57 studies. Int J Radiat Oncol Biol Phys. 2019;103(4):843–50.
136. Kuo B, Urma D. Esophagus-anatomy and development. GI Motility Online. 2006;
137. Fleming C, Cagney DN, O'Keeffe S, Brennan SM, Armstrong JG, McClean B. Normal tissue considerations and dose volume constraints in the moderately hypofractionated treatment of non-small cell lung cancer. Radiother Oncol. 2016;119(3):423–31.

138. Chapet O, Kong FM, Lee JS, Hayman JA, Ten Haken RK. Normal tissue complication probability modeling for acute esophagitis in patients treated with conformal radiation therapy for non-small cell lung cancer. Radiother Oncol. 2005;77(2):176–81.
139. Ahn SJ, Kahn D, Zhou S, Yu X, Hollis D, Shafman TD, et al. Dosimetric and clinical predictors for radiation-induced esophageal injury. Int J Radiat Oncol Biol Phys. 2005;61(2):335–47.
140. Dieleman EM, Senan S, Vincent A, Lagerwaard FJ, Slotman BJ, van Sornsen de Koste JR. Four-dimensional computed tomographic analysis of esophageal mobility during normal respiration. Int J Radiat Oncol Biol Phys. 2007;67(3):775–80.
141. Fairchild A, Harris K, Barnes E, Wong R, Lutz S, Bezjak A, et al. Palliative thoracic radiotherapy for lung cancer: a systematic review. J Clin Oncol. 2008;26(24):4001–11.
142. Bar-Ad V, Ohri N, Werner-Wasik M. Esophagitis, treatment-related toxicity in non-small cell lung cancer. Rev Recent Clin Trials. 2012;7(1):31–5.
143. Stevens R, Macbeth F, Toy E, Coles B, Lester JF. Palliative radiotherapy regimens for patients with thoracic symptoms from non-small cell lung cancer. Cochrane Database Syst Rev. 2015;1:CD002143.
144. Baker S, Fairchild A. Radiation-induced esophagitis in lung cancer. Lung Cancer (Auckl). 2016;7:119–27.
145. Palma DA, Senan S, Oberije C, Belderbos J, de Dios NR, Bradley JD, et al. Predicting esophagitis after chemoradiation therapy for non-small cell lung cancer: an individual patient data meta-analysis. Int J Radiat Oncol Biol Phys. 2013;87(4):690–6.
146. Sun Z, Li J, Lin M, Zhang S, Luo J, Tang Y. An RNA-seq-based expression profiling of radiation-induced esophageal injury in a rat model. Dose Response 2019;17(2):1559325819843373.
147. Epperly MW, Gretton JA, DeFilippi SJ, Greenberger JS, Sikora CA, Liggitt D, et al. Modulation of radiation-induced cytokine elevation associated with esophagitis and esophageal stricture by manganese superoxide dismutase-plasmid/liposome (SOD2-PL) gene therapy. Radiat Res. 2001;155(1 Pt 1):2–14.
148. Kim KS, Jeon SU, Lee CJ, Kim YE, Bok S, Hong BJ, et al. Radiation-induced esophagitis in vivo and in vitro reveals that epidermal growth factor is a potential candidate for therapeutic intervention strategy. Int J Radiat Oncol Biol Phys. 2016;95(3):1032–41.
149. Murro D, Jakate S. Radiation esophagitis. Arch Pathol Lab Med. 2015;139(6):827–30.
150. Hirota S, Tsujino K, Hishikawa Y, Watanabe H, Kono K, Soejima T, et al. Endoscopic findings of radiation esophagitis in concurrent chemoradiotherapy for intrathoracic malignancies. Radiother Oncol. 2001;58(3):273–8.
151. Emami B, Lyman J, Brown A, Coia L, Goitein M, Munzenrider JE, et al. Tolerance of normal tissue to therapeutic irradiation. Int J Radiat Oncol Biol Phys. 1991;21(1):109–22.
152. Seaman WB, Ackerman LV. The effect of radiation on the esophagus; a clinical and histologic study of the effects produced by the betatron. Radiology. 1957;68(4):534–41.
153. Hirota S, Tsujino K, Endo M, Kotani Y, Satouchi M, Kado T, et al. Dosimetric predictors of radiation esophagitis in patients treated for non-small-cell lung cancer with carboplatin/paclitaxel/radiotherapy. Int J Radiat Oncol Biol Phys. 2001;51(2):291–5.
154. Choy H, Akerley W, Safran H, Graziano S, Chung C, Williams T, et al. Multiinstitutional phase II trial of paclitaxel, carboplatin, and concurrent radiation therapy for locally advanced non-small-cell lung cancer. J Clin Oncol. 1998;16(10):3316–22.
155. Zhang Z, Xu J, Zhou T, Yi Y, Li H, Sun H, et al. Risk factors of radiation-induced acute esophagitis in non-small cell lung cancer patients treated with concomitant chemoradiotherapy. Radiat Oncol. 2014;9:54.
156. Maguire PD, Sibley GS, Zhou SM, Jamieson TA, Light KL, Antoine PA, et al. Clinical and dosimetric predictors of radiation-induced esophageal toxicity. Int J Radiat Oncol Biol Phys. 1999;45(1):97–103.
157. Bradley J, Deasy JO, Bentzen S, El-Naqa I. Dosimetric correlates for acute esophagitis in patients treated with radiotherapy for lung carcinoma. Int J Radiat Oncol Biol Phys. 2004;58(4):1106–13.
158. Werner-Wasik M, Pequignot E, Leeper D, Hauck W, Curran W. Predictors of severe esophagitis include use of concurrent chemotherapy, but not the length of irradiated esophagus: a

multivariate analysis of patients with lung cancer treated with nonoperative therapy. Int J Radiat Oncol Biol Phys. 2000;48(3):689–96.

159. Belderbos J, Heemsbergen W, Hoogeman M, Pengel K, Rossi M, Lebesque J. Acute esophageal toxicity in non-small cell lung cancer patients after high dose conformal radiotherapy. Radiother Oncol. 2005;75(2):157–64.

160. Wang S, Campbell J, Stenmark MH, Stanton P, Zhao J, Matuszak MM, et al. A model combining age, equivalent uniform dose and IL-8 may predict radiation esophagitis in patients with non-small cell lung cancer. Radiother Oncol. 2018;126(3):506–10.

161. Werner-Wasik M, Yorke E, Deasy J, Nam J, Marks LB. Radiation dose-volume effects in the esophagus. Int J Radiat Oncol Biol Phys. 2010;76(3 Suppl):S86–93.

162. Wada K, Kishi N, Kanayama N, Hirata T, Ueda Y, Kawaguchi Y, et al. Predictors of acute radiation esophagitis in non-small cell lung cancer patients treated with accelerated hyperfractionated chemoradiotherapy. Anticancer Res. 2019;39(1):491–7.

163. Zehentmayr F, Sohn M, Exeli AK, Wurstbauer K, Troller A, Deutschmann H, et al. Normal tissue complication models for clinically relevant acute esophagitis (>/= grade 2) in patients treated with dose differentiated accelerated radiotherapy (DART-bid). Radiat Oncol. 2015;10:121.

164. Uyterlinde W, Chen C, Kwint M, de Bois J, Vincent A, Sonke JJ, et al. Prognostic parameters for acute esophagus toxicity in intensity modulated radiotherapy and concurrent chemotherapy for locally advanced non-small cell lung cancer. Radiother Oncol. 2013;107(3):392–7.

165. Huang J, He T, Yang R, Ji T, Li G. Clinical, dosimetric, and position factors for radiation-induced acute esophagitis in intensity-modulated (chemo)radiotherapy for locally advanced non-small-cell lung cancer. Onco Targets Ther. 2018;11:6167–75.

166. Al-Halabi H, Paetzold P, Sharp GC, Olsen C, Willers H. A contralateral esophagus-sparing technique to limit severe esophagitis associated with concurrent high-dose radiation and chemotherapy in patients with thoracic malignancies. Int J Radiat Oncol Biol Phys. 2015;92(4):803–10.

167. Kao J, Pettit J, Zahid S, Gold KD, Palatt T. Esophagus and contralateral lung-sparing IMRT for locally advanced lung cancer in the community hospital setting. Front Oncol. 2015;5:127.

168. Ma L, Qiu B, Li Q, Chen L, Wang B, Hu Y, et al. An esophagus-sparing technique to limit radiation esophagitis in locally advanced non-small cell lung cancer treated by simultaneous integrated boost intensity-modulated radiotherapy and concurrent chemotherapy. Radiat Oncol. 2018;13(1):130.

169. Grant JD, Shirvani SM, Tang C, Juloori A, Rebueno NC, Allen PK, et al. Incidence and predictors of severe acute esophagitis and subsequent esophageal stricture in patients treated with accelerated hyperfractionated chemoradiation for limited-stage small cell lung cancer. Pract Radiat Oncol. 2015;5(4):e383–91.

170. Giuliani ME, Lindsay PE, Kwan JY, Sun A, Bezjak A, Le LW, et al. Correlation of dosimetric and clinical factors with the development of esophagitis and radiation pneumonitis in patients with limited-stage small-cell lung carcinoma. Clin Lung Cancer. 2015;16(3):216–20.

171. Kim JW, Kim TH, Kim JH, Lee IJ. Predictors of post-treatment stenosis in cervical esophageal cancer undergoing high-dose radiotherapy. World J Gastroenterol. 2018;24(7):862–9.

172. Atsumi K, Shioyama Y, Arimura H, Terashima K, Matsuki T, Ohga S, et al. Esophageal stenosis associated with tumor regression in radiotherapy for esophageal cancer: frequency and prediction. Int J Radiat Oncol Biol Phys. 2012;82(5):1973–80.

173. McDermott RL, Armstrong JG, Thirion P, Dunne M, Finn M, Small C, et al. Cancer trials Ireland (ICORG) 06-34: a multi-centre clinical trial using three-dimensional conformal radiation therapy to reduce the toxicity of palliative radiation for lung cancer. Radiother Oncol. 2018;127(2):253–8.

174. Granton PV, Palma DA, Louie AV. Intentional avoidance of the esophagus using intensity modulated radiation therapy to reduce dysphagia after palliative thoracic radiation. Radiat Oncol. 2017;12(1):27.

175. Duijm M, Schillemans W, Aerts JG, Heijmen B, Nuyttens JJ. Dose and volume of the irradiated main Bronchi and related side effects in the treatment of central lung tumors with stereotactic radiotherapy. Semin Radiat Oncol. 2016;26(2):140–8.

176. Yau V, Lindsay P, Le L, Lau A, Wong O, Glick D, et al. Low incidence of esophageal toxicity after lung stereotactic body radiation therapy: are current esophageal dose constraints too conservative? Int J Radiat Oncol Biol Phys. 2018;101(3):574–80.

177. Duijm M, Tekatli H, Oomen-de Hoop E, Verbakel W, Schillemans W, Slotman BJ, et al. Esophagus toxicity after stereotactic and hypofractionated radiotherapy for central lung tumors: normal tissue complication probability modeling. Radiother Oncol. 2018;127(2):233–8.

178. Wu AJ, Williams E, Modh A, Foster A, Yorke E, Rimner A, et al. Dosimetric predictors of esophageal toxicity after stereotactic body radiotherapy for central lung tumors. Radiother Oncol. 2014;112(2):267–71.

179. Stephans KL, Djemil T, Diaconu C, Reddy CA, Xia P, Woody NM, et al. Esophageal dose tolerance to hypofractionated stereotactic body radiation therapy: risk factors for late toxicity. Int J Radiat Oncol Biol Phys. 2014;90(1):197–202.

180. Senzer N. A phase III randomized evaluation of amifostine in stage IIIA/IIIB non-small cell lung cancer patients receiving concurrent carboplatin, paclitaxel, and radiation therapy followed by gemcitabine and cisplatin intensification: preliminary findings. Semin Oncol. 2002;29(6 Suppl 19):38–41.

181. Arquette M, Wasserman T, Govindan R, Garfield D, Senzer N, Gillenwater H, et al. Phase II evaluation of amifostine as an esophageal mucosal protectant in the treatment of limited-stage small cell lung cancer with chemotherapy and twice-daily radiation. Semin Radiat Oncol. 2002;12(1 Suppl 1):59–61.

182. Movsas B, Scott C, Langer C, Werner-Wasik M, Nicolaou N, Komaki R, et al. Randomized trial of amifostine in locally advanced non-small-cell lung cancer patients receiving chemotherapy and hyperfractionated radiation: radiation therapy oncology group trial 98-01. J Clin Oncol. 2005;23(10):2145–54.

183. Antonadou D, Throuvalas N, Petridis A, Bolanos N, Sagriotis A, Synodinou M. Effect of amifostine on toxicities associated with radiochemotherapy in patients with locally advanced non-small-cell lung cancer. Int J Radiat Oncol Biol Phys. 2003;57(2):402–8.

184. Koukourakis MI, Giatromanolaki A, Chong W, Simopoulos C, Polychronidis A, Sivridis E, et al. Amifostine induces anaerobic metabolism and hypoxia-inducible factor 1 alpha. Cancer Chemother Pharmacol. 2004;53(1):8–14.

185. Komaki R, Lee JS, Milas L, Lee HK, Fossella FV, Herbst RS, et al. Effects of amifostine on acute toxicity from concurrent chemotherapy and radiotherapy for inoperable non-small-cell lung cancer: report of a randomized comparative trial. Int J Radiat Oncol Biol Phys. 2004;58(5):1369–77.

186. Leong SS, Tan EH, Fong KW, Wilder-Smith E, Ong YK, Tai BC, et al. Randomized double-blind trial of combined modality treatment with or without amifostine in unresectable stage III non-small-cell lung cancer. J Clin Oncol. 2003;21(9):1767–74.

187. Sarna L, Swann S, Langer C, Werner-Wasik M, Nicolaou N, Komaki R, et al. Clinically meaningful differences in patient-reported outcomes with amifostine in combination with chemoradiation for locally advanced non-small-cell lung cancer: an analysis of RTOG 9801. Int J Radiat Oncol Biol Phys. 2008;72(5):1378–84.

188. Hensley ML, Hagerty KL, Kewalramani T, Green DM, Meropol NJ, Wasserman TH, et al. American Society of Clinical Oncology 2008 clinical practice guideline update: use of chemotherapy and radiation therapy protectants. J Clin Oncol. 2009;27(1):127–45.

189. Fogh SE, Deshmukh S, Berk LB, Dueck AC, Roof K, Yacoub S, et al. A randomized Phase 2 trial of prophylactic Manuka Honey for the reduction of chemoradiation therapy-induced esophagitis during the treatment of lung cancer: results of NRG oncology RTOG 1012. Int J Radiat Oncol Biol Phys. 2017;97(4):786–96.

190. Papanikolopoulou A, Syrigos KN, Drakoulis N. The role of glutamine supplementation in thoracic and upper aerodigestive malignancies. Nutr Cancer. 2015;67(2):231–7.

191. Topkan E, Yavuz MN, Onal C, Yavuz AA. Prevention of acute radiation-induced esophagitis with glutamine in non-small cell lung cancer patients treated with radiotherapy: evaluation of clinical and dosimetric parameters. Lung Cancer. 2009;63(3):393–9.

192. Topkan E, Parlak C, Topuk S, Pehlivan B. Influence of oral glutamine supplementation on survival outcomes of patients treated with concurrent chemoradiotherapy for locally advanced non-small cell lung cancer. BMC Cancer. 2012;12:502.
193. Algara M, Rodriguez N, Vinals P, Lacruz M, Foro P, Reig A, et al. Prevention of radiochemotherapy-induced esophagitis with glutamine: results of a pilot study. Int J Radiat Oncol Biol Phys. 2007;69(2):342–9.
194. Yoshida S, Matsui M, Shirouzu Y, Fujita H, Yamana H, Shirouzu K. Effects of glutamine supplements and radiochemotherapy on systemic immune and gut barrier function in patients with advanced esophageal cancer. Ann Surg. 1998;227(4):485–91.
195. Yoshida S, Kaibara A, Ishibashi N, Shirouzu K. Glutamine supplementation in cancer patients. Nutrition. 2001;17(9):766–8.
196. Hillman GG. Soy isoflavones protect normal tissues while enhancing radiation responses. Semin Radiat Oncol. 2019;29(1):62–71.
197. Fountain MD, Abernathy LM, Lonardo F, Rothstein SE, Dominello MM, Yunker CK, et al. Radiation-induced esophagitis is mitigated by Soy Isoflavones. Front Oncol. 2015;5:238.
198. Berkey FJ. Managing the adverse effects of radiation therapy. Am Fam Physician. 2010;82(4):381–8.. 94
199. Sasso FS, Sasso G, Marsiglia HR, de Palma G, Schiavone C, Barone A, et al. Pharmacological and dietary prophylaxis and treatment of acute actinic esophagitis during mediastinal radiotherapy. Dig Dis Sci. 2001;46(4):746–9.
200. Seres DS, Valcarcel M, Guillaume A. Advantages of enteral nutrition over parenteral nutrition. Ther Adv Gastroenterol. 2013;6(2):157–67.
201. Bamalan OA SMA, Thorax, Heart Great Vessels. [Updated 2019 Oct 4]. In: StatPearls [Internet]. Treasure Island (FL): StatPearls Publishing; 2019 Jan. Available from: https://www.ncbi.nlm.nih.gov/books/NBK547680/.
202. Shahoud JS BSA, Thorax, Heart Aorta. [Updated 2019 Feb 20]. In: StatPearls [Internet]. Treasure Island (FL): StatPearls Publishing; 2019 Jan. Available from: https://www.ncbi.nlm.nih.gov/books/NBK538140/.
203. Tucker WD BBA, Thorax, Heart Pulmonary Arteries. [Updated 2018 Dec 9]. In: StatPearls [Internet]. Treasure Island (FL): StatPearls Publishing; 2019 Jan. Available from: https://www.ncbi.nlm.nih.gov/books/NBK534812/.
204. White HJ SMA, Thorax, Superior Vena Cava. [Updated 2019 Aug 16]. In: StatPearls [Internet]. Treasure Island (FL): StatPearls Publishing; 2019 Jan. Available from: https://www.ncbi.nlm.nih.gov/books/NBK545255/.
205. Sundjaja JH BBA, Thorax, Lung Veins. [Updated 2019 Jul 29]. In: StatPearls [Internet]. Treasure Island (FL): StatPearls Publishing; 2019 Jan. Available from: https://www.ncbi.nlm.nih.gov/books/NBK545205/.
206. Nishimura S, Takeda A, Sanuki N, Ishikura S, Oku Y, Aoki Y, et al. Toxicities of organs at risk in the mediastinal and hilar regions following stereotactic body radiotherapy for centrally located lung tumors. J Thorac Oncol. 2014;9(9):1370–6.
207. Ichinose T, Nakazato Y, Miyano H, Kimura T, Yamashita H, Takizawa K, et al. Severe infundibular pulmonary stenosis and coronary artery stenosis with ventricular tachycardia 24 years after mediastinal irradiation. Intern Med. 2005;44(9):963–6.
208. Makker HK, Barnes PC. Fatal haemoptysis from the pulmonary artery as a late complication of pulmonary irradiation. Thorax. 1991;46(8):609–10.
209. Van Putten JW, Schlosser NJ, Vujaskovic Z, Leest AH, Groen HJ. Superior vena cava obstruction caused by radiation induced venous fibrosis. Thorax. 2000;55(3):245–6.
210. Kim JH, Jenrow KA, Brown SL. Mechanisms of radiation-induced normal tissue toxicity and implications for future clinical trials. Radiat Oncol J. 2014;32(3):103–15.
211. Lee CB, Stinchcombe TE, Moore DT, Morris DE, Hayes DN, Halle J, et al. Late complications of high-dose (>/=66 Gy) thoracic conformal radiation therapy in combined modality trials in unresectable stage III non-small cell lung cancer. J Thorac Oncol. 2009;4(1):74–9.
212. Yoo GS, Oh D, Pyo H, Ahn YC, Noh JM, Park HC, et al. Concurrent chemo-radiotherapy for unresectable non-small cell lung cancer invading adjacent great vessels on radiologic findings: is it safe? J Radiat Res. 2019;60(2):234–41.

213. Han CB, Wang WL, Quint L, Xue JX, Matuszak M, Ten Haken R, et al. Pulmonary artery invasion, high-dose radiation, and overall survival in patients with non-small cell lung cancer. Int J Radiat Oncol Biol Phys. 2014;89(2):313–21.
214. Ma JT, Sun L, Sun X, Xiong ZC, Liu Y, Zhang SL, et al. Is pulmonary artery a dose-limiting organ at risk in non-small cell lung cancer patients treated with definitive radiotherapy? Radiat Oncol. 2017;12(1):34.
215. Evans JD, Gomez DR, Amini A, Rebueno N, Allen PK, Martel MK, et al. Aortic dose constraints when reirradiating thoracic tumors. Radiother Oncol. 2013;106(3):327–32.
216. Trombetta MG, Colonias A, Makishi D, Keenan R, Werts ED, Landreneau R, et al. Tolerance of the aorta using intraoperative iodine-125 interstitial brachytherapy in cancer of the lung. Brachytherapy. 2008;7(1):50–4.
217. Peulen H, Karlsson K, Lindberg K, Tullgren O, Baumann P, Lax I, et al. Toxicity after reirradiation of pulmonary tumours with stereotactic body radiotherapy. Radiother Oncol. 2011;101(2):260–6.
218. Timmerman R, McGarry R, Yiannoutsos C, Papiez L, Tudor K, DeLuca J, et al. Excessive toxicity when treating central tumors in a phase II study of stereotactic body radiation therapy for medically inoperable early-stage lung cancer. J Clin Oncol. 2006;24(30):4833–9.
219. Bang A, Bezjak A. Stereotactic body radiotherapy for centrally located stage I non-small cell lung cancer. Transl Lung Cancer Res. 2019;8(1):58–69.
220. Xue J, Kubicek G, Patel A, Goldsmith B, Asbell SO, LaCouture TA. Validity of current stereotactic body radiation therapy dose constraints for aorta and major vessels. Semin Radiat Oncol. 2016;26(2):135–9.
221. Bezjak A, Paulus R, Gaspar LE, Timmerman RD, Straube WL, Ryan WF, et al. Safety and efficacy of a five-fraction stereotactic body radiotherapy schedule for centrally located non-small-cell lung cancer: NRG oncology/RTOG 0813 trial. J Clin Oncol. 2019;37(15):1316–25.
222. Ball M PDA, Airway. [Updated 2019 Apr 5]. In: StatPearls [Internet]. Treasure Island (FL): StatPearls Publishing; 2019 Jan-. Available from: https://www.ncbi.nlm.nih.gov/books/NBK459258/.
223. Taulelle M, Chauvet B, Vincent P, Felix-Faure C, Buciarelli B, Garcia R, et al. High dose rate endobronchial brachytherapy: results and complications in 189 patients. Eur Respir J. 1998;11(1):162–8.
224. Nomoto Y, Ii N, Murashima S, Yamashita Y, Ochiai S, Takada A, et al. Endobronchial brachytherapy with curative intent: the impact of reference points setting according to the bronchial diameter. J Radiat Res. 2017;58(6):849–53.
225. Reveiz L, Rueda JR, Cardona AF. Palliative endobronchial brachytherapy for non-small cell lung cancer. Cochrane Database Syst Rev. 2012;12:CD004284.
226. Mehta AC, Dweik RA. Necrosis of the bronchus. Role of radiation. Chest. 1995;108(5):1462–6.
227. Miller KL, Shafman TD, Anscher MS, Zhou SM, Clough RW, Garst JL, et al. Bronchial stenosis: an underreported complication of high-dose external beam radiotherapy for lung cancer? Int J Radiat Oncol Biol Phys. 2005;61(1):64–9.
228. Kelsey CR, Kahn D, Hollis DR, Miller KL, Zhou SM, Clough RW, et al. Radiation-induced narrowing of the tracheobronchial tree: an in-depth analysis. Lung Cancer. 2006;52(1):111–6.
229. Tekatli H, Senan S, Dahele M, Slotman BJ, Verbakel WF. Stereotactic ablative radiotherapy (SABR) for central lung tumors: plan quality and long-term clinical outcomes. Radiother Oncol. 2015;117(1):64–70.
230. Fakiris AJ, McGarry RC, Yiannoutsos CT, Papiez L, Williams M, Henderson MA, et al. Stereotactic body radiation therapy for early-stage non-small-cell lung carcinoma: four-year results of a prospective phase II study. Int J Radiat Oncol Biol Phys. 2009;75(3):677–82.
231. Bral S, Gevaert T, Linthout N, Versmessen H, Collen C, Engels B, et al. Prospective, risk-adapted strategy of stereotactic body radiotherapy for early-stage non-small-cell lung cancer: results of a Phase II trial. Int J Radiat Oncol Biol Phys. 2011;80(5):1343–9.
232. Park HS, Harder EM, Mancini BR, Decker RH. Central versus peripheral tumor location: influence on survival, local control, and toxicity following stereotactic body radiotherapy for primary non-small-cell lung cancer. J Thorac Oncol. 2015;10(5):832–7.

233. Xia T, Li H, Sun Q, Wang Y, Fan N, Yu Y, et al. Promising clinical outcome of stereotactic body radiation therapy for patients with inoperable Stage I/II non-small-cell lung cancer. Int J Radiat Oncol Biol Phys. 2006;66(1):117–25.
234. Roach MC, Robinson CG, DeWees TA, Ganachaud J, Przybysz D, Drzymala R, et al. Stereotactic body radiation therapy for central early-stage NSCLC: results of a prospective phase I/II trial. J Thorac Oncol. 2018;13(11):1727–32.
235. Song SY, Choi W, Shin SS, Lee SW, Ahn SD, Kim JH, et al. Fractionated stereotactic body radiation therapy for medically inoperable stage I lung cancer adjacent to central large bronchus. Lung Cancer. 2009;66(1):89–93.
236. Rowe BP, Boffa DJ, Wilson LD, Kim AW, Detterbeck FC, Decker RH. Stereotactic body radiotherapy for central lung tumors. J Thorac Oncol. 2012;7(9):1394–9.
237. Chang JY, Li QQ, Xu QY, Allen PK, Rebueno N, Gomez DR, et al. Stereotactic ablative radiation therapy for centrally located early stage or isolated parenchymal recurrences of non-small cell lung cancer: how to fly in a "no fly zone". Int J Radiat Oncol Biol Phys. 2014;88(5):1120–8.
238. Modh A, Rimner A, Williams E, Foster A, Shah M, Shi W, et al. Local control and toxicity in a large cohort of central lung tumors treated with stereotactic body radiation therapy. Int J Radiat Oncol Biol Phys. 2014;90(5):1168–76.
239. Kimura T, Nagata Y, Harada H, Hayashi S, Matsuo Y, Takanaka T, et al. Phase I study of stereotactic body radiation therapy for centrally located stage IA non-small cell lung cancer (JROSG10-1). Int J Clin Oncol. 2017;22(5):849–56.
240. Videtic GMM, Donington J, Giuliani M, Heinzerling J, Karas TZ, Kelsey CR, et al. Stereotactic body radiation therapy for early-stage non-small cell lung cancer: executive summary of an ASTRO evidence-based guideline. Pract Radiat Oncol. 2017;7(5):295–301.
241. Tekatli H, Haasbeek N, Dahele M, De Haan P, Verbakel W, Bongers E, et al. Outcomes of hypofractionated high-dose radiotherapy in poor-risk patients with "ultracentral" non-small cell lung cancer. J Thorac Oncol. 2016;11(7):1081–9.
242. Haseltine JM, Rimner A, Gelblum DY, Modh A, Rosenzweig KE, Jackson A, et al. Fatal complications after stereotactic body radiation therapy for central lung tumors abutting the proximal bronchial tree. Pract Radiat Oncol. 2016;6(2):e27–33.
243. Daly MNJ, Monjazeb A. Safety of stereotactic body radiotherapy for central, ultracentral and paramediastinal lung tumors. J Thorac Oncol. 2017;12:S1066.
244. Nguyen KNB, Hause DJ, Novak J, Monjazeb AM, Daly ME. Tumor control and toxicity after SBRT for ultracentral, central, and paramediastinal lung tumors. Pract Radiat Oncol. 2019;9(2):e196–202.
245. Lindberg KBP, Brustugun OT, et al. The nordic HILUS-trial – first report of a phase II trial of SBRT of centrally located lung tumors. J Thorac Oncol. 2017;12:S340.
246. Giuliani M, Mathew AS, Bahig H, Bratman SV, Filion E, Glick D, et al. SUNSET: stereotactic radiation for ultracentral non-small-cell lung Cancer-A safety and efficacy trial. Clin Lung Cancer. 2018;19(4):e529–e32.
247. Ito M, Niho S, Nihei K, Yoh K, Ohmatsu H, Ohe Y. Risk factors associated with fatal pulmonary hemorrhage in locally advanced non-small cell lung cancer treated with chemoradiotherapy. BMC Cancer. 2012;12:27.
248. Hapani S, Sher A, Chu D, Wu S. Increased risk of serious hemorrhage with bevacizumab in cancer patients: a meta-analysis. Oncology. 2010;79(1–2):27–38.
249. Topkan E, Selek U, Ozdemir Y, Besen AA, Guler OC, Yildirim BA, et al. Risk factors for fatal pulmonary hemorrhage following concurrent chemoradiotherapy in stage 3B/C squamous-cell lung carcinoma patients. J Oncol. 2018;2018:4518935.
250. Sandler AB, Schiller JH, Gray R, Dimery I, Brahmer J, Samant M, et al. Retrospective evaluation of the clinical and radiographic risk factors associated with severe pulmonary hemorrhage in first-line advanced, unresectable non-small-cell lung cancer treated with Carboplatin and Paclitaxel plus bevacizumab. J Clin Oncol. 2009;27(9):1405–12.
251. Dickhoff C, Dahele M, Hashemi SM, Senan S, Smit EF, Hartemink KJ, et al. Surgical treatment of complications after high-dose chemoradiotherapy for lung cancer. Ann Thorac Surg. 2017;104(2):436–42.

252. Murgu SD, Egressy K, Laxmanan B, Doblare G, Ortiz-Comino R, Hogarth DK. Central airway obstruction: benign strictures, tracheobronchomalacia, and malignancy-related obstruction. Chest. 2016;150(2):426–41.
253. Cho YC, Kim JH, Park JH, Shin JH, Ko HK, Song HY. Fluoroscopically guided balloon dilation for benign bronchial stricture occurring after radiotherapy in patients with lung cancer. Cardiovasc Intervent Radiol. 2014;37(3):750–5.
254. Jean-Baptiste E. Clinical assessment and management of massive hemoptysis. Crit Care Med. 2000;28(5):1642–7.
255. Khalil A, Fedida B, Parrot A, Haddad S, Fartoukh M, Carette MF. Severe hemoptysis: from diagnosis to embolization. Diagn Interv Imaging. 2015;96(7–8):775–88.
256. Swanson KL, Johnson CM, Prakash UB, McKusick MA, Andrews JC, Stanson AW. Bronchial artery embolization: experience with 54 patients. Chest. 2002;121(3):789–95.

Toxicity Management for Upper Abdomen Tumors in Radiation Oncology

5

Zumre Arican Alicikus and Barbaros Aydin

5.1 Liver

5.1.1 Anatomy

The liver is the largest organ and the mass of a healthy human liver is approximately 1.2–1.5 kg. Embryologically, the liver grows as a ventral diverticulum from the junction of foregut and the midgut into the ventral mesogastrium. The anterior portion of the hepatic diverticulum forms the intrahepatic biliary tree and the posterior portion forms the extrahepatic bile ducts and the gall bladder. The liver is a peritoneal organ positioned in the upper right-hand portion of the abdominal cavity, beneath the diaphragm, and on top of the stomach, right kidney, intestines, extending into the left hypochondrium and is partly protected by the rib cage. It is covered by a fibrous layer of connective tissue, named as Glisson's capsule.

The liver has two surfaces:

1. The diaphragmatic surface: The anterosuperior surface of the liver
2. The visceral surface: The posteroinferior surface of the liver

The liver is grossly divided into four lobes:

a. Right lobe: It is the largest lobe of the liver and is functionally separated from the left lobe by the middle hepatic vein. The functional right lobe is divided into the right medial and right lateral sectors by an oblique line that passes anteroposteriorly from the midpoint of the right lobe to the vena caval groove.

Z. A. Alicikus (✉) · B. Aydin
Department of Radiation Oncology, Dokuz Eylul University Faculty of Medicine, Izmir, Turkey

© Springer Nature Switzerland AG 2020
G. Ozyigit, U. Selek (eds.), *Prevention and Management of Acute and Late Toxicities in Radiation Oncology*, https://doi.org/10.1007/978-3-030-37798-4_5

b. Left lobe: It is smaller than the right lobe and is separated from the quadrate and caudate lobes by the fissure for the round and the venous ligament.

c. Quadrate lobe: It is located on the visceral surface of the liver between the gall-bladder and the fetal umbilical vein.

d. Caudate lobe: It is located on the upper aspect of the visceral surface of the liver between the inferior vena cava and the fetal ductus venosus.

Segments:

- Based on Couinaud classification, the functional lobes are divided into eight independent subsegments by a transverse plane through the bifurcation of the main portal vein [1].
- Consisting of the hepatic arterial branch, portal branch, and the bile duct with a separate hepatic venous branch that provides outflow, each segment has its own portal pedicle. The functional left lobe of the liver consists segments II, III, and IV. The anterior and posterior segments of the left lobe are named as segments II and III. In addition, segments V, VI, VII, VIII, the anterior segments, and the posterior segments make up the functional right lobe of the liver. The medial segment of the left lobe is named as segment IV and the caudate lobe which is located posteriorly of the liver is named as the segment I. The liver has a dual blood supply from the hepatic portal vein and hepatic arteries:
- Hepatic portal vein: It is the dominant blood supply (approximately 70–75% of the blood that passes through the liver) and is formed by the union of the superior mesenteric and splenic veins.
- Hepatic artery proper: It is a branch of the celiac truncus and supplies approximately 25% of the blood that passes through non-parenchymal structures of the liver.
- The hepatic vein collects the venous drainage of the liver. Multiple hepatic veins form the central veins of the hepatic lobule and open into the inferior vena cava.

5.1.2   Contouring

- The porta hepatis is the site of entry of the portal vein, hepatic artery, hepatic ducts, in addition to the hepatic nerve plexus and lymphatic vessels.
- The hepatic artery is a branch of the celiac artery. In some cases as a variant arise from the superior mesenteric artery (SMA).
- The right, middle, and the left hepatic veins collect blood from the liver to the inferior vena cava (IVC) just below the diaphragm.
- The plane extending vertically through the gallbladder fossa and middle hepatic vein separates the right and left lobe.

There are eight hepatic segments, beginning with the caudate lobe and moving clockwise on a coronal view (Fig. 5.1).

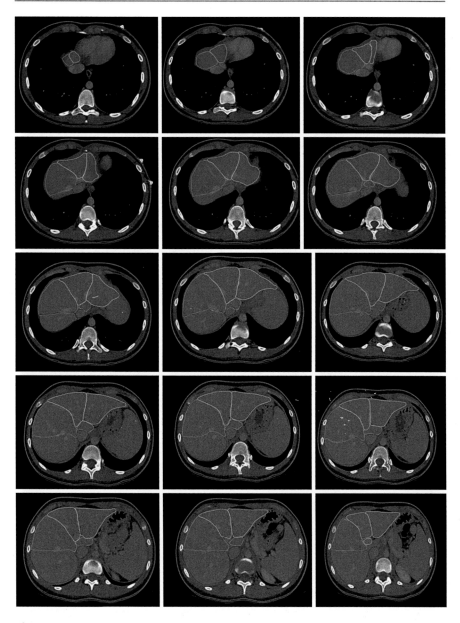

Fig. 5.1 The contouring of hepatic segments on computerized tomography (CT) images: white color: Gall Bladder, Portal vein, dark pink color: inferior vena cava (IVC), pink color: segment I, yellow color: segment II, light green: segment III, light blue color: segment IVa, orange color: segment IVb, dark blue color: segment V, purple color: segment VI, dark green color: segment VII, light green segment VIII

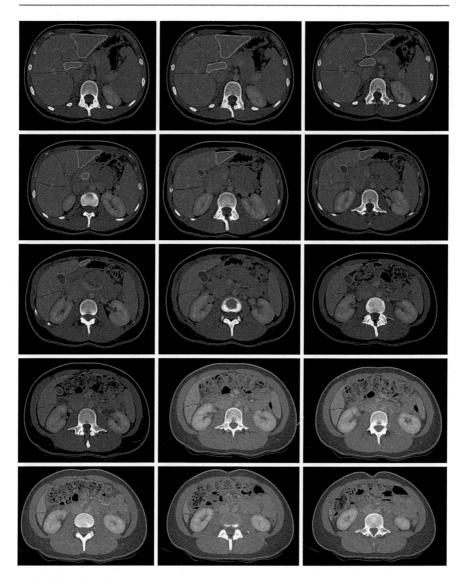

Fig. 5.1 (continued)

The left lobe of the liver includes:

a. Segment II (lateral superior)
b. Segment III (lateral inferior)
c. Segment IVA (medial superior)
d. Segment IVB (medial inferior)

The right lobe of the liver includes

a. Segment V (anterior inferior)
b. Segment VI (posterior inferior)
c. Segment VII (posterior superior)
d. Segment VIII (anterior superior)

The right anterior and posterior segments are divided by a vertical plane through the right hepatic vein (V and VIII anteriorly from VI and VII posteriorly).

The falciform ligament separates the left lateral and medial segments (II and III from IV). A plane of the main right and left portal vein demarcates superior from inferior segments (VII and VIII from V and VI). Gallbladder should be excluded. Inferior vena cava should be excluded when it is discrete from the liver.

The portal vein (PV) should be included in the liver contour when segment I (caudate lobe) is seen to the left of PV.

By the intersection of the superior mesenteric vein (SMV) and splenic vein (SV) the PV is formed. It is located posterior to the common bile duct and hepatic artery. The PV bifurcates into right posterior portal vein, right anterior portal vein and left portal vein. The left gastric vein enters the PV near its SV/PV confluence.

5.1.3 Pathophysiology

During RT treatment of gastrointestinal (GI) cancers, liver radiation exposure commonly occurs because of its large size and its proximity to the gastrointestinal organs.

Radiation-induced liver injuries (RILD) involve a complex cascade of radiobiological processes that occur as an acute response during or within a few weeks of RT or a late-response can happen months to years after completion of RT. Irradiation of the healthy tissue of the liver may cause cell damage resulting in loss of liver function.

Ingold et al. described the first report of a dose–complication relationship for RILD [2], but has not been investigated with its clinical findings so far. Radiation-induced liver injury is a major limitation of RT in the treatment of liver metastases or liver cancer due to consequence of liver cirrhosis and is accompanied by fatigue, rapid weight gain, and ascites. However, few patients develop liver insufficiency and treatment-associated mortality.

Following injury to the hepatic parenchyma after irradiation, production of growth factors and other cytokines such as tumor necrosis factor alpha (TNF-α) and transforming growth factor beta (TGF-β) occur. This cascade stimulates fibroblasts that would migrate to the regions of hepatic injury, causing collagen deposition. The early events is stellate cell proliferation in the affected sites and myofibroblastic transformation is thought to be responsible to liver damage in the pathogenesis of

Table 5.1 Clinical manifestations of radiation-induced liver toxicity

Classic RILD	Non-classic RILD
Clinical presentation: Weight gain, fatigue and abdominal right upper quadrant pain	Clinical presentation: Total bilirubin elevation and low albumin values
Alkaline phosphatase elevation	Transaminases elevation (up to five times)
Ascites	Increase ≥2 points in Child–Pugh (CP) score
Anicteric hepatomegaly	Absence of classic features

veno-occlusive disease [3–7]. The final and undesired scene of the veno-occlusive disease is the injury of sinusoidal endothelial cells causing a series of biologic processes leading to fibrosis and obstruction of liver blood flow [8, 9].

Some of the symptoms and signs of patients with classic RILD are abdominal pain, hepatomegaly, fatigue, anicteric ascites, increased abdominal girth, alkaline phosphatase (ALP) increases by more than twofold, whereas levels of transaminase and bilirubin remain normal 1–3 months after liver RT [10]. By complete obliteration of the central vein by erythrocytes with reticulin and collagen fibers the characterized hepatic veno-occlusive disease (VOD) of classic RILD occurs [11, 12].

Decreased oxygen delivery to the central zone results in the death of centrilobular hepatocytes (HCs) and atrophy of the inner hepatic plate, leading to hepatic dysfunction and hepatic fibrosis [13].

Non-classic RILD patients have usually chronic hepatic diseases, such as cirrhosis or with hepatitis B from a variety of causes, with hepatocellular loss, hepatic dysfunction, hepatic sinusoidal endothelial death, loss of regenerating hepatocytes and show more abnormal hepatic functions with jaundice like elevated serum transaminases (a more than fivefold increase compared to normal levels) rather than ALP [14, 15] (Table 5.1).

After hepatic irradiation in these patients, hepatocellular regeneration capacity breaks down and ends up with irreversible hepatic failure [16].

The use of Child–Pugh score helps us to characterize the outcomes of patients who develop non-classic RILD. Some published have identified studies various dose thresholds for the hepatic function. The most commonly used criterion in cirrhotic patients is an increase in Child–Pugh score ≥2.

5.1.4 Dose Constraints

Because of its rich blood supply metastases occur commonly in the liver and systemic therapy is often the preferred therapy. In selected patients and in some situations like limited involvement of the liver, surgical resection, focal ablation, or RT can be considered.

Ingold et al. described the classic RILD in 1 out of 8 patients (12.5%) who received 30–35 Gy and in 12 out of 27 patients (44%) who received 35 Gy [2]. In patients with normal liver function, conventionally fractionated RT doses above 30 Gy to the whole liver have a probability of 5–10% of developing classic RILD [14, 17]. The literature in subsequent years showed that partial liver irradiation to high doses is safe, as long as a sufficient volume of normal liver parenchyma is spared from high doses [18, 19]. Emami et al. estimated conventionally fractionated RT doses for one-third, two-third, and the whole liver to incur in a 5% risk of RILD at 5 years (TD5/5) were 50 Gy, 35 Gy, and 30 Gy, respectively [19].

By limiting the mean liver dose, the dose to the central liver, where the bile duct and venous vasculature fuse and sparing a sufficient amount of liver parenchyma may reduce the risk of RILD [20–22]. A dosimetric analysis conducted by Osmundson in 2015 demonstrated that a significant dose-dependent relationship was identified between the central hepatobiliary tract (cHBT) volumes and Grade ≥ 3 liver toxicities of 96 patients treated with liver SBRT. Biliary stricture or infection was the most common G3 toxicity observed in this study. V66 and V72 values were predictors for RILD on multivariable analysis [23]. In another study made by Toesca DA et al. with 130 patients, a significant dose–response relationship again was seen only for patients treated for HCC and CCA between the dose to the cHBT and the risk of RILD. V40 < 37 mL, V30 < 45 mL, and the mean cHBT dose <25 Gy were the predictors for RILD, while mean liver dose was not predictive on multivariate analysis. In this study to predict the probability of Grade ≥3 liver toxicity a nomogram was created including albumin–bilirubin (ALBI) score and primary liver cancer histology (HCC vs CCA) and cHBT15 V40. Compared with CP class the ALBI grade has been shown to more precisely predict worsening of liver function and survival in HCC patients following SBRT [24]. During treatment plan evaluation, the central hepatobiliary region needs special attention. The liver dose should be kept around 20–30 Gy and spare more of the normal liver while taking into account dose to other normal structures. The Stanford group recommends a central biliary tract dose of $V_{BED10}40 < 37$ cc, and $V_{BED10}30 < 45$ cc for patients treated with SBRT [24]. The dose constraint of sparing ≥700 cm³ from receiving >15 Gy in three fractions has been reported in many studies as a safe threshold for liver metastases treatment with the SBRT technique and with low toxicity rates [25, 26]. Lower radiation doses can induce liver toxicity for patients with underlying liver dysfunction [24–27]. Among 109 patients treated for primary liver cancer with hypofractionated 3DCRT, 9 out of 16 (56%) CP class B patients developed RILD, compared with 8 out of 93 (9%) CP class A patients, and severity of liver dysfunction was the only independent predictor of RILD on multivariable analysis [28]. Additionally, in a study patients with chronic hepatitis virus infection had worsened liver function, and had been associated with an increased sensitivity to radiation [29–31]. Dose–volume constraints for organs at risk with Biologic Equivalent Dose (BED) from selected studies are shown in Table 5.2.

Table 5.2 Dose–volume constraints for organs at risk with Biologic Equivalent Dose (BED) from selected studies

Organ at risk	Study	Dose—volume constraint (VGy)	Biologic equivalent dose
Liver	Herfarth [32]	V12 < 30%	V60 < 30%
	Wulf [33]	V7 < 30%	V29.3 < 50%
	Mendez Romero [34]	D30 < 7 Gy	3 fx
		D50 < 5 Gy	V12.4 < 30%
		V21 < 33%	V7.8 < 50%
		V15 < 50%	

Systemic therapy administration like immunotherapy or chemotherapy, prior liver directed therapies such as transarterial chemoembolization (TACE) or transarterial radio-embolization (TARE), small hepatic reserve and portal vein (PV) thrombosis are other factors that may increase the probability of RILD [28, 35–37]. In a study an increased risk for development of veno-occlusive disease was associated with the presence of tumors within healthy liver parenchyma [38]. Stereotactic body therapy, dose prescription, and local control rates from selected series are shown in Tables 5.3, 5.4, and 5.5.

Table 5.3 Stereotactic body therapy doses, local control rates, and toxicity rates from selected series

Study	Sample	Dose	Prescription	Local control	Toxicity
Blomgren et al. [39]	14 patients with metastases (mets)	7–45 Gy	ICRU point	50% response rate 1 hemorrhagic gastritis	50% response rate 1 hemorrhagic gastritis
Herfarth et al. [32]	37 patients with mets	1 × (14–26 Gy)	Isocenter 80% isodose surrounding PTV	71% 1 year 68% 2 years	None
Schefter et al. [40]	63 mets	3 × (12–20 Gy)	Isodose surrounding PTV	92% at 2 years	
Wulf et al. [33]	39 patients with mets 5 with HCC	3 × 10 Gy 3 × 12.5 Gy 1 × 26 Gy	65% isodose	100% HCC last follow up 66% 2 years mets	None
Mendez Romero et al. [34]	34 patients with mets, 11 with HCC	3 × 12.5 Gy At risk patients 5 × 5 Gy	65% isodose line	84% 2 years	1 classic RILD (liver failure and fatal infection, pt Child B initial) 1 portal hypertension with melena 2 elevation GGT Grade 3
McCammon et al. [41]	81 patients with mets and primaries	3 × 10 Gy to 3 × 20 Gy	Isodose surrounding PTV (80–90%)	100% (54–60 Gy) 89% (31.1–53.9 Gy) 100% (54–60 Gy) 89% (31.1–53.9 Gy)	None

Table 5.3 (continued)

Study	Sample	Dose	Prescription	Local control	Toxicity
Rusthoven et al. [42]	47 patients with 63 mets	3 × 12–20 Gy	80 or 90% isodose	92% 2 years	1 Grade 3 soft tissue toxicity
Goodman et al. [43]	26 patients with 40 lesions	18–30 Gy single dose cyber knife	Isodose surrounding PTV	77% 1 year	No limiting toxicity
Tse et al. [44]	47 HCC IHC	6 × 9–0 Gy	Not specified	65% 1 year	10 Grade 3 liver enzymes 1 bleeding from tumor duodenal connection (lethal) 1 SBO (lethal)
Andolino et al. [45]	60 HCC	3 × 14 (CTP) A 5 × 8 (CTP B)	80% isodose	90% 2 years	20% progression CTP class none non-hematologic toxicity ≥3 within 3 months
Andratschke et al. [46]	74 pts 91 mets	5–12.5 Gy 3–5 fns	60–95% surrounding isodose	Local control 74.7% 1 year	
Bujold et al. [47]	102 HCC	6 × 6 Gy (24–54)		Local control 87% 1 year	36% Grade ≥3 toxicity
Sanuki et al. [48]	185 HCC	5 × (30–40 Gy)		Local control 99% 1 year	13% Grade ≥3 toxicity
Jang et al. [49]	108 HCC	3 × 17 (33–60 Gy)		Local control 87% at 2 years	10% Grade ≥3 toxicity
Bujold et al. [47]	56 HCC (with vascular thrombosis)	6 × 6 (24–54) Median 36 Gy		1 year OS 44%	
Yoon et al. [50]	412 HCC (with vascular thrombosis)	2–5 Gy/fx Total 21–60 Gy		Median survival 10.6 months	10% Grade ≥3 toxicity
Lee et al. [51]	68 patients with mets	Median 41.8 Gy 6 fns 2 weeks	Isodose max in PTV 140%	71% 1 year	Grade 5 SBO + Grade 4 bleed (progression) SBO abdominal hernia Grade 3 gastritis/oesophagitis 2

Table 5.4 Summary of RILD according to radiation dose

Study	Fractionation	5% Risk of RILD			Cases of RILD	No of patients
		Whole liver (Gy)	2/3 liver (Gy)	1/3 liver (Gy)		
Austin-Seymour [18]	2–3 Gy daily	–	–	35	1	11
Emami [19]	2 Gy daily	30	35	50	27	407
Burman [52]	2 Gy daily	30	34	43	27	407
Lawrence [53]	1.5 Gy bid	35	45	72	9	79
Jackson [21]	1.5 Gy bid	35	52	–	9	93
Dawson [54]	1.5 Gy bid	31	47	90	19	183

Table 5.5 Liver dose limitation recommendations for hepatocellular carcinoma

	Conformal RT	SBRT	
Child–Pugh class	A	A	B
Mean non-GTV liver dose	≤28 Gy, in 1.8–2 Gy/fractions	<13 Gy in three fractions	<6 Gy in 4–6 Gy/fractions
		≤13 Gy if prescription dose is 50 Gy in five fractions	
		≤15 Gy if prescription dose is 40 Gy in five fractions	
		≤16 Gy if prescription dose is 30 Gy in five fractions	
Critical volume model		<18 Gy to 800 mL liver, in three fractions	

For treating primary hepatic tumors, and metastases SBRT is also an efficient alternative to local surgery, or chemoembolization. Using strict criteria to protect healthy organs, SBRT associated with IGRT offers a high therapeutic index.

The presented data and published results seem to be safe concerning both acute and late toxicity and demonstrate a potential for lasting local control achieved by stereotactic treatment of intrahepatic malignancy if restrictions to normal tissue dose and patient selection are respected. Nevertheless the most appropriate dose and fractionation scheme has not been determined yet.

5.1.5 Treatment

Stereotactic body radiation therapy (SBRT) is delivered in a curative intent to many primary and secondary tumors. Concerning liver metastasis, SBRT can be safely delivered using one to five fractions. An excellent local control is obtained with doses from 20 to 60 Gy. For primary hepatic tumors, results are also good, but the risk of hepatic toxicity related to liver preexistent pathology must be taken into account.

In summary, patients with Child–Pugh B or C scores have a higher risk of RT-related problems than those with Child–Pugh A scores. Impaired liver functions, hepatitis, prior transcatheter arterial chemoembolization, portal vein tumor thrombosis, concurrent chemotherapy, tumor stage [55], and male sex [28] cause a higher risk of RILD.

Various strategies are being investigated to prevent or minimize radiation-induced hepatotoxicity. Stem cell therapy has been shown to promote the regeneration of irradiated normal tissues [56, 57]. TGF-β showed a radiation dose-dependent increase, and suppression of TGF-β was reported to reduce hepatic fibrosis in the irradiated livers of experimental animal models [58, 59].

In addition, the Hedgehog (Hh) pathway in liver may also play a role in RILD progression [60, 61]. In irradiated mice the blockade of Hh reduced the hepatic toxicity and fibrogenic response by inhibiting myofibroblast accumulation [60]. These results suggest that the Hh pathway may be a potential target for therapeutic strategies for RILD.

In summary there is no clear and precise treatment after RILD has occurred.

5.1.6 Rx: Sample Prescriptions

To protect healthy liver tissue from radiation-induced damage some radioprotectors are used in combination therapy with RT.

- Protect HCs from radiation-induced damage: Amifostine [62].
- Decreasing oxidative stress: Melatonin [63].
- Fluid retention: Diuretics
- Ascites: Paracentesis
- Reducing hepatic congestion: Steroids [20].

Because of their intolerable side effects the use of such radioprotectors in routine clinical practice is still being investigated.

5.2 Kidney

5.2.1 Anatomy

The *kidneys* are the main organs of the urinary system. They are two bean-shaped organs and are located in retroperitoneal space. They typically locate between transvers processes of T12 and L3 vertebrae, although the right kidney is often located in the inferior position than the left due to the presence of the liver. The kidneys move few centimeters by respiration. The position of kidney is important due to surrounding organs. They are surrounded by adrenal glands in superior, the second part of the duodenum on the right side, the greater curvature of the stomach on the left side, the spleen in anterior, the colon in inferior, and the diaphragm in posterior. The peritoneum lies to fascia and helps to attach the kidneys to the posterior abdominal wall in a retroperitoneal space.

The kidneys are covered by the fibrous capsule that protects and holds their shape. The fibrous capsule is surrounded by adipose tissue called renal fat pad to protect them from trauma and turns a thin connective fascia called Gerota capsule. There is a region that is called renal hilum, for the entry and exit of kidney vessels, nerves, lymphatics, and also ureters. The renal pelvis emerging from the hilum is formed from the funnel-shaped expansion of the major and minor calyxes in the kidney. Urine is transported by peristaltic movements of smooth muscle in the renal hilum to the ureter. In the longitudinal section of the kidney, two main sites are seen: renal cortex and renal medulla. The renal cortex is the outer part of the kidney. Here, the capillary network called glomeruli is located. Each kidney has about one million glomeruli. The renal medulla is the inner part of the kidney and seen as 12–18 pyramid-shaped structures. These structures, called pyramids, are opened to 8–20 minor calyces. The place where the pyramids are opened to minor calyces is called papillae. The medulla is composed of tubules which are essentially extensions of the glomeruli and is free of glomeruli. The blood circulation of the medulla is poorer than the cortex. Therefore, it is very sensitive to ischemic damage.

The kidneys have important functions including filtration and excretion of urea and ammonium, regulation of fluid, electrolytes, acid–base balance, stimulation of red blood cell production, and regulation of some hormons. The nephrons are the "functional units" of the kidneys which have the important role for cleaning the blood and balancing the constituents of the circulation. There is an important issue: the kidneys are fully formed at birth, and no formation of nephrons is developed after that. There are adrenal glands on the superior of each kidney and cortex of the adrenal directly influences renal function through the production of the hormone aldosterone to stimulate sodium reabsorption.

5.2.2 Contouring

The kidneys are relatively easy to identify on the planning computerized tomography scan, even without intravenous contrast. Each kidney should be contoured as a whole organ. The renal pelvis is usually included in kidney contours. Ideally, the kidney parenchyma should be contoured separately because it is the "functional" component of kidney. In Fig. 5.2, the contouring of both the kidneys is presented on computerized tomography images.

5.2.3 Pathophysiology

The kidneys are the dose-limiting organs for radiotherapy to upper abdominal cancers and total body irradiation. The incidence of radiation-induced toxicity is probably underestimated due to its latency and confounding factors like chemotherapy.

The pathophysiology of radiation nephropathy is poorly understood. All histopathological knowledge of radiation damage in days to weeks after irradiation comes from animal studies [64, 65]. The human studies are limited and data comes from late or end-stage renal disease months or years after irradiation. In the past, the term nephritis was commonly used for terminology of radiation-induced kidney toxicity. Later, the terminology has changed to nephropathy, because inflammation is rarely associated with renal toxicity [66]. In radiation nephropathy, all

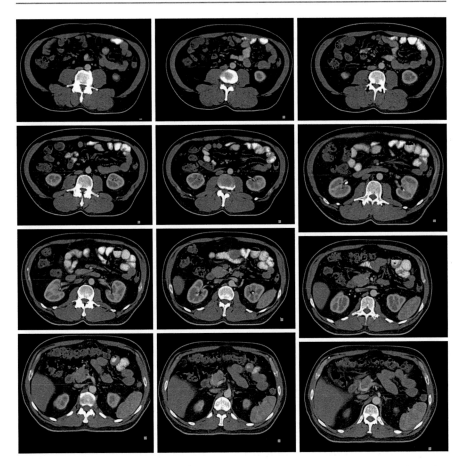

Fig. 5.2 The contouring of both the kidneys on computerized tomography images. Blue color: right and left kidney

components of kidney are affected, including the glomeruli, blood vessels, tubular epithelium, and interstitium. The architecture of the kidney is considered as subunits predominantly arranged "in parallel" while with some serial function. The nephrons are the "functional units" of the kidneys which have the important role for cleaning the blood and balancing the constituents of the circulation. The nephrons are arranged as parallel and consist of glomerulus with capillary network and a proximal and distal convoluted tubules. Although the nephron is considered as an organ which consists of cells in series, if one of these is functionally damaged, the parallel arrangement of many such units permit to developing significant cumulative damage without clinical or functional significance.

An intact vasculature of kidney is important for the kidney function. In radiation-induced nephropathy, the glomerular endothelial injury and mesangiolysis are characteristic on light and electron microscopy [64, 67]. After irradiation, the glomerular capillary endothelial cell damage which is important for nephropathy occurs first.

The glomerular capillary endothelial cell loss and increased permeability of remaining endothelial cells are seen within few weeks of irradiation. In this case, increased amount of protein and high molecular weight blood components escape from the capillaries and cause subendothelial transudate. The glomerular scarring starts to evoluate due to thrombotic microangiopathy. On the other hand, there is also mediator expression, such as TGFβ1 or activation of renin–angiotensin system, causing tubulointerstitial scarring. In addition, some mesangial changes, including hypercellularity, hypertrophy, increased mesangial matrix, mesangial sclerosis are seen. These endothelial changes consist atypism, and tubular necrosis that are temporary. Tubular injury appears to occur shortly after glomerular injury. However, the fibrosis of perivascular connective tissue is late toxicity and has progressive nature. This progressive nature of fibrosis may cause atrophy of tubules and reflects the significant degrees of interstitial fibrosis which is the late effect of irradiation [68–70]. Any injury to kidneys can affect glomerular filtration, salt and water balance, acid–base balance, water metabolism, the homeostasis of phosphorus and uric acid. The overall filtering function of kidneys may reduce with direct glomerular or tubular injuries. Additionally, the kidney has an important role for feedback control of red blood cell formation and blood pressure regulation.

Radiation-induced kidney damages are seen into subclinical and clinical. Acute kidney damage is usually subclinical. In subacute period, the signs of damage such as decreased glomerular filtration rate (GFR), increased serum b2-microglobulin occur. Finally, the characteristic signs and symptoms which are benign or malignant hypertension, elevated creatinine levels, anemia, and renal failure are seen in late period (3–18 months). Most toxicity occurs around 18 months. The long latency for clinical kidney toxicity was reported in Thompson et al.'s study [71]. However, if no changes in renal blood perfusion or GFR are developed within 2 years after irradiation subsequent chronic damage is rare [72, 73]. The hemolytic-uremic syndrome, which is characterized by microangiopathic hemolytic anemia and thrombocytopenia, is also seen after total body irradiation (TBI) [74].

5.2.4 Dose Constraints

The kidneys, which are highly radiosensitive organs, are dose-limiting structures in abdominal radiation. However, the existing published data mainly comes from patients treated without computerized tomography-based planning. Also, in the literature, there is limited data on dose–volume parameters for late renal toxicity. Because of the clinical practice, the irradiated kidney volume is tried to be minimized to avoid late toxicities [75]. Typically, the doses of receiving each kidney alone and combined should be evaluated. With modern CT-based planning, there are uncertainties about up to 3–7 cm movement or shifts of kidneys' position with breathing or supine/prone position [76, 77]. Therefore, the planned kidney doses would be different than actual kidney doses.

The kidneys are the dose-limiting organs for lymphomas, gastrointestinal and gynecological cancers, and during total body irradiation (TBI) [70]. The risk of radiation-induced kidney toxicity depends on the use of whole or partial volume to one or both kidneys. Additionally, the risk of radiation nephropathy may increase in using nephrotoxic chemotherapeutic agents. Total body irradiation is also one of the main risk factors to development of radiation nephropathy due to irradiation of both kidneys. In the comprehensive review of 12 studies reporting kidney toxicity after TBI in adult patients, Cheng et al. found the dose the only significant factor associated with kidney toxicity on multivariate analysis [78]. Chemotherapy can also increase radiotherapy-induced kidney injury in TBI or non-TBI.

The radiation-induced nephropathy is characterized by renal injury and loss of function. This will occur after sufficient irradiation of both kidneys [79]. In one of the earlier studies, Luxton RW described 23 Gy as the threshold dose for radiation nephropathy if both kidneys irradiated in abdominal radiotherapy with 20 fractions over 4 weeks [80]. In the TBI patients, single dose of 10 Gy or 14 Gy in three fractions was reported as a dose leading nephropathy [81]. More recently, in the review of Dawson et al., the dose volume constraints for radiation-induced kidney toxicity were evaluated in several studies of TBI and non-TBI [70]. In case of whole kidney irradiation for TBI patients the dose associated with a 5% risk of kidney toxicity, without nephrotoxic drugs, was defined as 9.8 Gy, regardless of fractionation regimens. In both kidney irradiation for non-TBI, this risk was seen with a 5% and 50% risk of injury at 5 years of 18–23 Gy and 28 Gy.

In unilateral kidney irradiation, there is still risk for renal toxicity after many years. There is a dose response for kidney atrophy, increase in serum creatinine and clinical signs. The scintigraphic changes can occur without clinical symptoms, and these can be observed at doses <10 Gy [82]. If ≥50 volume of one kidney is receiving ≥26 Gy, 10% of decreased creatinine clearance was found in 12–18 months after radiotherapy [71, 83, 84]. The relationship was also reported between the volume of kidney receiving >20 Gy or the mean kidney dose and increased risk of renal toxicity. The irradiation with 20 Gy results in an apparent size and activity reduction in the scintigraphy [82]. The partial kidney damage has been detected after even low doses such as 3–6 Gy in 15–30 fractions in scintigraphy. May KS et al. reported that the patients who received 25 Gy to 25% of the irradiated kidney and 40 Gy to 40% of irradiated kidney had ≥5% of decrease in relative renal functions [85]. When one kidney is irradiated with higher doses than threshold, radiation injury occurs in that kidney, but renal failure will not develop. But, the unirradiated volume of kidney is injured from the renin mediated hypertension due to unilateral renal scarring [86]. If the total irradiated renal volume is <30% of both kidneys, the small injury leading to hypertension may be occur in irradiated volume [87]. The importance of monitoring V5 and V10 kidney doses was reported in complex techniques such as intensity modulated radiation therapy (IMRT) era, due to low dose in a larger area. Diavolitsis et al. found the strongest correlations when using V5 and V10 of kidney treated to >20 Gy with decreased creatinine clearance more than expected [88].

There is limited data on dose–volume parameters to predict late renal toxicity. The tolerance doses of kidney for various end points were defined in studies. In the case of total body irradiation, the dose responsible for a 5% risk of toxicities is around 16 Gy in 2 Gy fractions over 2 weeks. Earlier, Rubin and Casarett described the 5% risk of complication within 5 years (TD 5/5) of 20 Gy and 50% risk of complication within 5 years (TD50/5) of 25 Gy in whole kidney irradiation with conventional fractions for nephrosclerosis while Cohen and Creditor defined TD 5/5 of 21–31 Gy [89, 90]. Flentje M et al. defined a median dose of 17.5–21.5 Gy and 22–26 Gy associated to a 5% and 50% late toxicity risk, respectively, such as anemia, azotemia, hypertension, and edema [75]. In 1991, Emami et al. published a landmark review about the tolerance dose of normal tissues. They recommended TD 5/5 of 50 Gy, 30 Gy, and 23 Gy for irradiation of one-third, two-third, and the entire kidney while TD 50/5 of 40 Gy and 28 Gy for irradiation of two-third and the entire kidney for clinical nephritis end point [91]. The TD 50/5 for one-third of organ irradiation was not recommended because this volume is routinely irradiated in many clinical cases without any major toxicity. Milano et al. updated the Emami normal tissue dose constraints [92]. Consequently due to limited published data renal dose tolerance limits could not be modified. In the more recent QUANTEC review, Marks LB et al. concluded the mean dose of bilateral whole organ volume <15–18 Gy for 5% and <28 Gy for 50% of clinically relevant renal dysfunction risk in three-dimensional conformal planning, except TBI. There are also some dose–volume suggestions that the risk of clinically relevant renal dysfunction will be <5% if the percent volume of kidney receiving <12 Gy (V12) is <55 and V20 < 32%, V23 < 30%, V28 < 20% [93].

When nephrotoxic chemotherapeutic agents are used with radiotherapy, tolerance dose limits should be reduced. In the case of cisplatin used before or after abdominal radiotherapy, the cumulative safe cisplatin dose of 200 mg/m^2 was reported when limiting 37.5% of the kidney volume to ≤12 Gy [94]. For the paraaortic irradiation of gynecological tumors with IMRT, the maximum dose of 45 Gy and V16 of 35% was used as a renal dose constraint [95]. May et al. observed correlation between pre-RT creatinine clearance, V10, mean dose of kidney and decline in creatinine clearance at 1 year after chemotherapy and abdominal radiotherapy [96]. This suggests that the dose response curve may be lower than proposed for chemoradiation-induced nephropathy. After injury in one kidney, a compensatory increase in kidney function of the spared kidney usually develops. The reserve capacity of unirradiated kidney is important to improve findings with time [70]. In Table 5.6 some recommendations for dose limits of kidney are presented.

Table 5.6 Kidney dose limitation recommendations for non-TBI

Treatment technique	Delineation of organ	Limits	End point
3D-CRT/IMRT (with conventional fractionation)	Whole kidney (combined)	Each kidney mean dose <15–18 Gy If one kidney mean dose >18 Gy, maximally spare other kidney (V6 Gy <30%) V12 < 55% V23 < 30% V28 < 20%	Renal toxicity <5%
Stereotactic body radiotherapy (with 3–5 ablative fractionation)	Whole kidney	Volume < 200 mL Dmax ≤ 14.4 Gy (3 fx) and ≤17.5 Gy (5 fx)	Basic renal function

5.2.5 Treatment

The clinical signs of radiation-induced nephropathy vary according to dose and volume of irradiation. The presentation can be acute and irreversible with progressive dysfunction over years. There is also latent period that is clinically silent until manifestation [87]. According to Luxton classification, the radiation nephropathy is grouped as acute, chronic, hypertensive forms with variants of the benign and malignant [81]. The clinical syndromes following renal irradiation are acute radiation nephropathy at 6–12 months, chronic radiation nephropathy at ≥18 months, malignant hypertension at 12–18 months, and benign hypertension at ≥18 months. The typical clinical presentation of acute radiation nephropathy is decreased kidney function, proteinuria, hypertension, and anemia. There is elevation in levels of serum creatinine and BUN. Fluid retention, edema, and hypertension are seen in the patients after receiving radiation dose to kidney. Severe cases have features of thrombotic microangiopathy. There are various degrees of normochromic normocytic anemia and features of intravascular hemolysis. If acute radiation nephropathy is left untreated, it may progress to renal failure and chronic dialysis.

First of all, if the radiation-induced renal toxicity has been seen, patients should be referred to a nephrologist. There is no treatment guide for radiation-induced nephropathy. Therefore, treatment is managed by the same principles of treatment of any hypertensive kidney disease with blood pressure and metabolic acidosis control. A dietary protein and salt restriction for renal workload may help to delay the progression of renal failure. Also, it is useful for managing of anemia, secondary hyperparathyroidism, and water–electrolyte balance.

Treatment of radiation-induced nephropathy may include angiotensin-converting enzyme (ACE) inhibitors or angiotensin II receptor blockers (ARBs). The mechanism of the benefit of ACE inhibitors or AII blockers in radiation nephropathy is not very well established. Angiotensin II is known as a renal cell growth facilitator [73]. The protection effect of ACE inhibitors and AII blockers could came from delay or inhibition of renal cell proliferation which occurs in the first few weeks of radiation nephropathy. Preventive use of these agents significantly attenuates the tubular component that is responsible for proliferative response. Animal models showed that angiotensin-converting enzyme inhibitors, dexamethasone, and acetylsalicylic acid can prevent and treat radiation-related kidney injuries [97, 98]. ACE inhibitors and AII receptor antagonists are more effective agents in the prevention and treatment of radiation nephropathy [99–101]. The angiotensin-converting enzyme inhibitors have been shown to reduce glomerular sclerosis more than other antihypertensive agents [102]. Therefore, ACE inhibitors are useful for slowing the progression of chronic renal failure [100]. They may improve kidney failure and reduce the incidence of nephropathy or hemolytic uremic syndrome in patients treated with TBI [99, 103]. The captopril which is the angiotensin-converting enzyme inhibitor was found to successfully mitigate radiation nephropathy caused by 18.8 Gy in six fractions when drug was used 3.5–10 weeks after TBI. The interval of 4–10 weeks after radiation is critical in the pathogenesis of radiation nephropathy; before and after this period there was less benefit [101, 104, 105]. Additionally, hypertension aggravates most forms of kidney disease [106]. The successful control of the blood pressure slows down the progression of kidney diseases. For high blood pressure, one of the several effective antihypertensive drugs can be used.

Severe cases may have features of thrombotic microangiopathy. In these patients, plasmapheresis may beneficial for hemolytic uremic syndrome and thrombocytopenia, but appears to have no benefit on the renal manifestations [107]. The blood transfusion and/or parenteral erythropoietin might be used for anemia.

Despite appropriate treatment, radiation nephropathy may evolve to complete renal failure and the need for dialysis or kidney transplant (i.e., end-stage renal disease). Unfortunately, the survival of such dialysis patients is poor [108]. Kidney transplantation may be possible.

5.2.6 Rx: Sample Prescriptions

There is a summary of recommendations for kidney toxicity below:

- Refer to a nephrologist
- Dietary protein restriction
- Salt restriction
- To reduce glomerular sclerosis (ACE inhibitors (Captopril), Angiotensin II blocker (losartan))
- Antihypertensive drugs (if benign/malign hypertension present)
- Plasmapheresis (if hemolytic uremic syndrome and thrombocytopenia present)
- Erythropoietin (if anemia is present)
- Dialysis and renal transplantation (if renal failure)

5.3 Stomach

Following irradiation of lower thoracic, abdominal, or pelvic malignancies early and late gastrointestinal (GI) injury of the stomach may occur that becasue the stomach is located within the radiation field. Therefore, stomach tolerance may limit radiation doses that can be delivered.

5.3.1 Anatomy

The stomach, is an intraperitoneal muscular digestive organ located between the esophagus and the duodenum and is located on the left side of the upper abdomen. The exact size, shape, and position of the stomach can vary from person to person and with position and respiration. It receives food from the esophagus through a muscular valve called the lower esophageal sphincter.

The stomach has many functions over digestion like hydrochloric acid, pepsin, intrinsic factor, and gastric lipase secretion. In addition, the stomach secretes gastrin into the blood stream which stimulates release of hydrochloric acid and pepsinogen in the stomach and by a thin layer of mucus secreted by mucus surface and neck cells, the gastric epithelial cells are protected from gastric acid.

The stomach wall is composed of four layers:

a. Mucosa
b. Submucosa
c. Muscularis
d. Serosa.

The muscularis layer is composed of three (outer-longitudinal, middle, inner-oblique) layer.

The stomach has four main anatomical divisions:

- Cardia: Surrounds the superior opening of the stomach at the T11 level.
- Fundus: Often gas filled portion of the stomach. It is located in superior left of the cardia.
- Body: The large central portion of the stomach.
- Pylorus: The connection part of the stomach to duodenum. It comprises the pyloric antrum, pyloric canal, and pyloric sphincter.

Greater and Lesser Curvatures
The lesser and greater curvatures form the medial and lateral borders of the stomach.

The anatomical relations of the stomach are as follows:

- *Superior*: Esophagus and left dome of the diaphragm
- *Anterior*: Diaphragm, greater omentum, anterior abdominal wall, left lobe of liver, gall bladder
- *Posterior*: Lesser sac, pancreas, left kidney, left adrenal gland, spleen, splenic artery, transverse mesocolon

There are two sphincters of the stomach, located at each orifice. They control the passage of materials entering and exiting the stomach.

- *Inferior Esophageal Sphincter*
- At the level of Torakal 10, the esophagus passes through the diaphragm and descends and forms the inferior esophageal sphincter at the T11 level. The inferior esophageal sphincter allows food to pass through the cardiac orifice into the stomach.
- *Pyloric Sphincter*
- The pyloric sphincter lies between the pylorus and the first part of the duodenum.
- It contains smooth muscle and is an anatomical sphincter.

5.3.2 Contouring

Gastroesophageal Junction (GEJ):

- The line between the squamous esophageal mucosa and the gastric columnar mucosa, the GEJ is marked on the mucosal surface by the Z line.
- The GEJ should include the most distal esophagus and its interface with the cardia of the stomach [109–111].

The stomach (contoured as one organ) includes (Fig. 5.3):

- Cardia: begins at the GEJ. The lesser and greater curvatures of the stomach intersect here.
- Fundus: the most inferior part, abuts the left hemidiaphragm, left and superior to cardia

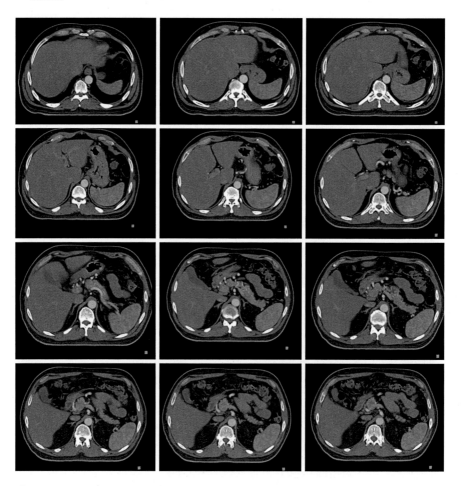

Fig. 5.3 The contouring of stomach on computerized tomography images

- Body: central, largest portion
- Antrum: gateway into the pylorus (the sphincter opening to the duodenum)

5.3.3 Pathophysiology

Radiation injury involves a complex cascade of radiobiological processes that occur as an acute response during or within a few weeks of RT or a late response can happen months to years after completion of RT. Stromal fibrosis occurs mostly as late RT injury and is related with the volume of tissue irradiated, total dose, dose per fraction, chemotherapy administration, and surgery.

It is known that, especially in some animal studies, radiation exposure the expression of tumor suppressor gene p53 after radiation exposure is increased in stem cell. After exposure to low-dose radiation programmed cell death (apoptosis) of GI crypts cells can be observed and the rate is dose dependent (stable at 1 Gy) [112–114].

A potent fibrogenic and pro-inflammatory cytokine TGF-β is activated by ionizing radiation by translation of the gene coding in the GI tract. The activation of TGF-β leads to hyperplasia of connective tissue mast cells and leukocyte migration into the GI wall. The expression of collagen and fibronectin genes are stimulated by TGF-β ending with chemotaxis of fibroblasts especially in regions with radiation damage [112–114]. There are three isoforms of TGF-β and are over-expressed in the early postradiation phase.

After radiation exposure in the early phase TGF-β1 messenger RNA is increased in fibroblasts and epithelial cells of the GI wall. Furthermore, increased TGF-β levels in pathological specimens of bowel patients undergoing surgery for radiation enteropathy were determined [115].

Another extracellular cytokine found to be responsible for the development of radiation injury by sustaining the activation of fibrogenesis in the irradiated GI tract is connective tissue growth factor (CTGF) which is increased in GI radiation fibrosis [116]. Mechanisms underlying the pathogenesis of radiation-induced GI damage remain an active area of investigation.

Following irradiation of patients with peptic ulcer, coagulation necrosis of chief and parietal cells with mucosal thinning, edema, and chronic inflammatory infiltration were reported [117, 118].

After an irradiation dose of 20–25 Gy endothelial swelling with gastric mucosal edema, nuclear pyknosis, and dilated capillaries occur. In higher doses, these changes appear more severely and may include mucosal erosion and capillary thrombosis resulting in symptomatic gastritis or gastric ulceration and the damage of mucosa results in loss of mucous, resulting in mucosal atrophy [119].

5.3.4 Dose Constraints

Goldstein et al. described 121 patients receiving 50 Gy to the para-aortic lymph nodes. This resulted in an ulceration rate of approximately 8% [120].

Table 5.7 Dose–volume constraints for stomach with biologic equivalent dose (BED) from selected studies

Organs at risk	Study	Dose–volume constraint (VGy)	Biologic equivalent dose
Stomach (alpha/beta 5)	Herfarth [32]	12 Gy max	40.8 Gy max
	Wulf [33]	D100 < 7 Gy	
	Mendez Romero [128]	D5 cc < 21 Gy	1 fx1 6.8 Gy max/3 fx10.3 Gy
	Tse [44]	V30 < 0.5 cc whole organ 50 Gy	max 3 fx V50.5 < 5 cc/5 fx V38.6 < 5 cc

In some studies acute gastric ulceration occurred at doses ranging from 43 to 49 Gy delivered over 5 weeks, with increased frequency observed at or above doses of 50 Gy delivered over a similar time period [121].

In some studies radiation therapy applied for Hodgkin's lymphoma or for testicular, gastric, or cervical cancers having tolerance limits for gastric irradiation were evaluated [122–125]. Gastric ulceration and gastric ulcer-associated perforation was reported in patients who received doses above 50 Gy at rates of 15% and 10%, respectively and these ulcers healed poorly. In a study conducted by Novak et al. after irradiation over 50 Gy to stomach eight patients required partial gastrectomy [126]. As a result of these studies doses above 55 Gy will result in gastric mucosal injury in 50% of patients.

In a study reported by Blomgren at higher doses per fraction, 20 Gy in four fractions or 21 Gy in three fractions, patients developed gastric ulceration [127].

Dose–volume constraints for stomach with biologic equivalent dose (BED) from selected studies are shown in Table 5.7.

5.3.5 Treatment

The incidence and severity of radiation-induced gastric injury depend on total radiation dose, radiation fraction size, treated volume, and the presence of other treatment modalities like systemic chemotherapy. The standard treatment method after radiation-induced gastric injury has not been established. After the occurrence of hemorrhagic gastritis antisecretory agents and H2 receptor antagonist drugs remained inadequate and all failed to control bleeding. Argon plasma coagulation had been reported for successful hemostasis of radiation-induced hemorrhagic gastritis or colitis [129–132]. Surgery may be necessary if other treatment fails, but it is associated with a high morbidity. Rectal steroids have often been recommended for the treatment of radiation-induced proctitis. Kochhar et al. [133] reported that steroids successfully treated radiation-induced proctosigmoiditis. But only few instances of Prednisolone can inhibit inflammation by a diverse array of mechanisms, including decreasing chemotaxis of monocytes and neutrophils, inhibiting adhesive molecule synthesis, and decreasing eicosanoid production.

5.3.6 Rx: Sample Prescriptions

- Gastric ulcer: Antisecretory agents and H2 receptor antagonist
- Hemorrhagic gastritis: Antisecretory agents, H2 receptor antagonist+argon plasma coagulation (APC)
- Gastric cramping/pain: Anticholinergic antispasmodic agents
- Perforation, fistula: Refer to surgeon

5.4 Duodenum

5.4.1 Anatomy

The small intestine including duodenum is a complex organ comprising a mucosa, a submucosa, a muscularis, and a serosa. The mucosa, a rapidly renewing tissue, is at the origin of the early radiation-induced toxicity. The other tunics, with slow renewal, are at the origin of the late toxicity. The intestinal tissue corollary gives sensitivity to fractionation and the risk of late toxicity.

5.4.2 Contouring

Duodenum (see Fig. 5.4)

- First portion: It is retroperitoneal and begins after the pylorus. It is suspended by hepatoduodenal ligament after an extension of 5 cm.
- Second (descending) portion: It is attached to the head of pancreas and the starting point is the superior duodenal flexure. It extends about 7.5 cm and is located to right of the IVC at levels L1–L3.
- Third (transverse) portion: Crosses in front of the aorta and inferior vena cava and is posterior to the superior mesenteric artery and superior mesenteric vein. It is about 10 cm, and marks the end of the C-loop of the duodenum.
- Fourth (ascending) portion: Travels superiorly until it is adjacent to the inferior pancreatic body, is about 2.5 cm long, lies anteriorly to the IMV until the IMV moves medially at the transition to the jejunum.

5.4.3 Pathophysiology

The intestinal mucosa is composed of crypts and villi and is completely renewed every 5 days. At the bottom of the crypts, the intestinal stem cells are multipotent and will give the progenitor cells, which themselves will turn into differentiated intestinal cells. They migrate along the crypts and then form the villi. The more a cell has a high proliferative potential, such as intestinal crypt cells, the more it is radiosensitive by radiation-induced mitotic death.

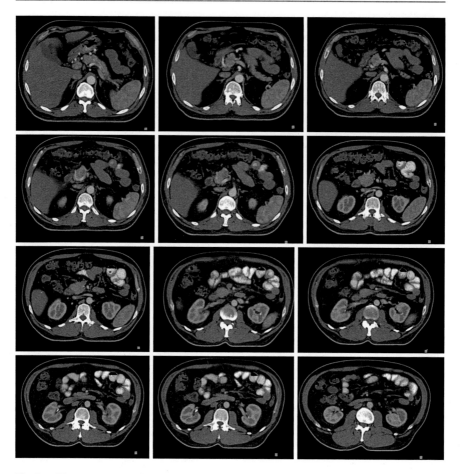

Fig. 5.4 The contouring of the duodenum on computerized tomography imaging

Irritable acute intestinal damage is mainly related to mitotic death of deep epithelial cells of intestinal crypts. However, irradiation does not inhibit cell migration from crypts to villi. This loss of mitotic activity, coupled with the continuous migration of cells leads to the denudation of the mucosal surface. The loss of the mucosal surface results in not only the loss of water, proteins, and electrolytes, but also the loss of the intestinal protection barrier that promotes the passage of antigens and bacteria responsible for an inflammatory reaction [134]. Radiotherapy also induces activation of myofibroblasts leading to collagen deposition and fibrosis of the submucosa. This phenomenon, added to the lesions of endothelial cells, leads to vascular degeneration, formation of neo-vessels with telangiectasia leading to chronic ischemia of the muscularis and serosa [135]. Detailed information about the intestinal pathophysiology is given in the previous section.

5.4.4 Dose Constraints

Today, radiotherapy indications under stereotaxic conditions are characterized by a prescription of high doses in a reduced volume, initially applied to the treatment of intracranial lesions, now extended to abdominal and pelvic lesions. The treatment of primary and secondary hepatic, pancreatic, adrenal, renal, prostatic, and abdominopelvic adenopathies is currently retained. For these locations, the main limitation to dose escalation allowing a better rate of tumor control is the dose constraint to organs at risk, including the small intestine. Defining these constraints optimally allows the optimization of high-precision radiotherapy, especially with the contribution of inverse planning for intensity modulated radiotherapy (IMRT) or in stereotaxic conditions.

The duodenum, considered as a serial organ, is sensitive at the maximum dose and volume receiving irradiation. Few studies have focused on reporting tolerance doses for the duodenum following conformal radiation therapy (Tables 5.8, 5.9, and 5.10).

In the treatment of abdominal tumors, intestinal toxicity remains the principal factor limiting the escalation of radiotherapy dose especially in SBRT treatment technique [148] (Table 5.10).

5.4.5 Treatment

The radiation induced duodenal toxicity is a new concept emerging with the introduction of stereotactic radiotherapy. In previous studies, evaluating the radiation induced gastrointestinal toxicity, duodenum was not seperately evaluated. In these studies, the treatment approach for duodenal toxicity is considered as the small bowel toxicity. Therefore, treatment approaches for duodenal toxicity will be described in the Sect. 5.5.5.

Table 5.8 Dosimetric parameters analyzed and correlation statistics with pathologic duodenal damage [136]

Parameter	Median (range)	P-value
Duodenal volume (cc)	90 (54–107)	0.06
Mean duodenal dose	20 (14–27)	0.003
Maximum duodenal dose	37 (28–44)	0.11
PTV volume (cc)	113 (71–249)	0.69
Mean PTV dose	37 (27–43)	0.03
Maximum PTV dose	39 (28–44)	0.03
Minimum PTV dose	33 (24–38)	0.07
Duodenal V5 (cc)	64 (45–87)	0.12
Duodenal V10 (cc)	62 (42–84)	0.10
Duodenal V15 (cc)	52 (40–79)	0.32
Duodenal V20 (cc)	39 (26–81)	0.05
Duodenal V25 (cc)	27 (10–50)	0.01
Duodenal V30 (cc)	14 (0–29)	0.01
Duodenal V35 (cc)	5 (0–20)	0.03

Gy gray, *PTV* planning target volume

Table 5.9 Details of publications and clinical trial cohorts with duodenum DVH data available, including those used in this analysis

Reference	Patients	mFU (months)	Cancer site	Radiotherapy dose-schedule (EQD25# where applicable)	Radiotherapy technique	Grade ≤ 3 toxicity (%)
Wilson [137]	23	14	LAPC	59.4 Gy in 33 fx (EQD25 fx = 55.4 Gy)	3D-CRT/IMRT	14
Xu [138]	76	19	Gynae (PA nodes)	45 ± 10 Gy boost in 25 fx	IMRT	4
Verma [139]	105	32	Gynae	64 Gy in 25 fx	IMRT	8
Poorvu [140]	53	17	Gynae	54 Gy in 30 fx (EQD25 fx = 51.6 Gy)	IMRT	7
Kelly [141]	106	12	LAPC	50.4 Gy in 28 fx (EQD25 fx = 49.0 Gy)	3D-CRT (5)	8
Cattaneo [142]	61	19	LAPC	45 ± 15 Gy boost in 15 fx (EQD25 fx = 51.9 ± 17.1 Gy)	IMRT	12
Mukherjee [143]	74	12	LAPC	50.4 Gy in 28 fx (EQD25 fx = 49.0 Gy)	3D-CRT	9
Xia [144]	33	6	Pancreas	PTV: 50 Gy, GTV: 70 Gy in 20 fx (EQD25 fx = PTV: 53.1 Gy, GTV: 75.0 Gy	IMRT (31) Tomo	0
Kim [145]	73	11	HCC	36 Gy in 12 fx	3D-CRT	12
Pan [146]	92	7.6	Hepatic	1.5 Gy per fx BD with chemo or 1.8–3 Gy per fx QDS without	3D-CRT	16

Table 5.10 Dose constraints (in grease) for 50%, 0.035–30 cm³ of the volume duodenal, based on the number of fractions and the estimated risk, by referring to data from Goldsmith et al. [147]

	Low risk (%)					High risk (%)				
	D50%	D30 cm³	D5 cm³	D1 cm³	D0.035 cm³	D50%	D30 cm³	D5 cm³	D1 cm³	D0.035 cm³
One fraction	12.5 32.3%	9.0 6.1%	11.2 0.6%	17.0 6.4%	16.0 5.3%	14.5 48.3%	13.8 11.0%	17.0 14.6%	23.0 21.4%	23.0 8.8%
Two fractions	14.0 19.3%	12.5 6.3%	16.1 0.9%	21.5 4.9%	25.0 6.2%	16.5 30.2%	18.8 11.0%	24.0 18.8%	31.0 19.5%	31.5 8.7%
Three fractions	15.0 15.2%	15.0 6.5%	21.0 1.8%	25.3 4.7%	30.0 6.2%	18.0 24.3%	22.3 11.0%	30.0 26.5%	37.4 19.8%	37.0 8.4%
Four fractions	15.5 12.7%	17.5 6.8%	23.4 1.7%	27.0 3.9%	31.0 5.6%	19.0 20.9%	25.1 11.0%	34.0 26.8%	39.0 14.2%	40.0 7.8%
Five fractions	16.0 11.4%	20.0 7.3%	25.8 1.8%	28.0 3.4%	32.0 5.2%	20.0 19.3%	27.4 11.0%	38.0 30.2%	40.0 10.9%	42.0 7.3%

5.4.6   Rx: Sample Prescriptions

There is a summary of recommendation for duodenum toxicity below:

- Severe diarrhea with fever, neutropenia, sepsis: Antibiotics
- Diarrhea: Antidiarrhetic agents (loperamide, octreotide)
- Dehydration: Adequate hydration (35 mL/kg/day)
- Bowel cramping/pain: Anticholinergic antispasmodic agents
- Dietary modifications: High protein, low lactose, low fat, nutritional support, TPN
- If stricture, perforation, fistula, and bleeding: Refer to a surgeon

5.5   Small Bowel

5.5.1   Anatomy

The small intestine (small bowel) is an organ in the gastrointestinal tract. It is an important part of GI tract because most of the end absorption of nutrients and minerals from food takes place. The small bowel is a hollow tube approximately 2.5 cm in diameter and 6–7 m in length and lies from the stomach at the pyloric sphincter to large bowel and can be divided into three parts: the duodenum, jejunum, and ileum. The difference between small and large bowels is that small bowel has smaller lumen diameter and longer length than large bowel. As mentioned before, the duodenum continues into the jejunum at the duodenojejunal junction which lies to the left of L2 vertebra and is fixed to the retroperitoneum by Treitz ligament. The jejunum and ileum are the distal two parts of the small intestine and are located intraperitoneally. No clear external demarcation exists between the jejunum and ileum. The ileum is the longest part of the small bowel and it is thicker, more vascular, and has more developed mucosal folds than the jejunum. The jejunum begins at the duodenojejunal flexure and lies primarily in the left upper quadrant of the abdomen. The ileum is the longest part of the small bowel, measuring about 1.8 m in length. It is thicker, more vascular, and has more developed mucosal folds than the jejunum. The ileum comprises the remainder of the small bowel and lies primarily in the right lower abdominal quadrant and terminates into the large bowel (cecum) at the ileocecal junction where the ileum invaginates into the cecum to form the ileocecal valve. The jejunum and ileum are intraperitoneal structures. The entire jejunum and ileum are tethered to the posterior abdominal wall by the mesentery. The mesentery is a double fold of peritoneum attached to the posterior abdominal wall. The mesenteric vessels and lymph nodes are located between these two leaves of the mesentery.

5.5.2   Contouring

The easiest way to contour the small bowel and colon is to follow the bowel slice by slice without mesentery from proximal to distal [149]. The second way to delineate intestines is "bowel bag" [150, 151]. In the absence of oral contrast, this technique is the simple and fast way to contouring the bowel. In this technique all portions of peritoneal cavity, except non-bowel structures, are contoured as a "bowel bag." The Radiation Therapy Oncology Group (RTOG) recommended that the small and large bowel should be contoured seperately in upper abdominal treatment planning, especially IMRT planning, due to importance of the maximal doses on the small and large bowel [149, 150]. Ideally, the best way to distinguish the small bowel from the colon requires administration of contrast. The small loops with contrast are contoured from end of the pylor until cecum is seen. The first part of small bowel is duodenum; if it is required to know the dose of the duodenum, it can be contoured separately. In Fig. 5.5, the contouring of the small bowel is presented on computerized tomography images.

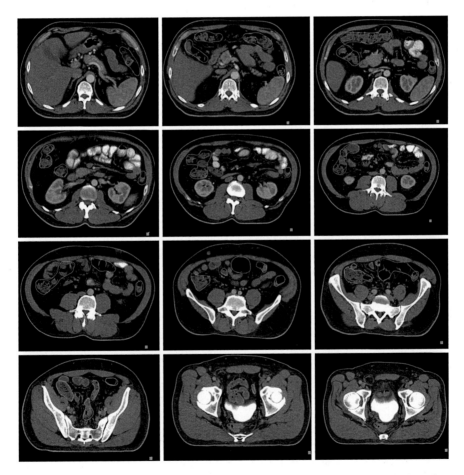

Fig. 5.5 The contouring of the small bowel on computerized tomography images (green color: colon; red color: small bowel)

5.5.3 Pathophysiology

During radiation therapy of upper abdominal malignancy, small bowel and colon are important normal tissues at risk. Intestinal radiation toxicity is grouped as acute when it occurs during the first days or within 3 months, or late (chronic) that occurs more than 3 months after radiotherapy. In acute radiation-related intestinal toxicity, the symptoms are generally mild to moderate and rarely severe, transient and cease after completion of radiation therapy. These symptoms make deterioration in the patient's quality of life during radiotherapy course. Severe acute symptoms may require discontinuation or alteration of treatment at the expense of the losing possibility of tumor control. Chronic radiation-related intestinal toxicity is important for survivors due to its progressive nature and risk of long-term morbidity and mortality. There is no effective treatment.

Radiation causes injuries in normal tissues in different ways, including direct cellular cytocidal and functional effects, indirect effects (reactive) [152–155]. The bowel is highly radiosensitive tissue. The main mechanisms of direct radiation effect are destruction of parenchymal cells (parenchymal hypoplasia). Histologically detectable alterations of the intestinal mucosa like injury, inflammation, edema and compensatory responses of the bowel wall can be found in several days after initiation of radiotherapy [156]. A typical microscopic finding of acute radiation damage is seen in the mucosa and includes mucosal atrophy, wall fibrosis, obliterative vascular sclerosis, and lymphatic dilation. The intestinal epithelium is a single layer of columnar cells containing crypt–villous units that increase the absorptive surface of the small intestine. There is a decrease in the number and height of villous leading to absorptive capacity reduction after radiation injury. The clonogenic and apoptotic cell death in the crypt epithelium of intestine causes insufficient replacement of the villus epithelium, breakdown of the mucosal barrier, mucositis, and proliferative reactions [154, 157]. Acute inflammatory reaction and leukocyte migration as well as increased microvascular permeability causing intestinal tissue damage and mucosal breakdown and development of ulceration occur [158]. Affecting the functioning of the intestinal mucosa causes protein, electrolyte, and water loss [159, 160]. In addition, decreased bowel surface causes insufficient absorption of conjugated bile salt in the small intestine, entering bile salts to the colon. Local bacterial flora deconjugates the bile salts leading to chologenic diarrhea [156, 161]. In some patients, lactose malabsorption was seen to contribute into radiation-related diarrhea [162]. Also, the reduced absorption of fats, carbohydrates, proteins, and vitamin B12 happens with damaged epithelium during radiation therapy [163]. The small bowel motility pattern also changes during radiation therapy due to mucosal injury, alterations of water–electrolyte and some neurotransmitters release [164]. Acute small bowel toxicity typically manifests as diarrhea, cramping, abdominal pain, steatorrhea, or bloating. During the abdominopelvic radiotherapy, intestinal permeability and histologic injury are seen at the maximum level in the middle of the radiotherapy course and the clinical symptoms of bowel injury increase toward the end of the radiotherapy.

The pathogenesis of chronic bowel toxicity involves changes in the whole intestinal wall [165]. Hydroxyl radicals are mediator for radiation injury. It induces transforming growth factor-$\beta 1$ which acts as a potent fibrogenic and proinflammatory cytokine and promotes fibrosis [166, 167]. Histologically, the main structural features are mucosal atrophy, submucosal fibrosis, and progressive vascular sclerosis [168–170]. Typical microscopic signs of chronic toxicity are seen in the submucosa. The stromal tissue of intestinal wall contains fibroblasts with collagen proliferation. Due to the proliferation of collagen within the intestinal wall, the intestinal motility is reduced. Increased fibrosis within the intestinal wall leads to narrowing of bowel segments and bowel obstruction. These cause bowel wall ischemia, mucosal ulcerations, and development of collateral vessels. The obstruction of the small intestinal arterioles can also lead to ulceration and necrosis of the intestinal wall. If this persists, perforation and peritonitis may develop. The malabsorption and dysmotility are the main functional changes in this situation. In some cases, life-threatening situations such as bleeding, obstruction or fistula may also develop.

5.5.4 Dose Constraints

Diarrhea, which is the common acute radiation-induced small bowel toxicity has been reported as Grade 2 in 12–34%, Grade 3–4 in 7–25% of patients and rarely causes death (1–2% of patients) [171, 172]. The late small bowel toxicity has been reported to be around 7–9%. Additionally, the concurrent chemoradiotherapy increases the risk of small bowel toxicity [173, 174].

In two-dimensional treatment planning era, the relationship between acute toxicity and irradiation of small bowel had been known but could not been well defined. The small bowel injury is affected from volume of the treatment field, fraction size, and total radiation dose and treatment technique. In most studies, the patients are treated by 1.8–2 Gy fraction dose in total of 45–50 Gy without significant incidence of toxicity. For postoperative patients, these doses are associated with a 5% incidence of severe small bowel toxicity such as obstruction, requiring surgery [175]. The incidence rises to 25–50% at higher doses than 50 Gy. With the improving technology, the dose–volume relationship for the small bowel has been shown in dosimetric studies based on computed tomography. These studies show that the total radiation dose and the volume of irradiated bowel are important factors for bowel toxicity.

The severe enteropathy and bowel injury is relatively rare with doses <50 Gy. The dose–volume relationship between volume of irradiated small bowel and severity of toxicity has been shown [176–179]. However, there are differences for contouring of small bowel between studies. In the landmark review of Emami, the dose that causes enteropathy in 5% of patients at 5 years ($TD_{5/5}$) was defined as 50 Gy for one-third of the small bowel volume and 40 Gy for the whole volume [91]. The dose that causes severe enteropathy in 50% of patients at 5 years ($TD_{50/5}$) is 60 Gy for a third of the volume and 55 Gy for the whole volume was also defined. In earlier series the average volume of small bowel receiving 100% of the prescription dose

(45 Gy) (VolSB,100) was reported as approximately 600 cc in standard whole pelvic radiotherapy while 300 cc in using intensity modulated whole pelvic radiation therapy [180]. They analyzed using normal tissue complication probability (NTCP) model, the 600 cc of small bowel volume would have 77% risk of clinically significant acute gastrointestinal toxicity in standard pelvic radiotherapy while 300 cc and 200 cc would have respectively 27% and 10% risk of clinically significant acute gastrointestinal toxicity in intensity modulated pelvic radiotherapy [179]. Roeske et al. evaluated the dose–volume relationship of acute grade 2–5 gastrointestinal toxicity in gynecologic cancers treated with whole pelvic intensity modulated radiotherapy (IMRT) [179]. The extent of contrast-enhanced small bowel loops were contoured as a single structure for delineation of the small bowel (neither as individual loops nor as peritoneal space). They found a significant correlation between grade 2 toxicity and the volume of small bowel receiving 100% of the prescribed dose (V100 or V45 Gy), and V45 should be restricted to <195 cc. Baglan et al. evaluated small bowel toxicity in patients treated for rectal cancer with 5-FU-based chemotherapy and radiation therapy [176]. The small bowel volume was defined by contouring both opaque and nonopaque loops. They found statistically significant relationship between ≥Grade 3 acute small bowel toxicity and the volume of small bowel irradiated to each 5-Gy dose level. The threshold volume was demonstrated at each dose level, below which no grade ≥3 toxicity was seen, whereas grade ≥3 toxicity developed in 50–60% of patients. Their detailed analyses supported a dose–volume relationship for doses below 15 Gy, which had a threshold of 150 cc. Robertson JM et al. confirmed highly significant relationship with small bowel dose–volume and grade 3 diarrhea in patients receiving pelvic radiotherapy for rectal cancer [181]. The grade 3 diarrhea was observed at a lower incidence in preoperative irradiation than in postoperative irradiation. The highly statistically significant relationship was found for the dose volumes of 15, 20, and 25 Gy. Huang et al. prospectively studied DVH correlation with acute toxicity in patients who underwent pelvic radiotherapy with or without prior abdominal surgery [178]. They contoured only small bowel loops within the irradiation field. Their results showed that abdominal surgery increased the grade ≥2 acute diarrhea. They reported that V15 (or 40% dose) predicts grade ≥2 acute diarrhea in patients without prior surgery and V40 (or 100% dose) for patients with prior surgery. Lee TF et al. developed NTCP model to analyze dose–volume effects for grade ≥2 acute diarrhea in gynecological patients with/without prior abdominal surgery [182]. They contoured the small bowel as small-bowel loops and suggested to keep the incidence of grade ≥2 acute small bowel toxicity below 10%, to receive 16 Gy of small bowel volume (V16) <290 cc (in patients without abdominal surgery) and V40 Gy <75 cc (in patients with abdominal surgery). However, this study has limited number of patients to obtain a model with high predictive power. Kavanagh BD et al. reviewed dose–volume and toxicity data from six papers which evaluated the dose–volume relationship with acute bowel toxicity. In this review, Quantitative Analyses of Normal Tissue Effects in the Clinic (QUANTEC) recommends minimizing small bowel to prevent acute toxicity [183]. The QUANTEC recommendation is that absolute volume of small bowel receiving ≥1500 cGy should be <120 cc. It is more

important when the individual loops of small bowel are contoured. If whole volume of peritoneal cavity contoured the recommendation is that the volume receiving >45 Gy should be <195 cc. There is no correlation for late bowel toxicity and the QUANTEC reviewers suggest that the same limits may apply to reduce late toxicity risk. There is also some dose–volume parameters for stereotactic radiotherapy that in a single fraction the small bowel volume receiving >12.5 Gy should be <30 cc and in 3–5 fractions the maximum point dose should be <30 Gy.

The treatment technique such as prone position, using belly-board, full bladder helps to reduce the small bowel volume in treatment field [184]. These all lead to less toxicity. There are also some data for improving doses with techniques such as intensity modulated planning [177, 185–187]. In the IMRT group as compared to the 3DCRT group, almost threefold fewer of patients might experience the grade ≥ 2 diarrhea (9.9% vs 22.4% 3DCRT) [187]. In a pooled analysis of Wee CW et al. which compared intensity modulated radiotherapy with three-dimensional conformal radiotherapy for acute toxicity in patients with rectal cancer, they concluded that significantly less grade 2–3 acute gastrointestinal toxicity are seen in IMRT patients compared to three-dimensional conformal technique (3D-CRT) [186]. They reported overall gastrointestinal grade ≥ 2 and grade ≥ 3 acute toxicity rate is 29% in IMRT group of patients compared to 55% in 3D-CRT and 3% in IMRT compared to 9% in 3D-CRT, respectively. The grade ≥ 2 diarrhea was separately reported as 12% in IMRT group compared to 36% in 3D-CRT and grade ≥ 3 diarrhea was 12% in IMRT compared to 36% in 3D-CRT, respectively. Tho LM et al. investigated the dose–volume relationship between volume of irradiated small bowel (VSB) and acute toxicity in patients with rectal cancer who were treated by preoperative concomitant 5-FU-based chemotherapy and 3D-CRT/IMRT [177]. They found that VSB correlated strongly with severity of diarrhea at each dose level with strongest correlation at lowest doses. The median VSBs were significantly greater in experiencing diarrhea $\geq$Grade 2 compared with diarrhea <Grade 2 at all dose levels. In that study, inverse planning significantly reduced the median dose to small bowel by 5.1 Gy and calculated late normal tissue complication probability by 67%. They also pointed a model using mathematical analysis to predict acute diarrhea occurring at V5 and V15. However, they were unable to identify any certain VSB thresholds for the diarrhea due to some confounding factor such as surgery.

The NRG Oncology Radiation Therapy Oncology Group 0822 Phase 2 study evaluated the bowel toxicity in patients treated with preoperative chemoradiation by using IMRT. In this study, the small bowel dose constraints were limited to V35 <180 cc, V40 <100 cc, and V45 <65 cc. The rate of grade ≥ 2 and grade ≥ 3 diarrhea were determined as 35% and 18%, respectively [188]. When the small bowel volume receiving 10–40 Gy at 5-Gy intervals were compared between patients who had grade <2–3 versus grade ≥ 2–3 gastrointestinal toxicity, no statistically significant difference was found at any dose. They also found no relation between grade ≥ 3 GI toxicity rates and V15 ≥ 150 cc as suggested by Baglan et al. or V15 ≥ 120 cc as suggested in the update by Robertson et al. [176, 181]. They did similar analyses for small bowel dose–volume parameters for grade 2–3 diarrhea and also found no correlations. In that study, gastrointestinal toxicity rates could not be decreased by

IMRT. Their explanation of IMRT's inability to reduce gastrointestinal toxicity was to use inadequate dosimetric constraints for small bowel dose. They also added that contouring the peritoneal cavity rather than loops for small bowel delineation may have contributed to negative results. However, contouring every bowel loop is very time consuming and difficult in routine practice. The small bowel except duodenum is mostly mobile and has day-to-day variation in abdomen. Different contouring methods of small bowel volume have led to different dose–toxicity relationships. There are data supporting the contouring of the entire peritoneal cavity as a bowel bag. In a recent study, researchers tried to determine whether peritoneal space can be used instead of individual small bowel loops to predict for grade ≥3 acute small bowel toxicity [189]. They found a significant dose–volume relationship between toxicity and small bowel volume in both contouring techniques. The strongest factor for predicting toxicity was the volume received between 15 and 25 Gy. The DVH analysis of the peritoneal space showed that it accurately predicted grade ≥3 bowel toxicity in patients with rectal cancer receiving neoadjuvant chemoradiotherapy. The authors concluded that if small bowel-V15 <275 cc and peritoneal space-V15 <830 cc, there is a <10% risk of grade ≥3 acute bowel toxicity. In Radiation Therapy Oncology Group (RTOG) protocols for external beam radiation therapy of gynecological malignancies require bowel contouring as entire peritoneal cavity through the pelvis and superiorly until 2 cm above the planning target volume. The dose constraint is that <30% of small bowel volume receives ≥40 Gy [190, 191]. The QUANTEC analysis recommended dose–volume constraints of V15 ≤120 cm³ when small bowel is contoured as bowel loops and V45 ≤195 cm³ when SB is contoured as a bowel bag for <10% of grade ≥3 acute toxicity [93].

Bleeding and bowel obstruction are serious late intestinal toxicity. The incidence of grade ≥3 late bowel toxicity is reported as approximately 10% [192, 193]. However, limited data are available regarding the relationship between dose volume effects and late small bowel toxicity. Gallagher MJ et al. reported that a greater volume of small bowel in the pelvis after surgery and the volume of small bowel receiving more than 45 Gy were related with late small bowel toxicity [194]. Letschert et al. found a volume effect in radiation-induced diarrhea at a dose of 50 Gy in 25 fractions while no volume effect for obstruction at this dose level [195]. In a prospective study, the dose volume predictors of grade ≥3 late bowel toxicity in patients undergoing postoperative radiation for cervical cancer were investigated [196]. Small and large bowel loops were contoured 2 cm above the target volume and V15 Gy (volume of the small and large bowel receiving 15 Gy) was found as a significant predictive factor and restricting small bowel—V15 <275 cc and large bowel—V15 <250 cc will reduce grade ≥3 late toxicity to <5%. On the other hand, in the widely used QUANTEC review, there is no clear recommendation regarding the dose–volume relationship for late small bowel toxicity [183]. It is known that maximum doses in the small bowel should be avoided during planning, but the maximum dose is not defined. Therefore, Stanic et al. focused on late toxicity in patients receiving para-aortic nodal irradiation for gynecologic malignancies and established dose constraint guidelines for late small bowel toxicity and the maximum tolerance dose of the small bowel [192]. After the analysis of prospective studies in the literature, they agreed to recommendation of Emami et al. for small bowel TD5/5 with maximum dose of 50 Gy. They estimated that for small bowel TD10/5 is the maximum point dose of 55 Gy. Their recommendation is trying to keep the maximum point dose (Dmax) to the small bowel at 55 Gy or less. Poorvu PD et al. assessed the rate of acute and late duodenal and bowel toxicities in patients who were treated by extended-field intensity modulated radiation therapy to the para-aortic and pelvic nodes due to cervical and endometrial cancers [140]. They analyzed the dose–volume relationships of GI toxicities. The bowel was contoured as both opacified and nonopacified small bowel loops. Only 6.5% of patients had both acute and late grade ≥3 GI toxicity. The median dose to para-aortic nodes was 54 Gy (range, 41.4–65 Gy). The mean D55 of small bowel was 5.3 cc (range 0–13) and the mean D60 was 1 cc (range, 0–6) in the patients with gastrointestinal toxicity. In dosimetric analysis of with and without toxicity, there were no differences between the mean volumes at any 5-Gy interval between 5 Gy and the maximum dose. They also found no association between concurrent chemotherapy and toxicity. They concluded that it is possible to increase the dose up to 65 Gy with adequate spare of the small bowel in IMRT patients, even with using of concurrent chemotherapy.

Recently, stereotactic body radiotherapy (SBRT) has been used frequently in primary or metastatic tumors. Gastric, duodenal, and small bowel toxicities were major concerns following SBRT planning for abdominal malignancies [197–200]. Studies have mainly focused on the toxicity of the duodenum which is relatively immobile than the small bowel and stomach, due to the proximity of the irradiated area. The mostly reported gastrointestinal toxicities were duodenal obstruction/ulceration, duodenal bleeding, hemorrhage, and gastric perforation [197, 198, 200]. Therefore, studies evaluating only small bowel toxicity of stereotactic radiotherapy are limited. In a Phase II study of SBRT for colorectal metastasis, the fractionation schema was 45 Gy in three fractions within 5–8 days [201]. The bowel dose was tried to be as low as possible. The grade ≥2 toxicity was observed in 48% of patients within 6 months after SBRT. This report was one of the first reports for high toxicity rates after SBRT in patients with pancreatic cancer. Kopek et al.'s study used same fractionation schema in patients with cholangiocarcinoma [202]. They found that the mean maximum dose to 1 cm³ of duodenum (Dmax 1 cc) was significantly higher in patients with grade ≥2 ulceration or stenosis (37.4 Gy vs 25.3 Gy). They suggested 1 cc of duodenum to receive no more than 21 Gy in three fractions (V21 Gy ≤1 cc) for all abdominal SBRT. In the study of Koong AC et al., a single fraction dose escalation from 15 to 20 or 25 Gy was evaluated in patients with locally advanced pancreatic cancer [203]. They suggested the mean dose to be 50% and 5% of the duodenum and bowel of 14.5 and 22.5 Gy, respectively, at the 25 Gy dose level. In a Korean series, severe gastroduodenal toxicity was reported in 15% of patients who were treated with stereotactic body radiotherapy (SBRT) using three fractions for abdominopelvic malignancies [204]. The median SBRT dose was 45 Gy (range, 33–60 Gy) with three fractions. They found the Dmax as the best dosimetric predictor for severe gastroduodenal toxicity. The Dmax of 35 Gy and 38 Gy were correlated with a 5% and 10% risk of severe gastroduodenal toxicity. Goldsmith et al. surveyed the literature for quantitative models of risk in 1–5 fractions and used their institutional data of 3–5 fractions of stereotactic body radiotherapy to create a DVH Risk Map for the duodenum [205]. Their logistic model of duodenal data in three fractions showed that D1 cc = 25.3 Gy had 4.7% risk of grade 3–4 hemorrhage or stricture and D1 cc = 37.4 Gy had 20% risk. For five fractions, the lower risk limit of toxicity were found that 3.4% for D1 cm^3 = 28 Gy and for D1 cm^3 = 40 Gy was 10.9%. They concluded that the 10% risk level was D1 cc = 31.4 Gy for 3–5 fractions of stereotactic body radiotherapy. In a recent study, 84 patients with solitary or oligometastatic abdominopelvic tumors were treated with mainly 48 Gy in six fractions or 45 Gy in five fractions of SBRT [206]. The stomach, duodenum, and bowel were contoured as separate structures, but they were summed together for analysis. The grade $\geq$2 acute and late gastrointestinal toxicity were observed in 15% and 10% of patients. There is also grade 3 toxicity in 4% of the patients. The volume irradiated by V30–V65 Gy was associated with acute grade $\geq$2 bowel toxicity. According to their NTCP model for V40 Gy, an irradiated bowel volume of 10 cm^3 of V40 Gy resulted in complication probability of grade $\geq$2 acute toxicity <10%.

In 2010 QUANTEC recommendations for dose constraints in SBRT were: the small bowel volume receiving >12.5 Gy to <30 mL if using single fraction and a maximum point dose of <30 Gy for 3–5 fraction SBRT [183]. More recently, La Couture et al. reviewed the literature regarding small bowel dose tolerance limits for stereotactic body radiation therapy and created a dose–volume histogram Risk Map, demonstrating low and high risk of dose limits for small bowel [207]. For all analyses, they considered that high-risk small bowel limits if the risk was $\leq$8.2% and the low-risk limits had $\leq$4% estimated risk. In this review, within 2 year before or after SBRT 30% of patients were treated with biological agents such as vascular endothelial growth factor inhibitors. They found that the small bowel—D5 cm^3 = 21 Gy in three fractions and D5 cm^3 = 16.2 Gy in five fractions has low toxicity with 6.5% and 2.5% estimated risk of grade $\geq$3 toxicity, respectively.

However, many other clinical factors such as prior ulcer and use of biological agents can influence the development of bowel toxicity [204, 207]. In Table 5.11, some recommendations for dose limits of small bowel are presented.

Table 5.11 The small bowel dose limitation recommendations

Treatment technique	Delineation of organ	Limits	End point
3D-CRT/IMRT (with conventional fractionation	Individual small bowel loops	V15 < 120 cc	Grade $\geq$ 3 acute toxicity <10%
3D-CRT/IMRT (with conventional fractionation)	Bowel bag within peritoneal cavity	V45 < 195 cc	Grade $\geq$ 3 acute toxicity <10%
Stereotactic body radiotherapy (with 3–5 ablative fractionation)	Individual small bowel loops (Jejunum/ileum)	V18 < 5 cc V40 Gy $\leq$ 10 cm^3 D2 cm^3 < 24.5 Gy (3 fx) and 30 Gy (5 fx) D5 cm^3 < 21 Gy (3 fx) and 16.2 (5 fx) Dmax $\leq$30 Gy	Grade $\geq$ 2 toxicity <10%

5.5.5 Treatment

Typically radiation-induced small bowel toxicity occur during the third week of fractionated radiotherapy in almost half of the patients. The incidence of those is higher with concomitant chemotherapy [181–183]. The acute small bowel toxicity is characterized by diarrhea and abdominal cramping. Nausea and vomiting may accompany. The treatment of radiation-induced small bowel toxicity varies according to various grades of symptoms. Acute toxicity, including diarrhea, nausea, vomiting, and abdominal cramping is treated symptomatically. The important point in the approach to radiation-induced diarrhea is to determine the severity of the diarrhea and the general condition of the patient. A mild diarrhea without any other important symptoms can be treated with dietary modifications, antidiarrheals, and antispasmodics in the outpatient setting. All patients with diarrhea should be examined every 24 h. Oral supplementation or intravenous hydration (35 mL/kg/day) may be indicated in patients according to their general condition, laboratory test results, and dehydration status.

Oral opiates are effective agent in mild symptoms. The classic treatment of radiotherapy-induced diarrhea includes loperamide and diphenoxylate with atropine. Loperamide is commonly used as a first-line antidiarheic agent. Loperamide is generally the preferred opioid because it has local activity in the bowel [208]. It is minimally absorbed; therefore, there is lack of systemic effects. Its main effect is on the reduction of stool weight, frequency of bowel movements, urgency, and fecal incontinence in diarrhea. Loperamide should be started at an initial dose of 4 mg followed by 2 mg every 4 h or after every unformed stool (not to exceed 16 mg/day) [209]. Treatment of loperamide should be continued during radiotherapy with standard dose. If the resolution of diarrhea happened with loperamide, the patients should make dietary modifications and add solid foods to their meal. If diarrhea is not resolved after 48 h on high-dose loperamide (increasing the dose 2 mg every 2 h, not to exceed 16 mg/day), loperamide should be discontinued and changed second-line treatment with octreotide [209]. The prescription dose of octreotide is 100–150 mg starting dose, with dose escalation as needed. The different agent octreotide is a somatostatin analog and has multiple antidiarrheal actions. It decreases the gastrointestinal motility and intestinal secretion of fluids and electrolytes. Octreotide seems to be more effective than diphenoxylate and atropine to reduce radiation-induced diarrhea [210, 211]. In preclinical studies, octreotide administration has been shown to effectively reduce acute mucosal changes after irradiation of the small intestine [212]. A randomized clinical trial of Yavuz MN et al. assessed the effectiveness of octreotide in patients with radiation-induced diarrhea [213]. They reported resolution of ≥grade 2 diarrhea within 3 days in octreotide (100 µg three times daily) group compared to a diphenoxylate hydrochloride plus atropine sulfate (2.5 mg four times daily) group. A microencapsulated, long-acting formulation of octreotide has been developed for once monthly intramuscular dosing. Martenson et al. in their study evaluated the use of long-acting octreotide depot (20 mg LAO) for the prevention of radiation-induced diarrhea [214]. However, the long-acting octreotide depot (20 mg LAO) was not found as an effective agent to reduce the severity or incidence of diarrhea during pelvic radiotherapy. In a current metanalysis, octreotide was accepted as a therapeutic anti-diarrheal agent rather than a prophylactic agent in radiotherapy- and chemo-therapy-induced diarrhea [215]. The prescription dose of octreotide is 100–150 mg subcutaneously (SC) three times daily starting dose, with dose escalation as needed [209]. It should keep in mind that opioid antidiarrheal agents are contraindicated in patients with obstructive symptoms. If mild to severe diarrhea is accompanied with fever, dehydration, neutropenia, oral antibiotics (e.g., fluoroquinolone) should be started as prophylaxis for infection [216].

There is some evidence of the benefit of acetylsalicylic acid (aspirin), an anti-inflammatory agent in radiation-induced small bowel toxicity whereas the other nonsteroidal anti-inflammatories are not effective [217, 218]. However, there are also studies showing that it may increase symptoms of acute toxicity [219]. Based on the role of prostaglandin in pathophysiology of diarrhea, inhibition of prosta-glandin biosynthesis by salicylates, including sulfasalazine and olsalazine, have been evaluated for prevention of radiation-induced diarrhea. Several studies reported that sulfasalazine moderately reduced acute radiation-induced small bowel toxic-ity compared to olsalazine. Even in some cases olsalazine increased diarrhea [220–222]. Due to these confounding results about two drugs which have same action mechanisms, until a confirmatory trial is conducted for these agents, sulfasalazine is not routinely recommended [223]. Sucralfate is a nonsystemically absorbed alumi-num hydroxide complex. It is thought to promote epithelial healing and provide a protective barrier on damaged mucosal surfaces [224]. Oral sucralfate was evalu-ated to decrease frequency and improvement in consistency of bowel movements in patients receiving pelvic irradiation. In several randomized studied there are mixed results for sucralfate. Some of them reported that receiving 1–2 g sucralfate (two to six times daily) during radiotherapy significantly decreased diarrhea while some showed no improvement in diarrhea and significant worsening of some gastrointes-tinal symptoms comparing with placebo [225–227]. Taken together, the results show that sucralfate is not effective in the prevention of radiation-induced diarrhea and may aggravate some symptoms. In radiation-induced diarrhea, decreased absorption of bile salts, vitamin B12, lactose, fat are developed [208]. A total of 95% of bile acids are absorbed in the terminal ileum, and radiation damage of this region can lead to the malabsorption of bile acid. The decreased absorption of bile salts is responsible for symptoms in 35–72% of patients with radiation-induced small bowel toxicity [134, 228]. Cholestyramine is a nonabsorbable high-molecular resin that binds bile salts irreversibly and shows some effect to treat absorption of bile acid. Some studies have supported cholestyramine's efficacy in the treatment of acute and chronic diarrhea in patients treated with radiation therapy [229]. A tran-sient lactose intolerance and fat malabsorption may occur in many patients [161, 209]. A lactose-free and low-fat diet may also improve symptoms. In radiation-induced acute small bowel toxicity, abdominal cramping may accompany diarrhea. An anticholinergic antispasmodic agent could relief bowel cramping. Nausea and vomiting, bloating, and loss of appetite may occur [209]. Anti-emetic agents are also used. Some diet modification such as adequate hydration, eating small, frequent high-protein food, avoiding chocolate, alcohol, caffeine, foods with insoluble fiber including skins of fruits and raw vegetables should be made.

For the late small bowel toxicity, most patients require only symptomatic therapy and can be treated symptomatically as above. Conservative management may include regulation of intestinal transit, correction of nutritional deficits, special diets, anti-inflammatory drugs, treatment of bile acid malabsorption and bacterial overgrowth. If malnutrition develops, total parenteral nutrition (TPN) can improve clinical outcome [230]. A cohort study with 24 patients showed that corticosteroid therapy (methylprednisolone) may enhance the effect of TPN and improved clinical symptoms [231]. More severe cases of radiation enteritis often require aggressive treatment such as surgery [232, 233]. Indications for surgery include intestinal obstruction, perforation, or fistula formation, severe bleeding or malabsorption. However, indications and timing of surgical intervention are controversial. Due to radiation-induced changes in the small bowel and mesentery, recovery after surgery is often poor and there is a high risk of anastomosis separation and fistula formation. However, surgical intervention may help to avoid progressive bowel necrosis, perforation, and sepsis control in selected patients.

5.5.6   Rx: Sample Prescriptions

There is a summary of recommendation for small bowel toxicity below:

- Diarrhea: Antidiarrhetic agents (loperamide, octreotide)
- Dehydration: Adequate hydration (35 mL/kg/day)
- Antibiotics: Severe diarrhea with fever, dehydration, neutropenia, sepsis
- Bowel cramping/pain: Anticholinergic antispasmodic agents
- Bile acid malabsorption: Cholestyramine
- Dietary modifications: High protein, low lactose, low fat, nutritional support, TPN
- Malabsorption: Nutritional support
- Needs surgery: Refer to a surgeon (if stricture, perforation, fistula, and bleeding)

5.6   Colon

5.6.1   Anatomy

The large bowel is the terminal part of the intestinal canal. The final absorption of nutrients and water, synthesize vitamins, form feces are its primary function. The large bowel starts from the appendix and continues until the anus. The large bowel lies partially in the mesentery, namely the cecum, appendix, transverse, and sigmoid colon that maintain vascular and lymphatic vessels, lymph nodes, and nerves. The diameter of the colon is larger than small bowels; however, its length is half of the small bowel. The main difference between the small and large bowel is the presence of taeniae coli which are three separate longitudinal bands of smooth muscle on the outside of the bowel below the serosa. The large bowel is subdivided in regions as the cecum, the appendix, the colon, the rectum, and the anal canal. The ileocecal valve is located between ileum and large bowel. The first part of the large bowel is the cecum. The cecum is a pouch-like structure suspended from the lower part of the ileocecal valve. Its length is about 6 cm. The appendix is a winding tube that attaches to the cecum. The cecum receives the contents of the ileum, and plays a role for absorption of water and salts. The appendix contains lymphoid tissue and is considered to have a role in immunologic function. The cecum and appendix both lie in the right lower quadrant within the iliac fossa and continues with the colon. The colon consists of ascending, transverse, descending, and sigmoid colon. The ascending colon starts after ileocecal valve, continues along the right side of the abdomen and turns to the right under liver (hepatic flexura) and then continues as a transverse colon. The transvers colon turns to down under the spleen (splenic flexura) and continues along the left side of the abdomen as descending colon and then enters the pelvis as a sigmoid colon. There is no clear anatomic demarcation of the transition between the sigmoid and rectum. The ascending and descending colon is located retroperitoneal while the transverse and sigmoid colon are connected by the mesocolon to the posterior abdominal wall intraperitoneally.

5.6.2 Contouring

The simplest way to delineate the colon is to track the bowel without mesentery slice by slice from the proximal to the distal bowel. Once the rectosigmoid or the cecum appears in the CT slice, non-contrast colon folds are seen easily visible and contoured by following up or down. Other option is to contour the "bowel bag," which includes all portions of the peritoneal cavity aside from non-bowel structures and encompasses all the small bowel and colon contours. This may be useful if no small bowel oral contrast was used. However, RTOG does not recommend bowel bag method for upper abdomen treatment planning [149]. In Fig. 5.6, the contouring of the colon is presented on computerized tomography images.

5.6.3 Pathophysiology

The histologic structure of the colon is similar to small bowel with the presence of the same structural subcomponents. The significant differences include the presence of taeniae coli instead of muscularis externa, as well as a significantly different mucosal structure. The colonic mucosa is flat and free of villus. This architectural difference relates to the primary function of the colon which is the absorption of water and electrolytes in the lumen.

Acute radiation-induced colon toxicity occurs in all layers of the mucosa, including epithelium, goblet cells, and lamina propria [154, 234, 235]. Mitotic arrest in

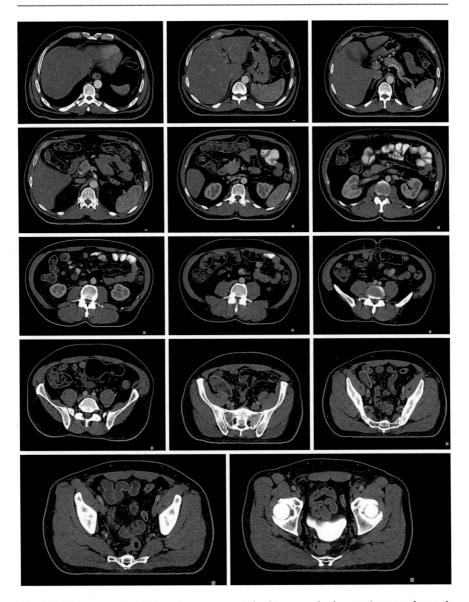

Fig. 5.6 The contouring of the colon on computerized tomography images (green: colon; red: small bowel)

rapidly proliferating epithelial cells in mucosal crypts causes cell loss, shortening and narrowing of crypt lengths, erosion and loss of integrity on the epithelial surface. Inflammatory response is triggered by the infiltration of inflammatory cells and followed by developing crypt abscesses, edema, and ulceration. All these in mucosal damage lead to capillary permeability. The extensive mucosal inflammation, eosinophilic infiltration of the submucosa, crypt atrophy, and abscesses are observed in histologically. This injury causes symptoms such as diarrhea, mucus discharge, cramping, bloating, and bleeding.

The main distinction of late colon toxicity is the obliterative enteritis with ulceration, fibrosis, and the presence of small vessel vasculopathy [234, 235]. In late radiation-induced colon toxicity, the submucosa is characterized by atypical fibroblasts and collagen proliferation. There may also be atypical vascular changes and small arteries may indicate intimal cell proliferation and thickening of the wall with fibrin thrombus in the lumen. Some telangiectatic changes might see in the mucosa. The mucosal layer may show abnormality, ulceration, or thickening with fibrosis. Additionally, there may develop focal stenosis, ulceration, and/or fistula formation. The clinical manifestations of late toxicity are characterized by pain, bleeding, mucous discharge, and strictures.

5.6.4   Dose Constraints

The tolerance of the small and large bowel is a major dose-limiting factor in the treatment of many cancers of the abdomen and pelvis. However, in the literature most of the series reported mainly small bowel toxicities. The volume of irradiated colon depends on the location of the tumor which is being treated in a close position to a segment of the colon. The rectosigmoid area is the area most commonly implicated, but depending on the field of radiation, injury can be more extensive/proximal.

The total colon is considered to be less radiosensitive than the small bowel [236, 237]. Therefore, the maximum tolerated dose of the colon is slightly higher than for the small intestine. In the landmark review of Emami et al., the tolerance doses for the colon are higher with a $TD_{5/5}$ of 55 Gy for a third of the volume and 45 Gy for the whole volume, whereas the $TD_{50/5}$ is 65 Gy for a third of the volume and 60 Gy for the whole volume of the colon [91]. The tolerance dose for each section of the colon is assumed to have the same order of magnitude.

There is limited data in the literature to evaluate the relationship between dose-volume and toxicity of large bowel. In a prospective study, the dose volume predictors of grade $\geq$ 3 late bowel toxicity in patients undergoing postoperative radiation for cervical cancer were investigated [196]. The small and large bowel loops were contoured as individual loops 2 cm above the target volume and V15 Gy (volume of the small and large bowel receiving 15 Gy) was found as a significant predictive factor for grade $\geq$3 toxicity. They suggested that restricting small bowel—V15 <275 cc and large bowel—V15 <250 cc will reduce grade $\geq$3 late toxicity to <5%. Their constraint are V15 <250 cc, V30 <100 cc, and V40 <90 cc to reduce grade $\geq$3 toxicity from 26.7 to 5.4%. Isohashi et al. evaluated dose–volume histogram predictors for the development of grade $\geq$2 chronic gastrointestinal complications in cervical cancer patients who underwent radical hysterectomy and postoperative concurrent platinum-based chemoradiotherapy [238]. The large bowel was contoured as a single loop continuing from end of sigmoid to ascending colon. The grade $\geq$2 toxicity were observed in 16.5% of patients. However, V40 of the small bowel was reported as independent predictors of chronic GI complications while no constraint were found for large bowel.

For the sigmoid colon Fonteyne V et al. aimed to find correlation between late radiation-induced bowel toxicity and volume parameters of the rectum, sigmoid colon and small bowel after intensity-modulated radiotherapy in prostate cancer patients [239]. The sigmoid was contoured from where the rectum sweeps anteriorly to one slice above aortic bifurcation. In their multivariate analyses the sigmoid V40 was found as a significant parameter for grade 1 diarrhea and blood loss while none of the small bowel volume parameters found significant. They recommended V40 <10% and V30 <16% of sigmoid to avoid grade 1–2 diarrhea. In a prospective series, acute and late toxicity data following IMRT for cervix cancer was evaluated [240]. All patients were treated with 50 Gy to the PTV1 (pelvis) and 60 Gy to the PTV2 (central pelvic disease and GTV nodes) concomitantly in 28 fractions, followed by a brachytherapy boost. For the small bowel, 50 Gy was the maximal dose, while V45 and V40 had to be <50 cc and 200 cc, respectively. For the sigmoid structures, 60 Gy was the maximal dose, and V45 and V40 had to be <20% and <50%. The anterior curvature of sigmoid colon to anterior abdominal wall was contoured as sigmoid. The rates of grade 1–3 diarrhea and "whole digestive toxicity" were 21.6% and 46%, respectively. The "whole late digestive toxicity" was found associated with sigmoid V30–40 Gy although no specific constraints were defined. Lind et al. analyzed the relationship between mean radiation dose to bowels/anal-sphincter and occurrence of "defecation into clothing without forewarning" which is specific and serious fecal incontinence symptom, in 519 gynecological cancer survivors who were treated with pelvic radiotherapy [241]. The sigmoid was contoured from where midposition of rectum deviation to where it turns cranially in left abdomen connecting to colon descendens. The defecation into clothing without warning was observed in 12% of patients. They reported that the mean dose above 50 Gy to small bowel or sigmoid was related with clinical symptoms, however the findings for individual organs were not clarified.

In summary, irradiation of the colon or large bowel is generally not considered an important risk factor for radiation-induced enteritis, but evidence is largely lacking. This may be due to irradiation of a smaller portion of the colon or a smaller surface area per length of the bowel or its own radioresistant nature. In Table 5.12, some recommendations for dose limits of colon are presented.

Table 5.12 Colon/large bowel dose limitation recommendations

Treatment technique	Delineation of organ	Limits	End point
3D-CRT/IMRT (with conventional fractionation)	Individual large bowel loops	V15 < 250 cc V40 Gy < 10% Dmax ≤ 60 Gy Mean dose < 50 Gy	Grade ≥ 2 toxicity <10%
Stereotactic body radiotherapy (with 3–5 ablative fractionation)	Individual large bowel loops	V25 < 20 cc Dmax ≤30 Gy (3 fx) and ≤38 Gy (5 fx)	Grade ≥ 2 toxicity <10%

5.6.5 Treatment

Acute radiation-induced colon toxicity appears mucosal necrosis which may manifest as bowel dysmotility, diarrhea, abdominal cramps, tenesmus, or hematochezia. In colonoscopy, mucosal edema, erosions, and ulcerations may be observed. The symptoms are generally self-limited. In general, at the beginning of toxicity treatment, any predisposing factor should be identified and be eliminated and then each treatment should be individualized. Once toxicity develops, the most conservative method should be preferred. Management of radiation-induced colon toxicities is symptomatic as discussed in detail in the small bowel section.

Late radiation-induced colon toxicity is the result of chronic ischemia and fibrosis [242, 243]. This may lead to dysmotility and changing in bowel habits from constipation to diarrhea. Mild cases of chronic radiation toxicity of the large bowel can be managed conservatively with stool softeners and a low residue diet. The stenosis or stricture also may develop and cause an inability to evacuate the bowel. It is kept in mind that fiber supplementation may not be useful because increasing the fecal caliber makes it more difficult to pass through the stenotic segment of colon [243]. An emollient such as small doses of mineral oil makes soft fecal matter that can be passed easily through stenotic segment [243]. Lactulose can be effective; however, it causes excessive gassiness/bloating that may cause abdominal pain and incontinence [243].

Bleeding from telangiectasias is chronic complication of radiation-induced colonic toxicity. Argon plasma coagulation (APC) via flexible sigmoidoscopy or colonoscopy is the primary therapeutic approach. High success rates were reported [242, 243].

Colonic fibrosis or stenosis and fistulous formation are also seen in patients. In these cases, endoscopic dilation can be considered, and stenting may be useful for short or distal strictures. The surgical approaches for stricture and fistulous tracts have high risk and associated with poor outcomes due to underlying chronic ischemia and fibrosis [244–246]. In more severe cases, the malnutrition may develop because of malabsorption. It has been reported that the total parenteral nutrition can resolve malabsorption from radiation enteritis in multiple reports [230, 247–250].

5.6.6 Rx: Sample Prescriptions

There is a summary of recommendation for colon/large bowel toxicity below:

- Diarrhea: Antidiarrhetic agents (loperamide, octreotide)
- Dehydration: Adequate hydration
- Antibiotics: Severe diarrhea with fever, dehydration, neutropenia, sepsis
- Bowel cramping/pain: Anticholinergic antispasmodic agents
- Dietary modifications: Adequate soluble fiber, nutritional support, TPN

- Stenosis/stricture: Emollients, lactulose
- Malabsorption: Nutritional support
- Bleeding: Refer to a gastroenterologist (Endoscopic manipulations, APC)
- Needs surgery: Refer to a surgeon (if fistulous tracts, strictures, obstruction)

Acknowledgment We specially thank Volkan Semiz, MD from Dokuz Eylul University Medical School Department of Radiation Oncology for data processing of computerized tomography scans.

References

1. The University of Iowa College of Medicine University of Iowa. College of medicine: couinaud classification. http://dpi.radiology.uiowa.edu/nlm/app/livertoc/liver/8seg.html.
2. Ingold JA, Reed GB, Kaplan HS, Bagshaw MA. Radiation hepatitis. Am J Roentgenol Radium Therapy, Nucl Med. 1965;93:200–8.
3. Clement B, Grimaud JA, Campion JP, et al. Cell types involved in collagen and fibronectin production in normal and fibrotic human liver. Hepatology. 1986;6:225–34.
4. Lee UE, Friedman SL. Mechanisms of hepatic fibrogenesis. Best Pract Res Clin Gastroenterol. 2011;25:195–206. https://doi.org/10.1016/j.bpg.2011.02.005.
5. Anscher MS, Cracker IR, Jirtle RL. Transforming growth factor-β1 expression in irradiated liver. Radiat Res. 1990;122:77–85.
6. Castilla A, Prieto J, Fausto N. Transforming growth factor β I and alpha in chronic liver disease—effects of interferon alpha therapy. N Engl J Med. 1991;324:993–40. https://doi.org/10.1056/NEJM199104043241401.
7. Seidensticker M, Seidensticker R, Damm R, et al. Prospective randomized trial of enoxaparin, pentoxifylline and ursodeoxycholic acid for prevention of radiation-induced liver toxicity. PLoS One. 2014;9:e112731. https://doi.org/10.1371/journal.pone.0112731.
8. Christiansen H, Saile B, Neubauer-Saile K, et al. Irradiation leads to susceptibility of hepatocytes to TNF-alpha mediated apoptosis. Radiother Oncol. 2004;72:291–6. https://doi.org/10.1016/j.radonc.2004.07.001.
9. DeLeve LD, Shulman HM, McDonald GB. Toxic injury to hepatic sinusoids: sinusoidal obstruction syndrome (venoocclusive disease). Semin Liver Dis. 2002;22:27–42. https://doi.org/10.1055/s-2002-23204.
10. Lawrence TS, Robertson JM, Anscher MS, Jirtle RL, Ensminger WD, Fajardo LF. Hepatic toxicity resulting from cancer treatment. Int J Radiat Oncol Biol Phys. 1995;31:1237–48. https://doi.org/10.1016/0360-3016(94)00418-K.
11. Ogata K, Hizawa K, Yoshida M, Kitamuro T, Akagi G, Kagawa K, et al. Hepatic injury following irradiation–a morphologic study. Tokushima J Exp Med. 1963;10:240–51.
12. Reed GB Jr, Cox AJ Jr. The human liver after radiation injury. A form of veno-occlusive disease. Am J Pathol. 1966;48:597–11.
13. Sempoux C, Horsmans Y, Geubel A, Fraikin J, Van Beers BE, Gigot JF, et al. Severe radiation-induced liver disease following localized radiation therapy for biliopancreatic carcinoma: activation of hepatic stellate cells as an early event. Hepatology. 1997;26:128–34. https://doi.org/10.1002/hep.510260117.
14. Pan CC, Kavanagh BD, Dawson LA, Li XA, Das SK, Miften M, et al. Radiation-associated liver injury. Int J Radiat Oncol Biol Phys. 2010;76:S94–100. https://doi.org/10.1016/j.ijrobp.2009.06.092.
15. Cheng JC, Wu JK, Lee PC, Liu HS, Jian JJ, Lin YM, et al. Biologic susceptibility of hepatocellular carcinoma patients treated withradiotherapy to radiation-induced liver disease. Int J Radiat Oncol Biol Phys. 2004;60:1502–9. https://doi.org/10.1016/j.ijrobp.2004.05.048.

16. Guha C, Sharma A, Gupta S, Alfieri A, Gorla GR, Gagandeep S, et al. Amelioration of radiation-induced liver damage in partially hepatectomized rats by hepatocyte transplantation. Cancer Res. 1999;59:5871–4.

17. Lawrence TS, Robertson JM, Anscher MS, et al. Hepatic toxicity resulting from cancer treatment. Int J Radiat Oncol Biol Phys. 1995;31:1237–48. https://doi.org/10.1016/0360-3016(94)00418-K.

18. Austin-Seymour MM, Chen GT, Castro JR, et al. Dose volume histogram analysis of liver radiation tolerance. Int J Radiat Oncol Biol Phys. 1986;12:31–5.

19. Emami B, Lyman J, Brown A, et al. Tolerance of normal tissue to therapeutic irradiation. Int J Radiat Oncol Biol Phys. 1991;21:109–22. https://doi.org/10.1016/0360-3016(91)90171-y.

20. Guha C, Kavanagh BD. Hepatic radiation toxicity: avoidance and amelioration. Semin Radiat Oncol. 2011;21:256–63. https://doi.org/10.1016/j.semradonc.2011.05.003.

21. Jackson A, Ten Haken RK, Robertson JM, et al. Analysis of clinical complication data for radiation hepatitis using a parallel architecture model. Int J Radiat Oncol Biol Phys. 1995;31:883–91. https://doi.org/10.1016/0360-3016(94)00471-4.

22. Shaffer JL, Osmundson EC, Visser BC, et al. Stereotactic body radiation therapy and central liver toxicity: a case report. Pract Radiat Oncol. 2015;5:282–5. https://doi.org/10.1016/j.prro.2015.04.011.

23. Osmundson EC, Wu Y, Luxton G, et al. Predictors of toxicity associated with stereotactic body radiation therapy to the central hepatobiliary tract. Int J Radiat Oncol Biol Phys. 2015;91:986–94. https://doi.org/10.1016/j.ijrobp.2014.11.028.

24. Toesca DA, Osmundson EC, Eyben RV, et al. Central liver toxicity after SBRT: an expanded analysis and predictive nomogram. Radiother Oncol. 2017;122:130–6. https://doi.org/10.1016/j.radonc.2016.10.024.

25. Schefter TE, Kavanagh BD, Timmerman RD, et al. A phase I trial of stereotactic body radiation therapy (SBRT) for liver metastases. Int J Radiat Oncol Biol Phys. 2005;62:1371–8.

26. Penna C, Nordlinger B. Colorectal metastasis (liver and lung). Surg Clin North Am. 2002;82:1075–90. https://doi.org/10.1016/j.ijrobp.2005.01.002.

27. Xu ZY, Liang SX, Zhu J, et al. Prediction of radiation-induced liver disease by Lyman normal-tissue complication probability model in three-dimensional conformal radiation therapy for primary liver carcinoma. Int J Radiat Oncol Biol Phys. 2006;65:189–95. https://doi.org/10.1016/j.ijrobp.2005.11.034.

28. Liang SX, Zhu XD, Xu ZY, et al. Radiation-induced liver disease in three-dimensional conformal radiation therapy for primary liver carcinoma: the risk factors and hepatic radiation tolerance. Int J Radiat Oncol Biol Phys. 2006;65:426–34. https://doi.org/10.1016/j.ijrobp.2005.12.031.

29. Kim JH, Park JW, Kim TH, et al. Hepatitis B virus reactivation after three-dimensional conformal radiotherapy in patients with hepatitis B virus-related hepatocellular carcinoma. Int J Radiat Oncol Biol Phys. 2007;69:813–9. https://doi.org/10.1016/j.ijrobp.2007.04.005.

30. Chou CH, Chen PJ, Lee PH, et al. Radiation-induced hepatitis B virus reactivation in liver mediated by the bystander effect from irradiated endothelial cells. Clin Cancer Res. 2007;13:851–7. https://doi.org/10.1158/1078-0432.CCR-06-2459.

31. Huang W, Zhang W, Fan M, et al. Risk factors for hepatitis B virus reactivation after conformal radiotherapy in patients with hepatocellular carcinoma. Cancer Sci. 2014;105:697–703. https://doi.org/10.1111/cas.12400.

32. Herfarth KK, Debus J, Wannenmacher M. Stereotactic radiation therapy of liver metastases: update of the initialphase-I/II trial. Front Radiat Ther Oncol. 2004;38:100–5.

33. Wulf J, Hädinger U, Oppitz U, Olshausen B, Flentje M. Stereotactic radiotherapy of extracranial targets: CT-simulation and accuracy of treatment in the stereotacticbody frame. Radiother Oncol. 2000;57(2):225–36. https://doi.org/10.1016/S0167-8140(00)00226-7.

34. Mendez Romero A, Bakri L, Seppenwoolde Y, et al. Inter- and intraobserver variability in daily tumor setup usingcontrast-enhanced CT scans for patient positioning duringstereotactic body radiation therapy for liver metastases. Int J Radiat Oncol. 2013;87(2 Suppl):S318. https://doi.org/10.1016/j.ijrobp.2013.06.836.

35. Wu DH, Liu L, Chen LH. Therapeutic effects and prognostic factors in three-dimensional conformal radiotherapy combined with transcatheter arterial chemoembolization for hepatocellular carcinoma. World J Gastroenterol. 2004;10:2184–9. https://doi.org/10.3748/wjg.v10.i15.2184.
36. Shim SJ, Seong J, Lee IJ, et al. Radiation-induced hepatic toxicity after radiotherapy combined with chemotherapy for hepatocellular carcinoma. Hepatol Res. 2007;37:906–13. https://doi.org/10.1111/j.1872-034X.2007.00149.x.
37. Yu JI, Park JW, Park HC, et al. Clinical impact of combined transarterial chemoembolization and radiotherapy for advanced hepatocellular carcinoma with portal vein tumor thrombosis: an external validation study. Radiother Oncol. 2016;118:408–15. https://doi.org/10.1016/j.radonc.2015.11.019.
38. Robinson SM, Mann DA, Manas DM, et al. The potential contribution of tumour-related factors to the development of FOLFOX-induced sinusoidal obstruction syndrome. Br J Cancer. 2013;109:2396–403. https://doi.org/10.1038/bjc.2013.604.
39. Blomgren H, Lax I, Näslund I, Svanström R. Stereotactic highdose fraction radiation therapy of extracranial tumors usingan accelerator. Clinical experience of the first thirty-onepatients. Acta Oncol. 1995;34(6):861–70. https://doi.org/10.3109/02841869509127197.8.
40. Schefter TE, Kavanagh BD, Timmerman RD, Cardenes HR, Baron A, Gaspar LE. A phase I trial of stereotactic bodyradiation therapy (SBRT) for liver metastases. Int J Radiat Oncol Biol Phys. 2005;62(5):1371–8. https://doi.org/10.1016/j.ijrobp.2005.01.002.18.
41. McCammon R, Schefter TE, Gaspar LE, Zaemisch R, Gravdahl D, Kavanagh B. Observation of a dose-control relationship forlung and liver tumors after stereotactic body radiationtherapy. Int J Radiat Oncol Biol Phys. 2009;73(1):112–8. https://doi.org/10.1016/j.ijrobp.2008.03.062.19.
42. Rusthoven KE, Kavanagh BD, Cardenes H, et al. Multi-institutional phase I/II trial of stereotactic bodyradiation therapy for liver metastases. J Clin Oncol. 2009;27(10):1572–8. https://doi.org/10.1200/JCO.2008.19.6329.
43. Goodman KA, Wiegner EA, Maturen KE, et al. Dose-escalationstudy of single-fraction stereotactic body radiotherapy forliver malignancies. Int J Radiat Oncol Biol Phys. 2010;78(2):486–93. https://doi.org/10.1016/j.ijrobp.2009.08.020.
44. Tse RV, Hawkins M, Lockwood G, et al. Phase I study ofindividualized stereotactic body radiotherapy forhepatocellular carcinoma and intrahepaticcholangiocarcinoma. J Clin Oncol. 2008;26(4):657–64. https://doi.org/10.1200/JCO.2007.14.3529.
45. Andolino DL, Forquer JA, Henderson MA, et al. Chest walltoxicity after stereotactic body radiotherapy for malignantlesions of the lung and liver. Int J Radiat Oncol Biol Phys. 2011;80(3):692–7. https://doi.org/10.1016/j.ijrobp.2010.03.020.
46. Andratschke NH, Nieder C, Heppt F, Molls M, Zimmermann F. Stereotactic radiation therapy for liver metastases: factorsaffecting local control and survival. Radiat Oncol. 2015;10:69. https://doi.org/10.1186/s13014-015-0369-9.11.
47. Bujold A, Massey CA, Kim JJ, Brierley J, Cho C, Wong RK, et al. Sequential phase I and II trials of stereotactic body radiotherapy for locally advanced hepatocellular carcinoma. J Clin Oncol. 2013;31(13):1631–9. https://doi.org/10.1200/JCO.2012.44.1659.
48. Sanuki N, Takeda A, Oku Y, et al. Threshold doses for focalliver reaction after stereotactic ablative body radiationtherapy for small hepatocellular carcinoma depend on liverfunction: evaluation on magnetic resonance imaging withGd-EOB-DTPA. Int J Radiat Oncol Biol Phys. 2014;88(2):306–11. https://doi.org/10.1016/j.ijrobp.2013.10.045.
49. Jang WI, Kim MS, Bae SH, Cho CK, Yoo HJ, Seo YS, et al. High-dose stereotactic body radiotherapy correlates increased local control and overall survival in patients with inoperable hepatocellular carcinoma. Radiat Oncol. 2013;8:250. https://doi.org/10.1186/1748-717X-8-250.
50. Yoon SM, Lim YS, Park MJ, Kim SY, Cho B, Shim JH, et al. Stereotactic body radiation therapy as an alternative treatment for small hepatocellular carcinoma. PLoS One. 2013;8(11):e79854. https://doi.org/10.1371/journal.pone.0079854.
51. Lee MT, Kim JJ, Dinniwell R, et al. Phase I study ofindividualized stereotactic body radiotherapy of livermetastases. J Clin Oncol. 2009;27(10):1585–91. https://doi.org/10.1200/JCO.2008.20.0600.

52. Burman C, Kutcher GJ, Emami B, et al. Fitting of normal tissue tolerance data to an ana-lytic function. Int J Radiat Oncol Biol Phys. 1991;21:123–35. https://doi.org/10.1016/0360-3016(91)90172-z.
53. Lawrence TS, Ten Haken RK, Kessler ML, et al. The use of 3-D dose volume analysis to predict radiation hepatitis. Int J Radiat Oncol Biol Phys. 1992;23:781–8.
54. Dawson LA, Ten Haken RK, Lawrence TS. Partial irradiation of the liver. Semin Radiat Oncol. 2001;11:240–6.
55. Lee IJ, Seong J, Shim SJ, Han KH. Radiotherapeutic parameters predictive of liver complications induced by liver tumor radiotherapy. Int J Radiat Oncol Biol Phys. 2009;73:154–8. https://doi.org/10.1016/j.ijrobp.2008.04.035.
56. Chen YX, Zeng ZC, Sun J, Zeng HY, Huang Y, Zhang ZY. Mesenchymal stem cell-conditioned medium prevents radiation-induced liver injury by inhibiting inflammation and protecting sinusoidal endothelial cells. J Radiat Res. 2015;56:700–8.
57. Mouiseddine M, Francois S, Souidi M, Chapel A. Intravenous human mesenchymal stem cells transplantation in NOD/SCID mice preserve liver integrity of irradiation damage. Methods Mol Biol. 2012;826:179–88.
58. Anscher MS, Crocker IR, Jirtle RL. Transforming growth factor-beta 1 expression in irradiated liver. Radiat Res. 1990;122:77–85.
59. Du SS, Qiang M, Zeng ZC, Zhou J, Tan YS, Zhang ZY, et al. Radiation-induced liver fibrosis is mitigated by gene therapy inhibiting transforming growth factor-beta signaling in the rat. Int J Radiat Oncol Biol Phys. 2010;78:1513–23.
60. Wang S, Lee Y, Kim J, Hyun J, Lee K, Kim Y, et al. Potential role of hedgehog pathway in liver response to radiation. PLoS One. 2013;8:e74141.
61. Wang S, Hyun J, Youn B, Jung Y. Hedgehog signaling regulates the repair response in mouse liver damaged by irradiation. Radiat Res. 2013;179:69–75.
62. Symon Z, Levi M, Ensminger WD, Smith DE, Lawrence TS. Selective radioprotection of hepatocytes by systemic and portal vein infusions of amifostine in a rat liver tumor model. Int J Radiat Oncol Biol Phys. 2001;50:473–8. https://doi.org/10.1016/s0360-3016(01)01522-x.
63. Taysi S, Koc M, Buyukokuroglu ME, Altinkaynak K, Sahin YN. Melatonin reduces lipid peroxidation and nitric oxide during irradiation-induced oxidative injury in the rat liver. J Pineal Res. 2003;34:173–7. https://doi.org/10.1034/j.1600-079X.2003.00024.x.
64. Glatstein E, Fajardo LF, Brown JM. Radiation injury in the mouse kidney-I. Sequential light microscopic study. Int J Radiat Oncol Biol Phys. 1977;2(9–10):933–43. https://doi.org/10.1016/0360-3016(77)90191-2.
65. Moulder JE, Fish BL. Late toxicity of total body irradiation with bone marrow transplantation in a rat model. Int J Radiat Oncol Biol Phys. 1989;16(6):1501–9. https://doi.org/10.1016/0360-3016(89)90955-3.
66. Rubenstone AI, Fitch LB. Radiation nephritis. A clinicopathologic study. Am J Med. 1962;33:545–54. https://doi.org/10.1016/0002-9343(62)90265-6.
67. Jaenke RS, Robbins ME, Bywaters T, Whitehouse E, Rezvani M, Hopewell JW. Capillary endothelium. Target site of renal radiation injury. Lab Investig. 1993;68(4):396–405.
68. Keane WF, Crosson JT, Staley NA, Anderson WR, Shapiro FL. Radiation-induced renal disease. A clinicopathologic study. Am J Med. 1976 Jan;60(1):127–37. https://doi.org/10.1016/0002-9343(76)90541-6.
69. Krochak RJ, Baker DG. Radiation nephritis. Clinical manifestations and pathophysiologic mechanisms. Urology. 1986;27(5):389–93. https://doi.org/10.1016/0090-4295(86)90399-7.
70. Dawson LA, Kavanagh BD, Paulino AC, Das SK, Miften M, Li XA, et al. Radiation-associated kidney injury. Int J Radiat Oncol Biol Phys. 2010;76(3 Suppl):S108–15. https://doi.org/10.1016/j.ijrobp.2009.02.089.
71. Thompson PL, Mackay IR, Robson GS, et al. Late radiation nephritis after gastric x-irradiation for peptic ulcer. Q J Med. 1971;40:145–57.
72. Verheij M, Dewit LG, Valdés Olmos RA, Arisz L. Evidence for a renovascular component in hypertensive patients with late radiation nephropathy. Int J Radiat Oncol Biol Phys. 1994;30(3):677–83. https://doi.org/10.1016/0360-3016(92)90955-h.

73. Cohen EP, Robbins ME. Radiation nephropathy. Semin Nephrol. 2003;23:486–99.
74. Cruz DN, Perazella MA, Mahnensmith RL. Bone marrow transplant nephropathy: a case report and review of the literature. J Am Soc Nephrol. 1997;8(1):166–73.
75. Flentje M, Hensley F, Gademann G, Menke M, Wannenmacher M. Renal tolerance to non-homogenous irradiation: comparison of observed effects to predictions of normal tissue complication probability from different biophysical models. Int J Radiat Oncol Biol Phys. 1993;27(1):25–30. https://doi.org/10.1016/0360-3016(93)90417-t.
76. Ahmad NR, Huq MS, Corn BW. Respiration-induced motion of the kidneys in whole abdominal radiotherapy: implications for treatment planning and late toxicity. Radiother Oncol. 1997;42:87–90. https://doi.org/10.1016/s0167-8140(96)01859-2.
77. Reiff JE, Werner-Wasik M, Valicenti RK, Huq MS. Changes in the size and location of kidneys from the supine to standing positions and the implications for block placement during total body irradiation. Int J Radiat Oncol Biol Phys. 1999;45(2):447–9. https://doi.org/10.1016/s0360-3016(99)00208-4.
78. Cheng J, Schultheiss T, Wong J. Impact of drug therapy, radiation dose and dose rate on renal toxicity following bone marrow transplantation. Int J Radiat Oncol Biol Phys. 2008;71(5):1436–43. https://doi.org/10.1016/j.ijrobp.2007.12.009.
79. Cohen EP. Radiation nephropathy after bone marrow transplantation. Kidney Int. 2000;58:903–18. https://doi.org/10.1046/j.1523-1755.2000.00241.x.
80. Luxton RW. Radiation nephritis: along termstudy of 54 patients. Lancet. 1961;2(7214):1221–4. https://doi.org/10.1016/s0140-6736(61)92590-9.
81. Luxton RW. Radiation nephritis. Q J Med. 1953;22(86):215–42.
82. Köst S, Dörr W, Keinert K, Glaser FH, Endert G, Herrmann T. Effect of dose and dose-distribution in damage to the kidney following abdominal radiotherapy. Int J Radiat Biol. 2002;78(8):695–702. https://doi.org/10.1080/09553000210134791.
83. Willett CG, Tepper JE, Orlow EL, Shipley WU. Renal complications secondary to radiation treatment of upper abdominal malignancies. Int J Radiat Oncol Biol Phys. 1986;12(9):1601–4. https://doi.org/10.1016/0360-3016(86)90284-1.
84. Jansen EP, Saunders MP, Boot H, Oppedijk V, Dubbelman R, Porritt B, et al. Prospective study on late renal toxicity following postoperative chemoradiotherapy in gastric cancer. Int J Radiat Oncol Biol Phys. 2007;67(3):781–5. https://doi.org/10.1016/j.ijrobp.2006.09.012.
85. May KS, Yang GY, Khushalani NI, Chandrasekhar R, Wilding GE, Flaherty L, et al. Association of Technetium(99m) MAG-3 renal scintigraphy with change in creatinine clearance following chemoradiation to the abdomen in patients with gastrointestinal malignancies. J Gastrointest Oncol. 2010;1(1):7–15. https://doi.org/10.3978/j.issn.2078-6891.2010.001.
86. Crummy AB, Hellman S, Stansel HC, Hukill PB. Renal hypertension secondary to unilateral radiation damage relieved by nephrectomy. Radiology. 1965;84:108–11. https://doi.org/10.1148/84.1.108.
87. Kala J. Radiation-induced kidney injury. J Onco-Nephrol. 2019;3(3):160–7. https://doi.org/10.1177/2399369319865271.
88. Diavolitsis VM, Rademaker A, Boyle J, Kang Z, Kiel K, Mulcahy M, et al. Change in creatinine clearance over time following upper abdominal irradiation: a dose-volume histogram multivariate analysis. Am J Clin Oncol. 2011;34(1):53–7. https://doi.org/10.1097/COC.0b013e3181d27080.
89. Rubin P, Casarett G. Radiation effect and tolerance of normal tissue. Front Radiat Ther Oncol. 1971;5:1–16.
90. Cohen L, Creditor M. Iso-effect tables for tolerance of irradiated normal human tissues. Int J Radiat Oncol Biol Phys. 1983;9(2):233–41. https://doi.org/10.1016/0360-3016(83)90105-0.
91. Emami B, Lyman J, Brown A, Coia L, Goitein M, Munzenrider JE, et al. Tolerance of normal tissue to therapeutic irradiation. Int J Radiat Oncol Biol Phys. 1991;21(1):109–22. https://doi.org/10.1016/0360-3016(91)90171-y.
92. Milano MT, Constine LS, Okunieff P. Normal tissue tolerance dose metrics for radiation therapy of major organs. Semin Radiat Oncol. 2007;17(2):131–40. https://doi.org/10.1016/j.semradonc.2006.11.009.

93. Marks LB, Yorke ED, Jackson A, Ten Haken RK, Constine LS, Eisbruch A, et al. Use of normal tissue complication probability models in the clinic. Int J Radiat Oncol Biol Phys. 2010;76(3 Suppl):S10–9. https://doi.org/10.1016/j.ijrobp.2009.07.1754.

94. Welz S, Hehr T, Kollmannsberger C, Bokemeyer C, Belka C, Budach W. Renal toxicity of adjuvant chemoradiotherapy with cisplatin in gastric cancer. Int J Radiat Oncol Biol Phys. 2007;69(5):1429–35. https://doi.org/10.1016/j.ijrobp.2007.05.021.

95. Varlotto JM, Gerszten K, Heron DE, Comerci J, Gautam S, Selvaraj R, et al. The potential nephrotoxic effects of intensity modulated radiotherapy delivered to the para-aortic area of women with gynecologic malignancies: preliminary results. Am J Clin Oncol. 2006;29(3):281–9. https://doi.org/10.1097/01.coc.0000217828.95729.b5.

96. May KS, Khushalani NI, Chandrasekhar R, Wilding GE, Iyer RV, Ma WW, et al. Analysis of clinical and dosimetric factors associated with change in renal function in patients with gastrointestinal malignancies after chemoradiation to the abdomen. Int J Radiat Oncol Biol Phys. 2010;76(4):1193–8. https://doi.org/10.1016/j.ijrobp.2009.03.002.

97. Moulder JE, Fish BL, Cohen EP. Treatment of radiation nephropathy with ACE inhibitors and AII type-1 and type-2 receptor antagonists. Curr Pharm Des. 2007;13:1317–25. https://doi.org/10.2174/138161207780618821.

98. Cohen EP, Fish BL, Sharma M, et al. Role of the angiotensin II type-2 receptor in radiation nephropathy. Transl Res. 2007;150:106–15. https://doi.org/10.1016/j.trsl.2007.03.004.

99. Cohen EP, Hussain S, Moulder JE. Successful treatment of radiation nephropathy with angiotensin II blockade. Int J Radiat Oncol Biol Phys. 2003;55:190–3. https://doi.org/10.1016/s0360-3016(02)03793-8.

100. Jafar TH, Stark PC, Schmid CH, Landa M, Maschio G, de Jong PE, AIPRD Study Group, et al. Progression of chronic kidney disease: the role of blood pressure control, proteinuria, and angiotensin-converting enzyme inhibition: a patient-level meta-analysis. Ann Intern Med. 2003;139(4):244–52. https://doi.org/10.7326/0003-4819-139-4-200308190-00006.

101. Cohen EP, Fish BL, Moulder JE. Mitigation of radiation injuries via suppression of the renin-angiotensin system: emphasis on radiation nephropathy. Curr Drug Targets. 2010;11:1423–9. https://doi.org/10.2174/1389450111009011423.

102. Juncos LI, Carrasco Dueñas S, Cornejo JC, Broglia CA, Cejas H. Long-term enalapril and hydrochlorothiazide in radiation nephritis. Nephron. 1993;64(2):249–55. https://doi.org/10.1159/000187322.

103. Verheij M, Stewart FA, Oussoren Y, Weening JJ, Dewit L. Amelioration of radiation nephropathy by acetylsalicylic acid. Int J Radiat Biol. 1995;67(5):587–96. https://doi.org/10.1080/09553009514550701.

104. Moulder JE, Fish BL, Cohen EP. Noncontinuous use of angiotensin converting enzyme inhibitors in the treatment of experimental bone marrow transplant nephropathy. Bone Marrow Transplant. 1997;19(7):729–35. https://doi.org/10.1038/sj.bmt.1700732.

105. Cohen EP, Fish BL, Moulder JE. Successful brief captopril treatment in experimental radiation nephropathy. J Lab Clin Med. 1997;129(5):536–47. https://doi.org/10.1016/S0022-2143(97)90008-1.

106. Sarnak MJ, Greene T, Wang X, Beck G, Kusek JW, Collins AJ, et al. The effect of a lower target blood pressure on the progression of kidney disease: long-term follow-up of the modification of diet in renal disease study. Ann Intern Med. 2005;142(5):342–51. https://doi.org/10.7326/0003-4819-142-5-200503010-00009.

107. Sarode R, McFarland JG, Flomenberg N, Casper JT, Cohen EP, Drobyski WR, et al. Therapeutic plasma exchange does not appear to be effective in the management of thrombotic thrombocytopenic purpura/hemolytic uremic syndrome following bone marrow transplantation. Bone Marrow Transplant. 1995;16(2):271–5.

108. Cohen EP, Piering WF, Kabler-Babbitt C, Moulder JE. End-stage renal disease (ESRD) after bone marrow transplantation: poor survival compar ed to other causes of ESRD. Nephron. 1998;79(4):408–12. https://doi.org/10.1159/000045085.

109. Federle MP, Rosado-de-Christenson ML, Woodward PJ, et al. Diagnostic and surgical imaging anatomy: chest, abdomen, pelvis. 1st ed. Philadelphia: Lippincott Williams & Wilkins; 2006.

110. Moore KA. Clinically oriented anatomy. 3rd ed. Philadelphia: Williams & Wilkins; 1992.
111. Gray H. Anatomy of the human body. Edited by Warren H. Lewis, 20th edition. Philadelphia: Lea & Febiger, 1918. New York: Barlteby.com; 2000.
112. Potten C, Booth C. The role of radiation induced and spontaneous apoptosis in the homeostasis of the gastrointestinal epithelium. Comp Biochem Physiol. 1997;3:473.
113. Richter K, Langberg C, Sung C, et al. Increased transforming growth factor β (TGF-β) immunoreactivity is independently associated with chronic injury in both consequential and primary radiation enteropathy. Int J Radiat Oncol Biol Phys. 1997;19:187.
114. Landberg C, Hauer-Jensen M, Sung C, et al. Expression of fi brogenic cytokines in rat small intestine after fractionated irradiation. Radiother Oncol. 1994;32:29.
115. Richter K, Fink L, Hughes B, et al. Is the loss of endothelial thrombomodulin involved in the mechanism of chronicity in late radiation enteropathy? Radiother Oncol. 1997;44:65.
116. Vozenin-Brotons M-C, Fabien M, Sabourin J-C, et al. Fibrogenic signals in patients with radiation enteritis are associated with increased connective tissue growth factor expression. Int J Radiat Oncol Biol Phys. 2003;56:561.
117. Coia LR, Myerson RJ, Tepper JE. Late effects of radiation therapy on the gastrointestinal tract. Int J Radiat Oncol Biol Phys. 1995;31:1213–36.
118. Goldgraber MB, Rubin CE, Palmer WL, et al. The early gastric response to irradiation; a serial biopsy study. Gastroenterology. 1954;27:1–20.
119. Fajardo L, Berthrong M, Anderson R. Radiation pathology. New York: Oxford University Press; 2001.
120. Goldstein H, Rogers L, Fletcher G, et al. Radiological manifestations of radiation-induced injury to the normal upper gastrointestinal tract. Radiology. 1975;227:135–40.
121. Sylven B, Vikterlof K, Schnurer L. Gastric ulceration following cobalt teletherapy Estimation of the tolerance dose. Acta Radiol. 1969;8:183.
122. Hamilton CR, Horwich A, Bliss JM, et al. Gastrointestinal morbidity of adjuvant radiotherapy in stage I malignant teratoma of the testis. Radiother Oncol. 1987;10:85–90.
123. Cosset JM, Henry-Amar M, Burgers JM, et al. Late radiation injuries of the gastrointestinal tract in the H2 and H5 EORTC Hodgkin's disease trials: emphasis on the role of explor-atory laparotomy and fractionation. Radiother Oncol. 1988;13:61–8.
124. Pearson JG. The present status and future potential of radiotherapy in the management of esophageal cancer. Cancer. 1977;39:882–90.
125. Gunderson LL, Hoskins RB, Cohen AC, et al. Combined modality treatment of gastric cancer. Int J Radiat Oncol Biol Phys. 1983;9:965–75.
126. Novak JM, Collins JT, Donowitz M, et al. Effects of radiation on the human gastrointestinal tract. J Clin Gastroenterol. 1979;1:9–39.
127. Blomgren H. Radiosurgery for tumors in the body: clinical experience using a new method. J Radiosurg. 1998;160:63–74.
128. Mendez Romero A, Bakri L, Seppenwoolde Y, et al. Inter-andintraobserver variability in daily tumor setup usingcontrast-enhanced CT scans for patient positioning duringstereotactic body radiation therapy for liver metastases. Int J Radiat Oncol. 2013;87(2 Suppl):S318. https://doi.org/10.1016/j.ijrobp.2013.06.836.
129. Wada S, Tamada K, Tomiyama T, Yamamoto H, Nakazawa K, Sugano K. Endoscopic hemostasis for radiation-induced gastritis using argon plasma coagulation. J Gastroenterol Hepatol. 2003;18:1215–8.
130. Shukuwa K, Kume K, Yamasaki M, Yoshikawa I, Otsuki M. Argon plasma coagulation therapy for a hemorrhagic radiation-induced gastritis in patient with pancreatic cancer. Intern Med. 2007;46:975–7.
131. Taïeb S, Rolachon A, Cenni JC, Nancey S, Bonvoisin S, Descos L, Fournet J, Gérard JP, Flourié B. Effective use of argon plasma coagulation in the treatment of severe radiation proctitis. Dis Colon Rectum. 2001;44:1766–71.
132. Venkatesh KS, Ramanujam P. Endoscopic therapy for radiation proctitis-induced hemorrhage in patients with prostatic carcinoma using argon plasma coagulator application. Surg Endosc. 2002;16:707–10.

133. Kochhar R, Patel F, Dhar A, Sharma SC, Ayyagari S, Aggarwal R, Goenka MK, Gupta BD, Mehta SK. Radiationinduced proctosigmoiditis. Prospective, randomized, double-blind controlled trial of oral sulfasalazine plus rectal steroids versus rectal sucralfate. Dig Dis Sci. 1991;36:103–7.
134. Theis VS, Sripadam R, Ramani V, Lal S. Chronic radiation enteritis. Clin Oncol (R Coll Radiol). 2010;22:70–83.
135. Kennedy GD, Heise CP. Radiation colitis and proctitis. Clin Colon Rectal Surg. 2007;20:64–72.
136. Vivek V, Audrey JL, Dandan Z, Abhijeet RB, Quan PL, Chandrakanth A, et al. Dosimetric parameters correlate with duodenal histopathologic damage after stereotactic body radiotherapy for pancreatic cancer: secondary analysis of a prospective clinical trial. Radiother Oncol. 2017;122:464–9. https://doi.org/10.1016/j.radonc.2016.12.030.
137. Wilson JM, Fokas E, Dutton SJ, et al. ARCII: a phase II trial of the HIV protease inhibitor Nelfinavir in combination with chemoradiation for locally advanced inoperable pancreatic cancer. Radiother Oncol. 2016;119:306–11.
138. Xu KM, Rajagopalan MS, Kim H, Beriwal S. Extended field intensity modulated radiation therapy for gynecologic cancers: is the risk of duodenal toxicity high? Pract Radiat Oncol. 2015;5:e291–7.
139. Verma J, Sulman EP, Jhingran A, et al. Dosimetric predictors of duodenal toxicity after intensity modulated radiation therapy for treatment of the para-aortic nodes in gynecologic cancer. Int J Radiat Oncol Biol Phys. 2014;88:357–62.
140. Poorvu PD, Sadow CA, Townamchai K, Damato AL, Viswanathan AN. Duodenal and other gastrointestinal toxicity in cervical and endometrial cancer treated with extended-field intensity modulated radiation therapy to paraaortic lymph nodes. Int J Radiat Oncol Biol Phys. 2013;85:1262–8.
141. Kelly P, Das P, Pinnix CC, et al. Duodenal toxicity after fractionated chemoradiation for unresectable pancreatic cancer. Int J Radiat Oncol Biol Phys. 2013;85:e143–9.
142. Cattaneo GM, Passoni P, Longobardi B, et al. Dosimetric and clinical predictors of toxicity following combined chemotherapy and moderately hypofractionated rotational radiotherapy of locally advanced pancreatic adenocarcinoma. Radiother Oncol. 2013;108:66–71.
143. Mukherjee S, Hurt CN, Bridgewater J, et al. Gemcitabine-based or capecitabine-based chemoradiotherapy for locally advanced pancreatic cancer (SCALOP): a multicentre, randomised, phase 2 trial. Lancet Oncol. 2013;14:317–26.
144. Xia T, Chang D, Wang Y, Li J, Wu W, Zhu F. Dose escalation to target volumes of helical tomotherapy for pancreatic cancer in the phase 1–2 clinical trial. Int J Radiat Oncol Biol Phys. 2013;87:S303.
145. Kim H, Lim DH, Paik SW, et al. Predictive factors of gastroduodenal toxicity in cirrhotic patients after three-dimensional conformal radiotherapy for hepatocellular carcinoma. Radiother Oncol. 2009;93:302–6.
146. Pan CC, Dawson LA, McGinn CJ, Lawrence TS, Ten Haken RK. Analysis of radiation-induced gastric and duodenal bleeds using the Lyman-Kutcher-Burman model. Int J Radiat Oncol Biol Phys. 2003;57:S217–8.
147. Goldsmith C, Price P, Cross T, Loughlin S, Cowley I, et al. Dose–volume histogram analysis of stereotactic body radiotherapy treatment of pancreatic cancer: a focus on duodenal dose constraints. Semin Radiat Oncol. 2016;26:149–56.
148. Ben-Josef E, Schipper M, Francis IR, et al. A phase I/II trial of intensity modulated radiation (IMRT) dose escalation with concurrent fixed-dose rate gemcitabine (FDR-G) in patients with unresectable pancreatic cancer. Int J Radiat Oncol Biol Phys. 2012;84:1166–71.
149. Jabbour SK, Hashem SA, Bosch W, Kim TK, Finkelstein SE, Anderson BM, et al. Upper abdominal normal organ contouring guidelines and atlas: a Radiation therapy oncology group consensus. Pract Radiat Oncol. 2014;4(2):82–9. https://doi.org/10.1016/j.prro.2013.06.004.
150. Gay HA, Barthold HJ, O'Meara E, Bosch WR, El Naqa I, Al-Lozi R, et al. Pelvic normal tissue contouring guidelines for radiation therapy: a Radiation Therapy Oncology Group Consensus Panel Atlas. Int J Radiat Oncol Biol Phys. 2012;83(3):e353–62. https://doi.org/10.1016/j.ijrobp.2012.01.023.

151. Sanguineti G, Little M, Endres EJ, Sormani MP, Parker BC. Comparison of three strategies to delineate the bowel for whole pelvis IMRT of prostate cancer. Radiother Oncol. 2008;88(1):95–101. https://doi.org/10.1016/j.radonc.2008.01.015.

152. Citrin DE, Mitchell JB. Mechanisms of normal tissue injury from irradiation. Semin Radiat Oncol. 2017;27(4):316–24. https://doi.org/10.1016/j.semradonc.2017.04.001.

153. Denham JW, Hauer-Jensen M. The radiotherapeutic injury--a complex 'wound'. Radiother Oncol. 2002;63(2):129–45. https://doi.org/10.1016/s0167-8140(02)00060-9.

154. Hauer-Jensen M, Wang J, Denham JW. Bowel injury: current and evolving management strategies. Semin Radiat Oncol. 2003;13(3):357–71. https://doi.org/10.1016/s1053-4296(03)00032-8.

155. Rotolo JA, Maj JG, Feldman R, Ren D, Haimovitz-Friedman A, Cordon-Cardo C, et al. Bax and Bak do not exhibit functional redundancy in mediating radiation-induced endothelial apoptosis in the intestinal mucosa. Int J Radiat Oncol Biol Phys. 2008;70(3):804–15. https://doi.org/10.1016/j.ijrobp.2007.11.043.

156. Zimmerer T, Böcker U, Wenz F, Singer MV. Medical prevention and treatment of acute and chronic radiation induced enteritis: is there any proven therapy? A short review. Z Gastroenterol. 2008;46(5):441–8. https://doi.org/10.1055/s-2008-1027150.

157. Nicholas S, Chen L, Choflet A, Fader A, Guss Z, Hazell S, et al. Pelvic radiation and normal tissue toxicity. Semin Radiat Oncol. 2017;27(4):358–69. https://doi.org/10.1016/j.semradonc.2017.04.010.

158. Carr KE. Effects of radiation damage on intestinal morphology. Int Rev Cytol. 2001;208:1–119. https://doi.org/10.1016/s0074-7696(01)08002-0.

159. Hagemann RF. Intestinal cell proliferation during fractionated abdominal irradiation. Br J Radiol. 1976;49(577):56–61. https://doi.org/10.1259/0007-1285-49-577-56.

160. Maj JG, Paris F, Haimovitz-Friedman A, Venkatraman E, Kolesnick R, Fuks Z. Microvascular function regulates intestinal crypt response to radiation. Cancer Res. 2003;63(15):4338–41.

161. Wedlake L, Thomas K, McGough C, Andreyev HJ. Small bowel bacterial overgrowth and lactose intolerance during radical pelvic radiotherapy: an observational study. Eur J Cancer. 2008;44(15):2212–7. https://doi.org/10.1016/j.ejca.2008.07.018.

162. Andreyev J. Gastrointestinal symptoms after pelvic radiotherapy: a new understanding to improve management of symptomatic patients. Lancet Oncol. 2007;8(11):1007–17. https://doi.org/10.1016/S1470-2045(07)70341-8.

163. Berthrong M, Fajardo LF. Radiation injury in surgical pathology. Part II. Alimentary tract. Am J Surg Pathol. 1981;5(2):153–78. https://doi.org/10.1097/00000478-198103000-00006.

164. Otterson MF, Sarna SK, Moulder JE. Effects of fractionated doses of ionizing radiation on small intestinal motor activity. Gastroenterology. 1988;95(5):1249–57. https://doi.org/10.1016/0016-5085(88)90358-7.

165. Husebye E, Skar V, Høverstad T, Iversen T, Melby K. Abnormal intestinal motor patterns explain enteric colonization with gram-negative bacilli in late radiation enteropathy. Gastroenterology. 1995;109(4):1078–89. https://doi.org/10.1016/0016-5085(95)90565-0.

166. Martin M, Lefaix JL, Delanian S. TGF-1 and radiation fibrosis: a master switch and a specific therapeutic target? Int J Radiat Oncol Biol Phys. 2000;47:277–90. https://doi.org/10.1016/s0360-3016(00)00435-1.

167. Nguyen NP, Antoine JE, Dutta S, Karlsson U, Sallah S. Current concepts in radiation enteritis and implications for future clinical trials. Cancer. 2002;95(5):1151–63. https://doi.org/10.1002/cncr.10766.

168. Donner CS. Pathophysiology and therapy of chronic radiation-induced injury to the colon. Dig Dis. 1998;16(4):253–61. https://doi.org/10.1159/000016873.

169. Haboubi NY, Schofield PF, Rowland PL. The light and electron microscopic features of early and late phase radiation-induced proctitis. Am J Gastroenterol. 1988;83:1140–4.

170. Regimbeau JM, Panis Y, Gouzi JL. Fagniez PL; operative and long term results after surgery for chronic radiation enteritis. Am J Surg. 2001;182(3):237–42. https://doi.org/10.1016/s0002-9610(01)00705-x.

171. Hamad A, Fragkos CK, Forbes A. A systematic review and meta-analysis of probiotics for the management of radiation induced bowel disease. Clin Nutr. 2013;32:353–60. https://doi.org/10.1016/j.clnu.2013.02.004.

172. Jadon R, Higgins E, Hanna L, Evans M, Coles B, Staffurth J. A systematic review of dose-volume predictors and constraints for late bowel toxicity following pelvic radiotherapy. Radiat Oncol. 2019;14(1):57. https://doi.org/10.1186/s13014-019-1262-8.

173. Macdonald JS, Smalley SR, Benedetti J, Hundahl SA, Estes NC, Stemmermann GN, et al. Chemoradiotherapy after surgery compared with surgery alone for adenocarcinoma of the stomach or gastroesophageal junction. N Engl J Med. 2001;345(10):725–30. https://doi.org/10.1056/NEJMoa010187.

174. Bosset JF, Collette L, Calais G, Mineur L, Maingon P, Radosevic-Jelic L, et al. Chemotherapy with preoperative radiotherapy in rectal cancer. N Engl J Med. 2006;355(11):1114–23. https://doi.org/10.1056/NEJMoa060829.

175. Hauer-Jensen M. Late radiation injury of the small intestine: clinical, pathophysiologic, and radiobiologic aspects. A review. Acta Oncol. 1990;29(4):401–15. https://doi.org/10.3109/02841869009090022.

176. Baglan KL, Frazier RC, Yan D, Huang RR, Martinez AA, Robertson JM. The dose-volume relationship of acute small bowel toxicity from concurrent 5-FU-based chemotherapy and radiation therapy for rectal cancer. Int J Radiat Oncol Biol Phys. 2002;52(1):176–83. https://doi.org/10.1016/s0360-3016(01)01820-x.

177. Tho LM, Glegg M, Paterson J, Yap C, MacLeod A, McCabe M, et al. Acute small bowel toxicity and preoperative chemoradiotherapy for rectal cancer: investigating dose-volume relationships and role for inverse planning. Int J Radiat Oncol Biol Phys. 2006;66(2):505–13. https://doi.org/10.1016/j.ijrobp.2006.05.005.

178. Huang EY, Sung CC, Ko SF, Wang CJ, Yang KD. The different volume effects of small-bowel toxicity during pelvic irradiation between gynecologic patients with and without abdominal surgery: a prospective study with computed tomography-based dosimetry. Int J Radiat Oncol Biol Phys. 2007;69(3):732–9. https://doi.org/10.1016/j.ijrobp.2007.03.060.

179. Roeske JC, Bonta D, Mell LK, Lujan AE, Mundt AJ. A dosimetric analysis of acute gastrointestinal toxicity in women receiving intensity-modulated whole-pelvic radiation therapy. Radiother Oncol. 2003;69(2):201–7. https://doi.org/10.1016/j.radonc.2003.05.001.

180. Roeske JC, Lujan A, Rotmensch J, Waggoner SE, Yamada D, Mundt AJ. Intensity-modulated whole pelvic radiation therapy in patients with gynecologic malignancies. Int J Radiat Oncol Biol Phys. 2000;48(5):1613–21. https://doi.org/10.1016/s0360-3016(00)00771-9.

181. Robertson JM, Lockman D, Yan D, Wallace M. The dose-volume relationship of small bowel irradiation and acute grade 3 diarrhea during chemoradiotherapy for rectal cancer. Int J Radiat Oncol Biol Phys. 2008;70(2):413–8. https://doi.org/10.1016/j.ijrobp.2007.06.066.

182. Lee TF, Huang EY. The different dose-volume effects of normal tissue complication probability using LASSO for acute small-bowel toxicity during radiotherapy in gynecological patients with or without prior abdominal surgery. Biomed Res Int. 2014;2014:143020. https://doi.org/10.1155/2014/143020.

183. Kavanagh BD, Pan CC, Dawson LA, Das SK, Li XA, Ten Haken RK, et al. Radiation dose-volume effects in the stomach and small bowel. Int J Radiat Oncol Biol Phys. 2010;76(3 Suppl):S101–7. https://doi.org/10.1016/j.ijrobp.2009.05.071.

184. Martin J, Fitzpatrick K, Horan G, McCloy R, Buckney S, O'Neill L, et al. Treatment with a belly-board device significantly reduces the volume of small bowel irradiated and results in low acute toxicity in adjuvant radiotherapy for gynecologic cancer: results of a prospective study. Radiother Oncol. 2005;74(3):267–74. https://doi.org/10.1016/j.radonc.2004.11.010.

185. Kölbl O, Richter S, Flentje M. Influence of treatment technique on dose-volume histogram and normal tissue complication probability for small bowel and bladder. A prospective study using a 3-D planning system and a radiobiological model in patients receiving postoperative pelvic irradiation. Strahlenther Onkol. 2000;176(3):105–11. https://doi.org/10.1007/pl00002334.

186. Wee CW, Kang HC, Wu HG, Chie EK, Choi N, Park JM, et al. Intensity-modulated radiotherapy versus three-dimensional conformal radiotherapy in rectal cancer treated with neoadjuvant concurrent chemoradiation: a meta-analysis and pooled-analysis of acute toxicity. Jpn J Clin Oncol. 2018;48(5):458–66. https://doi.org/10.1093/jjco/hyy029.

187. Ng SY, Colborn KL, Cambridge L, Hajj C, Yang TJ, Wu AJ, et al. Acute toxicity with intensity modulated radiotherapy versus 3-dimensional conformal radiotherapy during preoperative chemoradiation for locally advanced rectal cancer. Radiother Oncol. 2016;121(2):252–7. https://doi.org/10.1016/j.radonc.2016.09.010.

188. Hong TS, Moughan J, Garofalo MC, Bendell J, Berger AC, Oldenburg NB, et al. NRG oncology radiation therapy oncology group 0822: a phase 2 study of preoperative chemoradiation therapy using intensity modulated radiation therapy in combination with capecitabine and oxaliplatin for patients with locally advanced rectal cancer. Int J Radiat Oncol Biol Phys. 2015;93(1):29–36. https://doi.org/10.1016/j.ijrobp.2015.05.005.

189. Banerjee R, Chakraborty S, Nygren I, Sinha R. Small bowel dose parameters predicting grade ≥ 3 acute toxicity in rectal cancer patients treated with neoadjuvant chemoradiation: an independent validation study comparing peritoneal space versus small bowel loop contouring techniques. Int J Radiat Oncol Biol Phys. 2013;85(5):1225–31. https://doi.org/10.1016/j.ijrobp.2012.09.036.

190. Jhingran A, Winter K, Portelance L, Miller B, Salehpour M, Gaur R, et al. A phase II study of intensity modulated radiation therapy to the pelvis for postoperative patients with endometrial carcinoma: radiation therapy oncology group trial 0418. Int J Radiat Oncol Biol Phys. 2012;84(1):e23–8. https://doi.org/10.1016/j.ijrobp.2012.02.044.

191. Klopp AH, Yeung AR, Deshmukh S, Gil KM, Wenzel L, Westin SN, et al. Patient-reported toxicity during pelvic intensity-modulated radiation therapy: NRG oncology-RTOG 1203. J Clin Oncol. 2018;36(24):2538–44. https://doi.org/10.1200/JCO.2017.77.4273.

192. Stanic S, Mayadev JS. Tolerance of the small bowel to therapeutic irradiation: a focus on late toxicity in patients receiving para-aortic nodal irradiation for gynecologic malignancies. Int J Gynecol Cancer. 2013;23(4):592–7. https://doi.org/10.1097/IGC.0b013e318286aa68.

193. Beriwal S, Gan GN, Heron DE, Selvaraj RN, Kim H, Lalonde R, et al. Early clinical outcome with concurrent chemotherapy and extended-field, intensity-modulated radiotherapy for cervical cancer. Int J Radiat Oncol Biol Phys. 2007;68(1):166–71. https://doi.org/10.1016/j.ijrobp.2006.12.023.

194. Gallagher MJ, Brereton HD, Rostock RA, Zero JM, Zekoski DA, Poyss LF, et al. A prospective study of treatment techniques to minimize the volume of pelvic small bowel with reduction of acute and late effects associated with pelvic irradiation. Int J Radiat Oncol Biol Phys. 1986;12(9):1565–73. https://doi.org/10.1016/0360-3016(86)90279-8.

195. Letschert JG, Lebesque JV, Aleman BM, Bosset JF, Horiot JC, Bartelink H, et al. The volume effect in radiation-related late small bowel complications: results of a clinical study of the EORTC radiotherapy cooperative group in patients treated for rectal carcinoma. Radiother Oncol. 1994;32(2):116–23. https://doi.org/10.1016/0167-8140(94)90097-3.

196. Chopra S, Dora T, Chinnachamy AN, Thomas B, Kannan S, Engineer R, et al. Predictors of grade 3 or higher late bowel toxicity in patients undergoing pelvic radiation for cervical cancer: results from a prospective study. Int J Radiat Oncol Biol Phys. 2014;88(3):630–5. https://doi.org/10.1016/j.ijrobp.2013.11.214.

197. Lee J, Yoon WS, Koom WS, Rim CH. Efficacy of stereotactic body radiotherapy for unresectable or recurrent cholangiocarcinoma: a meta-analysis and systematic review. Strahlenther Onkol. 2019;195(2):93–102. https://doi.org/10.1007/s00066-018-1367-2.

198. Buwenge M, Macchia G, Arcelli A, Frakulli R, Fuccio L, Guerri S, et al. Stereotactic radiotherapy of pancreatic cancer: a systematic review on pain relief. J Pain Res. 2018;11:2169–78. https://doi.org/10.2147/JPR.S167994.

199. Taniguchi CM, Murphy JD, Eclov N, Atwood TF, Kielar KN, Christman-Skieller C, et al. Dosimetric analysis of organs at risk during expiratory gating in stereotactic body radiation therapy for pancreatic cancer. Int J Radiat Oncol Biol Phys. 2013;85(4):1090–5. https://doi.org/10.1016/j.ijrobp.2012.07.2366.

200. Barney BM, Olivier KR, Macdonald OK, Fong de Los Santos LE, Miller RC, Haddock MG. Clinical outcomes and dosimetric considerations using stereotactic body radiotherapy for abdominopelvic tumors. Am J Clin Oncol. 2012;35(6):537–42. https://doi.org/10.1097/COC.0b013e31821f876a.

201. Hoyer M, Roed H, Traberg Hansen A, Ohlhuis L, Petersen J, Nellemann H, et al. Phase II study on stereotactic body radiotherapy of colorectal metastases. Acta Oncol. 2006;45(7):823–30. https://doi.org/10.1080/02841860600904854.

202. Kopek N, Holt MI, Hansen AT, Høyer M. Stereotactic body radiotherapy for unresectable cholangiocarcinoma. Radiother Oncol. 2010;94(1):47–52. https://doi.org/10.1016/j.radonc.2009.11.004.

203. Koong AC, Le QT, Ho A, Fong B, Fisher G, Cho C, et al. Phase I study of stereotactic radiosurgery in patients with locally advanced pancreatic cancer. Int J Radiat Oncol Biol Phys. 2004;58(4):1017–21. https://doi.org/10.1016/j.ijrobp.2003.11.004.

204. Bae SH, Kim MS, Cho CK, Kang JK, Lee SY, Lee KN, et al. Predictor of severe gastroduodenal toxicity after stereotactic body radiotherapy for abdominopelvic malignancies. Int J Radiat Oncol Biol Phys. 2012;84(4):e469–74. https://doi.org/10.1016/j.ijrobp.2012.06.005.

205. Goldsmith C, Price P, Cross T, Loughlin S, Cowley I, Plowman N. Dose-volume histogram analysis of stereotactic body radiotherapy treatment of pancreatic cancer: a focus on duodenal dose constraints. Semin Radiat Oncol. 2016;26(2):149–56. https://doi.org/10.1016/j.semradonc.2015.12.002.

206. Frelinghuysen M, Schillemans W, Hol L, Verhoef C, Hoogeman M, Nuyttens JJ. Acute toxicity of the bowel after stereotactic robotic radiotherapy for abdominopelvic oligometastases. Acta Oncol. 2018;57(4):480–4. https://doi.org/10.1080/0284186X.2017.1378432.

207. LaCouture TA, Xue J, Subedi G, Xu Q, Lee JT, Kubicek G, et al. Small bowel dose tolerance for stereotactic body radiation therapy. Semin Radiat Oncol. 2016;26(2):157–64. https://doi.org/10.1016/j.semradonc.2015.11.009.

208. Yeoh E, Horowitz M, Russo A, Muecke T, Robb T, Maddox A, et al. Effect of pelvic irradiation on gastrointestinal function: a prospective longitudinal study. Am J Med. 1993;95(4):397–406. https://doi.org/10.1016/0002-9343(93)90309-d.

209. Stacey R, Green JT. Radiation-induced small bowel disease: latest developments and clinical guidance. Ther Adv Chronic Dis. 2014;5(1):15–29. https://doi.org/10.1177/2040622313510730.

210. Ruskoné A, René E, Chayvialle JA, Bonin N, Pignal F, Kremer M, et al. Effect of somatostatin on diarrhea and on small intestinal water and electrolyte transport in a patient with pancreatic cholera. Dig Dis Sci. 1982;27(5):459–66. https://doi.org/10.1007/bf01295657.

211. Szilagyi A, Shrier I. Systematic review: the use of somatostatin or octreotide in refractory diarrhoea. Aliment Pharmacol Ther. 2001;15(12):1889–97. https://doi.org/10.1046/j.1365-2036.2001.01114.x.

212. Sukhotnik I, Khateeb K, Krausz MM, Sabo E, Siplovich L, Coran AG, et al. Sandostatin impairs postresection intestinal adaptation in a rat model of short bowel syndrome. Dig Dis Sci. 2002;47(9):2095–102. https://doi.org/10.1023/a:1019641416671.

213. Yavuz MN, Yavuz AA, Aydin F, Can G, Kavgaci H. The efficacy of octreotide in the therapy of acute radiation-induced diarrhea: a randomized controlled study. Int J Radiat Oncol Biol Phys. 2002;54(1):195–202. https://doi.org/10.1016/s0360-3016(02)02870-5.

214. Martenson JA, Halyard MY, Sloan JA, Proulx GM, Miller RC, Deming RL, et al. Phase III, double-blind study of depot octreotide versus placebo in the prevention of acute diarrhea in patients receiving pelvic radiation therapy: results of north central Cancer treatment group N00CA. J Clin Oncol. 2008;26(32):5248–53. https://doi.org/10.1200/JCO.2008.17.1546.

215. Sun JX, Yang N. Role of octreotide in post chemotherapy and/or radiotherapy diarrhea: prophylaxis or therapy? Asia Pac J Clin Oncol. 2014;10(2):e108–13. https://doi.org/10.1111/ajco.12055.

216. Cherny NI. Evaluation and management of treatment-related diarrhea in patients with advanced cancer: a review. J Pain Symptom Manag. 2008;36(4):413–23. https://doi.org/10.1016/j.jpainsymman.2007.10.007.
217. Mennie AT, Dalley VM, Dinneen LC, Collier HO. Treatment of radiation-induced gastrointestinal distress with acetylsalicylate. Lancet. 1975;2(7942):942–3. https://doi.org/10.1016/s0140-6736(75)90358-x.
218. Stryker JA, Demers LM, Mortel R. Prophylactic ibuprofen administration during pelvic irradiation. Int J Radiat Oncol Biol Phys. 1979;5(11–12):2049–52. https://doi.org/10.1016/0360-3016(79)90958-1.
219. Gibson RJ, Keefe DM, Lalla RV, Bateman E, Blijlevens N, Fijlstra M, et al. Systematic review of agents for the management of gastrointestinal mucositis in cancer patients. Support Care Cancer. 2013;21(1):313–26. https://doi.org/10.1007/s00520-012-1644-z.
220. Kiliç D, Egehan I, Ozenirler S, Dursun A. Double-blinded, randomized, placebo-controlled study to evaluate the effectiveness of sulphasalazine in preventing acute gastrointestinal complications due to radiotherapy. Radiother Oncol. 2000;57(2):125–9. https://doi.org/10.1016/s0167-8140(00)00254-1.
221. Martenson JA Jr, Hyland G, Moertel CG, Mailliard JA, O'Fallon JR, Collins RT, et al. Olsalazine is contraindicated during pelvic radiation therapy: results of a double-blind, randomized clinical trial. Int J Radiat Oncol Biol Phys. 1996;35(2):299–303. https://doi.org/10.1016/0360-3016(96)00016-8.
222. Resbeut M, Marteau P, Cowen D, Richaud P, Bourdin S, Dubois JB, et al. A randomized double blind placebo controlled multicenter study of mesalazine for the prevention of acute radiation enteritis. Radiother Oncol. 1997;44(1):59–63. https://doi.org/10.1016/s0167-8140(97)00064-9.
223. Benson AB, Ajani JA, Catalano RB, Engelking C, Kornblau SM, Martenson JA Jr, et al. Recommended guidelines for the treatment of cancer treatment-induced diarrhea. J Clin Oncol. 2004;22(14):2918–26. https://doi.org/10.1200/JCO.2004.04.132.
224. van de Wetering FT, Verleye L, Andreyev HJ, Maher J, Vlayen J, Pieters BR, et al. Nonsurgical interventions for late rectal problems (proctopathy) of radiotherapy in people who have received radiotherapy to the pelvis. Cochrane Database Syst Rev. 2016;4:CD003455. https://doi.org/10.1002/14651858.
225. Valls A, Pestchen I, Prats C, Pera J, Aragón G, Vidarte M, et al. Multicenter double-blind clinical trial comparing sucralfate vs placebo in the prevention of diarrhea secondary to pelvic irradiation. Med Clin (Barc). 1999;113(18):681–4.
226. Kneebone A, Mameghan H, Bolin T, Berry M, Turner S, Kearsley J, et al. The effect of oral sucralfate on the acute proctitis associated with prostate radiotherapy: a double-blind, randomized trial. Int J Radiat Oncol Biol Phys. 2001;51(3):628–35. https://doi.org/10.1016/s0360-3016(01)01660-1.
227. Martenson JA, Bollinger JW, Sloan JA, Novotny PJ, Urias RE, Michalak JC, et al. Sucralfate in the prevention of treatment-induced diarrhea in patients receiving pelvic radiation therapy: a north central cancer treatment group phase III double-blind placebo-controlled trial. J Clin Oncol. 2000;18(6):1239–45. https://doi.org/10.1200/JCO.2000.18.6.1239.
228. Andreyev HJ, Vlavianos P, Blake P, Dearnaley D, Norman AR, Tait D. Gastrointestinal symptoms after pelvic radiotherapy: role for the gastroenterologist? Int J Radiat Oncol Biol Phys. 2005;62(5):1464–71. https://doi.org/10.1016/j.ijrobp.2004.12.087.
229. Heusinkveld RS, Manning MR, Aristizabal SA. Control of radiation-induced diarrhea with cholestyramine. Int J Radiat Oncol Biol Phys. 1978;4(7–8):687–90. https://doi.org/10.1016/0360-3016(78)90194-3.
230. Scolapio JS, Ukleja A, Burnes JU, Kelly DG. Outcome of patients with radiation enteritis treated with home parenteral nutrition. Am J Gastroenterol. 2002;97(3):662–6. https://doi.org/10.1111/j.1572-0241.2002.05546.x.
231. Loiudice TA, Lang JA. Treatment of radiation enteritis: a comparison study. Am J Gastroenterol. 1983;78(8):481–7.

232. Onodera H, Nagayama S, Mori A, Fujimoto A, Tachibana T, Yonenaga Y. Reappraisal of surgical treatment for radiation enteritis. World J Surg. 2005;29(4):459–63. https://doi.org/10.1007/s00268-004-7699-3.
233. Dietz DW, Remzi FH, Fazio VW. Strictureplasty for obstructing small-bowel lesions in diffuse radiation enteritis--successful outcome in five patients. Dis Colon Rectum. 2001;44(12):1772–7. https://doi.org/10.1007/bf02234454.
234. Hovdenak N, Fajardo LF, Hauer-Jensen M. Acute radiation proctitis: a sequential clinico-pathologic study during pelvic radiotherapy. Int J Radiat Oncol Biol Phys. 2000;48(4):1111–7. https://doi.org/10.1016/s0360-3016(00)00744-6.
235. Hauer-Jensen M, Wang J, Boerma M, Fu Q, Denham JW. Radiation damage to the gastrointestinal tract: mechanisms, diagnosis, and management. Curr Opin Support Palliat Care. 2007;1(1):23–9. https://doi.org/10.1097/SPC.0b013e3281108014.
236. Trott KR, Tamou S, Sassy T, Kiszel Z. The effect of irradiated volume on the chronic radiation damage of the rat large bowel. Strahlenther Onkol. 1995;171(6):326–31.
237. Frykholm GJ, Isacsson U, Nygård K, Montelius A, Jung B, Påhlman L, et al. Preoperative radiotherapy in rectal carcinoma--aspects of acute adverse effects and radiation technique. Int J Radiat Oncol Biol Phys. 1996;35(5):1039–48. https://doi.org/10.1016/0360-3016(96)00229-5.
238. Isohashi F, Yoshioka Y, Mabuchi S, Konishi K, Koizumi M, Takahashi Y, et al. Dose-volume histogram predictors of chronic gastrointestinal complications after radical hysterectomy and postoperative concurrent nedaplatin-based chemoradiation therapy for early-stage cervical cancer. Int J Radiat Oncol Biol Phys. 2013;85(3):728–34. https://doi.org/10.1016/j.ijrobp.2012.05.021.
239. Fonteyne V, De Neve W, Villeirs G, De Wagter C, De Meerleer G. Late radiotherapy-induced lower intestinal toxicity (RILIT) of intensity-modulated radiotherapy for prostate cancer: the need for adapting toxicity scales and the appearance of the sigmoid colon as co-responsible organ for lower intestinal toxicity. Radiother Oncol. 2007;84(2):156–63. https://doi.org/10.1016/j.radonc.2007.06.013.
240. Mouttet-Audouard R, Lacornerie T, Tresch E, Kramar A, Le Tinier F, Reynaert N, et al. What is the normal tissues morbidity following helical intensity modulated radiation treatment for cervical cancer? Radiother Oncol. 2015;115(3):386–91. https://doi.org/10.1016/j.radonc.2015.02.010.
241. Lind H, Alevronta E, Steineck G, Waldenström AC, Nyberg T, Olsson C, et al. Defecation into clothing without forewarning and mean radiation dose to bowel and anal-sphincter among gynecological cancer survivors. Acta Oncol. 2016;55(11):1285–93. https://doi.org/10.1080/0284186X.2016.1176247.
242. Sarin A, Safar B. Management of radiation proctitis. Gastroenterol Clin N Am. 2013;42(4):913–25. https://doi.org/10.1016/j.gtc.2013.08.004.
243. Qadeer MA, Vargo JJ. Approaches to the prevention and management of radiation colitis. Curr Gastroenterol Rep. 2008;10(5):507–13. https://doi.org/10.1007/s11894-008-0093-9.
244. Paquette IM, Vogel JD, Abbas MA, Feingold DL, Steele SR, Clinical Practice Guidelines Committee of The American Society of Colon and Rectal Surgeons. The American society of colon and rectal surgeons clinical practice guidelines for the treatment of chronic radiation proctitis. Dis Colon Rectum. 2018;61(10):1135–40. https://doi.org/10.1097/DCR.0000000000001209.
245. Haddad GK, Grodsinsky C, Allen H. The spectrum of radiation enteritis. Surgical considerations. Dis Colon Rectum. 1983;26(9):590–4. https://doi.org/10.1007/bf02552969.
246. Tabibian N, Umbreen A, Swehli E, Boyd A, Tabibian JH. Radiation therapy: managing GI tract complications. J Fam Pract. 2017;66(8):E1–7.
247. Silvain C, Besson I, Ingrand P, Beau P, Fort E, Matuchansky C, et al. Long-term outcome of severe radiation enteritis treated by total parenteral nutrition. Dig Dis Sci. 1992;37:1065–71. https://doi.org/10.1007/bf01300288.

248. McGough C, Baldwin C, Frost G, Andreyev HJ. Role of nutritional intervention in patients treated with radiotherapy for pelvic malignancy. Br J Cancer. 2004;90:2278–87. https://doi.org/10.1038/sj.bjc.6601868.

249. Yeoh E. Radiotherapy: long-term effects on gastrointestinal function. Curr Opin Support Palliat Care. 2008;2(1):40–4. https://doi.org/10.1097/SPC.0b013e3282f4451f.

250. Kountouras J, Zavos C. Recent advances in the management of radiation colitis. World J Gastroenterol. 2008;14(48):7289–301. https://doi.org/10.3748/wjg.14.7289.

Toxicity Management for Pelvic Tumors in Radiation Oncology

Nilufer Kılıc Durankus, Duygu Sezen, Ugur Selek, and Yasemin Bolukbasi

6.1 Pelvic Anatomy

6.1.1 Normal Sectional Anatomy with CT and MRI Images

Understanding the diagnostic imaging studies of the pelvis requires a comprehensive knowledge of the normal and variant anatomy of this region.

Computerized tomography (CT) and magnetic resonance imaging (MRI) can be useful for cases with sonographically complicated or discordant clinical findings.

Magnetic resonance imaging has advantages in pelvis because of its superior tissue contrast and nonionizing technique.

Right and left coxae, sacrum, and coccyx form the bone boundaries of the pelvis and it involves the structures of gastrointestinal and genitourinary system such as rectum, ureters, and bladder. Prostate, vesicula seminales, prostatic urethra, ductus deferens, ductus ejaculatorius in males; uterus, ovaries, tuba uterina, and vagina in females are the other structures located in the pelvis.

N. Kılıc Durankus (✉) · D. Sezen
Department of Radiation Oncology, Faculty of Medicine, Koc University, Istanbul, Turkey
e-mail: ndurankus@kuh.ku.edu.tr

U. Selek · Y. Bolukbasi (✉)
Department of Radiation Oncology, Faculty of Medicine, Koc University, Istanbul, Turkey

Department of Radiation Oncology, MD Anderson Cancer Center, University of Texas, Houston, TX, USA

MD Anderson Radiation Treatment Center, American Hospital, Istanbul, Turkey
e-mail: ugurs@amerikanhastanesi.org; yaseminb@amerikanhastanesi.org, Ybolukbasi@kuh.ku.edu.tr

© Springer Nature Switzerland AG 2020
G. Ozyigit, U. Selek (eds.), *Prevention and Management of Acute and Late Toxicities in Radiation Oncology*, https://doi.org/10.1007/978-3-030-37798-4_6

Pelvic diaphragm is the structure that separates the peritoneum and pelvic cavity. Pelvic diaphragm is formed by the levator ani and coccygeus muscles. Levator ani is in the central part of the pelvic diaphragm and has two parts called as medial pubo-coccygeus muscle and the lateral iliococcygeus muscles. The levator ani is the muscle that surrounds the vagina, urethra, and rectum. Paired coccygeus muscle constitutes the posterior region of the pelvic diaphragm. Additionally the piriformis muscle lies at the posterior wall of the minor pelvis and covers most of the greater sciatic notch before passing through it to insert on the greater trochanter of the femur.

The obturator internus muscle arises from the obturator fossa and covers the lateral pelvic wall. It passes inferiorly to exit the pelvis through the lesser sciatic foramen. The midlevel of the obturator internus muscle can be defined as the location of obturator artery, obturator vein, and obturator lymph nodes.

Each psoas muscle originates from the transverse processes of the lumbar vertebrae and they connect lomber spines to femur. Afterwards psoas muscle comes together with the iliacus muscle to form the iliopsoas. The external iliac artery and vein cross the iliopsoas at the level of the sacroiliac joint. The rectus muscles located bilateral of the midline of the lower abdominal wall.

6.1.2   Male Pelvis

The rectum is the lower segment of gastrointestinal tract and it connects sigmoid colon to anus. The rectum lies between the level of S2–S3 superiorly and the perineum inferiorly. It is approximately 15 cm (12–16 cm) and subdivided into three segments. The upper third is intraperitoneal, the middle third is retroperitoneal, and the lower third is extraperitoneal part of the rectum. The arterial circulation of rectum is provided by the superior rectal artery (branch of the inferior mesenteric artery), middle rectal artery (branch of the internal iliac artery), and inferior rectal artery (branch of the internal pudendal artery from the internal iliac artery). The superior, middle, and inferior rectal veins supply the venous drainage of rectum. The superior rectal veins drain the upper part of the rectum through the inferior mesenteric vein into the portal venous system; however, venous drainage of the lower segment of the rectum is carried out into the systematic circulation (internal iliac vein) via the middle and inferior rectal vein.

Bladder is a muscular sac located at the superior and posterior of the pubis. The muscular triangular region bounded laterally by the ureter orifices extending posteriorly to the urethra called as trigon [1]. Superior and inferior vesical branches of internal iliac arteries are the main arterial supply. Venous drainage and lymphatic drainage are carried out via internal iliac vein and via common and internal iliac chain, respectively. The urine within the bladder has low signal on T1-weighted images. The bladder wall has also low signal intensity but relatively higher than urine. However, intraluminal liquid has high signal intensity and the bladder wall still has low signal intensity on T2-weighted images [2].

The urethra arises from the bladder base and has three segments such as the prostatic, membranous, and penile urethra.

Prostate is an exocrine gland located at the base of the urinary bladder. The main function of prostate gland is to secrete alkaline fluid that is one of the components of semen. Proximal urethra is surrounded by the prostate. There are clinically important three zones called central zone, transitional zone, and peripheral zone.

The seminal vesicles are paired glands located posterior and superior of prostate. They produce reservoirs for seminal fluid. Denonvilliers' fascia separates prostate and seminal vesicles from the rectum. Seminal vesicles carry sperm from the testicles by vas deferens.

Imaging of the prostate with MRI has an important role in order to interpret any malignancy appropriately. The anatomy is better defined on T2-weighted images compared to T1-weighted images. Dynamic contrast-enhanced MRI, diffusion-weighted imaging, spectroscopy are different techniques for further evaluation.

The neurovascular bundles are located posterolateral of the prostate and pass through the pelvic floor. They contain nerve fibers and blood vessels for the corpora cavernosa.

The testes are paired ovoid-shaped structures in the male reproductive system. They are located in the scrotal sac. Testicles produce sperm, testosterone, and other androgens. They have also an important role for storage of sperm. Vessels, nerves, and ducts travel from the deep inguinal ring to the testes by spermatic cord. Homogeneous intermediate signal intensity on T1-weighted images and high signal intensity in regard to skeletal muscle on T2-weighted images are characteristics for normal testes.

The penis is an external organ of the male reproductive system. The penis has three compartments: the two corpora cavernosa and the corpus spongiosum covered by a connective tissue called the tunica albuginea.

The bulb of the penis (PB) is the posterior expanded portion of the corpus spongiosum attached to the perineal membrane that extends from the perineum and surrounded by the bulbo-cavernosus muscle. Urethra extends from the bulb. The PB can be seen as an ovoid-shaped structure on CT imaging, it is surrounded by the levator ani muscle and corpus spongiosum while it has an hyperintense appearance on T2-weighted MR images [3].

Delineation of normal structures in male pelvis is shown in Figs. 6.1 and 6.2.

6.1.3 Female Pelvis

The bladder is located anterior to the uterus and the vagina while the rectum is in the posterior pelvic compartment.

The uterus is a muscular organ located between the base of the bladder and the rectum. Broad ligaments are the lateral borders of uterus that have fallopian tubes superiorly and vagina inferiorly. Uterus is divided into body and cervix regions that are connected with the isthmus. The shape of the uterus varies with physiologic state as well as age and parity. In comparison with the uterus of multiparous women, the uterus may regress to the preadolescent size after the menopause as a result of atrophy of the myometrium.

Internal os separates the uterine body from the cervix. Different layers of cervix can be evaluated better with high resolution T2-weighted images compared with T1-weighted images.

The fallopian tubes are musculomembranous structures that vary from 7 to 14 cm in length. They are commonly divided into intramural, isthmic, and ampullary segments.

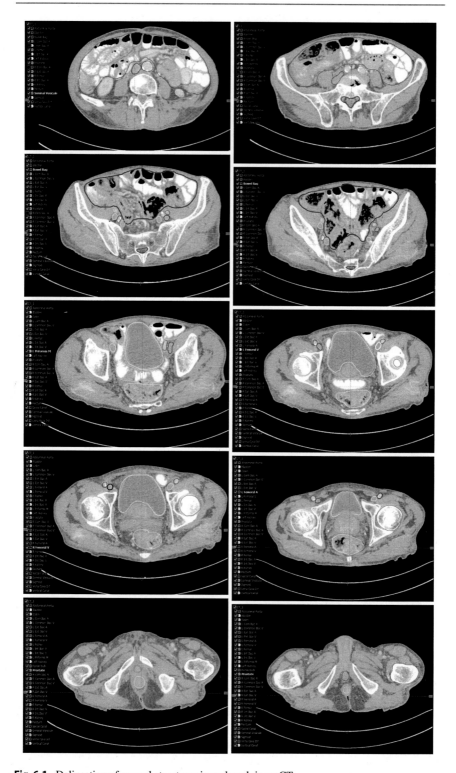

Fig. 6.1 Delineation of normal structures in male pelvis on CT

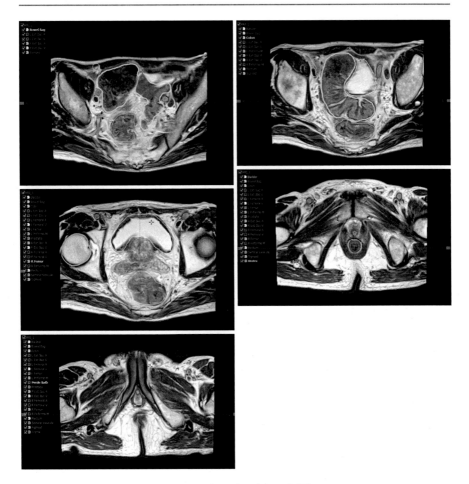

Fig. 6.2 Delineation of normal structures in male pelvis on MRI

The ovaries are between the uterus by the utero-ovarian ligament and the side walls of the minor pelvis by infundibulopelvic ligament bilaterally. They are communicated with fallopian tubes. The ovaries have physiological changes during the menstrual cycle. Ovarian artery is one of the main branches of abdominal aorta and it supplies the ovaries. Right and left gonadal are responsible for venous drainage. T2-weighted images are more demonstrative for ovary in premenopausal women compared with postmenopausal women because of the factors related with age [4].

The vagina is a fibromuscular canal that extends between the cervix superiorly and the vestibule of the external genitalia inferiorly. It is in the midline almost at the level of the lower sacrum and joins with the cervix above. It is connected to levator ani muscle at the level of urogenital diaphragm. Vagina is divided into three parts, upper third is defined as fornices of the vagina while middle third is located at the level of bladder base. The section below the level of bladder base and the level of urethra is the lower third of vagina. The branches of internal iliac artery are the main arterial source. Additionally internal pudendal artery and middle rectal artery support mid and lower third of vagina. Venous drainage is supplied by the venous plexuses into the internal iliac veins.

Vulva is the external section of the female genitalia. Mons pubis, labia majora and minora, Bartholin's glands, clitoris, urethral meatus, and vestibule of the vagina are the main structures. The region between vulva and anus is called as perineum. Bilateral internal and external pudendal arteries of internal iliac artery and pudendal veins constitute the vascular network, while the pudendal nerve and superficial inguinal lymph nodes are the components of innervation and lymphatic drainage. The vulva shows higher signal intensity on T2-weighted imaging compared to T1-weighted imaging.

Uterus also has three layers from inner to outer part called as endometrium, junctional zone, and myometrium. Endometrium is the innermost layer of the uterus and it may be seen different throughout the phases of menstrual cycle. Its thickness is more in the secretory phase while it became narrower during follicular phase or menstruation. Endometrium has high signal on T2-weighted images and low signal intensity on precontrast T1-weighted images. Myometrium has intermediate increased signal intensity on T2-weighted images, while generally no clear demarcation can be seen between different layers of uterus on T1-weighted images.

Female urethra is a tubular muscular channel extending from the internal urethral orifice at bladder trigone to the external urethral orifice located anterior of the vagina. Urethra is supported by ureteropelvic ligaments.

The obturator internus muscles lie medial to the side walls of the pelvis. The external iliac vessels cross the anterior surface of the iliopsoas muscle. Also all these structures were defined by RTOG group (Table 6.1) [5].

Delineation of normal structures in female pelvis is shown in Figs. 6.3 and 6.4.

Table 6.1 RTOG male and female pelvis normal tissue consensus definitions [5]

Organ	Standardized TPS name	Tumor category	Consensus definition
Rectum	Rectum	GU	Inferiorly from the lowest level of the ischial tuberosities (right or left). Contouring ends superiorly before the rectum loses its round shape in the axial plane and connects anteriorly with the sigmoid. The Rectum is used with the BowelBag
Anus + rectum	AnoRectum	GYN	Inferiorly from the anal verge as marked with a radiopaque marker at the time of simulation. Contouring ends superiorly before the rectum loses its round shape in the axial plane and connects anteriorly with the sigmoid. The AnoRectum is used with the Sigmoid and BowelBag

Table 6.1 (continued)

Organ	Standardized TPS name	Tumor category	Consensus definition
Sigmoid	Sigmoid	GYN	Bowel continuing where the AnoRectum contour ended. Stops before connecting to the ascending colon laterally. Contoured when a brachytherapy applicator rests in the uterus. Any sigmoid adjacent or above the uterus, as well as the brachytherapy applicator, should be contoured
Bowel bag	BowelBag	GU, GYN	Inferiorly from the most inferior small or large bowel loop or above the Rectum (GU) or AnoRectum (GYN), whichever is most inferior. If, when following the bowel loop rule, the Rectum or AnoRectum is present in that axial slice, it should be included as part of the bag; otherwise, it should be excluded
			Tips: Contour the abdominal contents excluding muscle and bones. Contour every other slice when the contour is not changing rapidly, and interpolate and edit as necessary. Finally, subtract any overlapping non-GI normal structures. If the TPS does not allow subtraction, leave as is
Small bowel	SmallBowel	GI	To distinguish from large bowel, the use of oral contrast is encouraged.* After administration of contrast (e.g., 3 oz of Gastrografin (Bracco Diagnostics Inc., Princeton, NJ) and 3 oz of water–barium mixture) 30 min before scanning, the small bowel can be outlined as loops containing contrast
Colon	Colon	GI	Large bowel continuing where the AnoRectumSig contour ended.* Depending on the volume treated, this will include portions or all of the ascending, transverse, descending, and sigmoid colon

(continued)

Table 6.1 (continued)

Organ	Standardized TPS name	Tumor category	Consensus definition
Anus + rectum + rectosigmoid (target)	AnoRectumSig	GI	Target structure. Inferiorly from the anal verge as marked with a radiopaque marker at time of simulation. Contouring ends superiorly at the rectosigmoid flexure after the mesorectum disappears. The AnoRectumSig is used with the SmallBowel and Colon
Mesorectum (target)	Mesorectum	GI	Target structure for anal and rectal cancer. The rectum inferiorly below where the mesorectal fat disappears, continuing superiorly, and encompassing the mesorectal fat until the mesorectal fascia disappears. For these entities, the AnoRectoSig (anus + rectum + rectosigmoid), unlike the rest of the alimentary canal, is not an avoidance structure. In cases where it is difficult to visualize the mesorectum, the anatomic borders of the mesorectum include the following: cranial, the level of the rectosigmoid junction; caudal, the anorectal junction defined by where the levator muscles fuse with the external sphincter muscles (or where the mesorectal fat/space can no longer be seen tapering inferiorly); posterior, pre-sacral space; anterior, GU/GYN organs with an internal margin of 10 mm to the anterior mesorectal border on the axial slices of the bladder to account for bladder volume variation on this boundary; and lateral, medial edge of the levator ani in the lower pelvis and pelvic brim in upper (excluding any non-target muscle)
			Tip: Adjusting the windowing level may facilitate visualizing the mesorectum
Bladder	Bladder	GU, GYN, GI	Inferiorly from its base and superiorly to the dome

Table 6.1   (continued)

Organ	Standardized TPS name	Tumor category	Consensus definition
Uterus + cervix	UteroCervix	GYN	The uterus and cervix as one structure
			Tip: Fuse with MRI to help identify it
Ovaries + fallopian tubes	Adnexa_R Adnexa_L	GYN	Right and left ovaries and fallopian tubes
			Tip: Fuse with MRI to help identify these.
Prostate	Prostate	GU	Inferiorly from its apex and superiorly to its base. If the capsule is visible, the muscles and soft tissues abutting the capsule are not included as "prostate"
			Tips: The apex is above the hourglass or a slit shape that results from the in-bowing of the levator ani just below.
Seminal vesicles	SeminalVesc	GU	Entire seminal vesicles including those slices that also have prostate identified
Penile bulb	PenileBulb	GU	That portion of the bulbous spongiosum of the penis immediately inferior to the GU diaphragm. Do not extend this structure anteriorly into the shaft or pendulous portion of the penis
			Tips: The penile bulb is best identified with MRI (bright on T2) or CT scan when there is contrast in the urethra. On CT scan, the penile bulb will be posterior to the urethra and has a round shape.
Proximal femurs	Femur_R Femur_L	GU, GYN, GI	The proximal femur inferiorly from the lowest level of the ischial tuberosities (right or left) and superiorly to the top of the ball of the femur, including the trochanters
			Tips: Auto-contouring threshold parameters with bone can facilitate this process but requires editing any auto-contouring artifacts

CT computed tomography, *GI* gastrointestinal, *GU* genitourinary, *MRI* magnetic resonance imaging, *PTV* planning target volume, *RTOG* radiation therapy oncology group, *TPS* treatment planning software

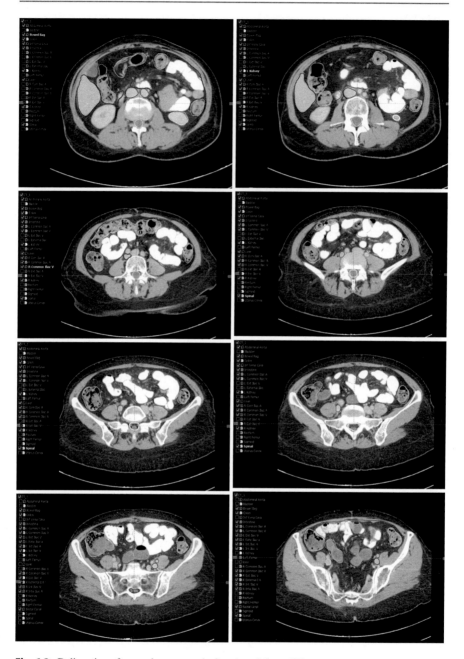

Fig. 6.3 Delineation of normal structures in female pelvis on CT

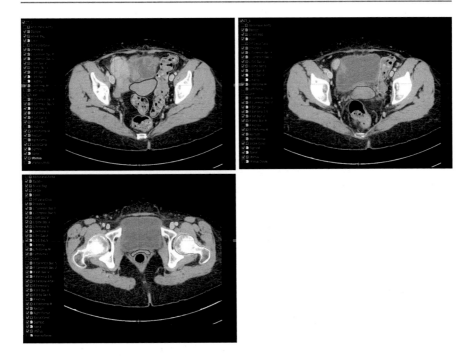

Fig. 6.3 (continued)

6.2 Concurrent Chemotherapy Drugs

6.2.1 Bevacizumab

VEGF is one of the most effective and critical regulators of normal and pathologic angiogenesis. The biological special effects of VEGF could be listed as endothelial cell mitogenesis and migration, increased vascular permeability, induction of proteinases leading to remodeling of the extracellular matrix, and suppression of dendritic cell maturation [6]. The mechanism of action of bevacizumab in combination with chemotherapy and radiation therapy may lead inhibition of the formation of new vessels, regression of newly formed blood vessels, normalization of vasculature leading to improved delivery of systemic therapy or enhanced oxygen delivery, or direct effects on tumor cells [7]. Recommended dose schedules of 5 mg/kg every 2 weeks, 10 mg/kg every 2 weeks, or 15 mg/kg every 3 weeks are used in clinical trials.

The most common adverse events are asthenia, pain, headache, hypertension, diarrhea, stomatitis, constipation, epistaxis, dyspnea, dermatitis, leukopenia, proteinuria, arterial thromboembolic events, hemorrhage, congestive heart failure (CHF), gastrointestinal perforations, and wound healing complications [6]. Hypertension related to bevacizumab can generally be controlled with routine oral drugs during treatment. The risk of arterial thromboembolic events is increased with

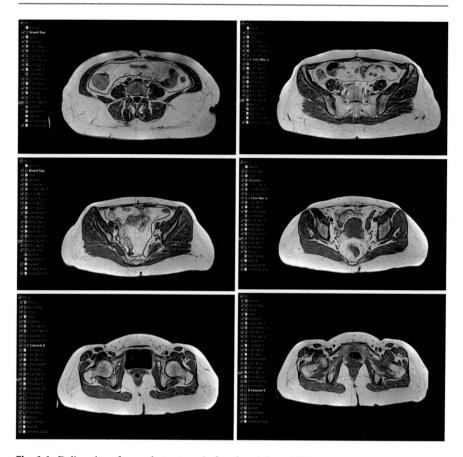

Fig. 6.4 Delineation of normal structures in female pelvis on MRI

bevacizumab therapy; such events included cerebral infarction, transient ischemic attack (TIA), myocardial infarction (MI), and other peripheral or visceral arterial thrombosis. Aspirin is a standard therapy for primary and secondary prophylaxis of ATE in patients at high risk of such events. Gastrointestinal perforation (GI perforation)/fistula was rare but more frequent among patients whose therapy included bevacizumab. The interval between surgery and initiation of bevacizumab required to be at least 28 days following major surgery or bevacizumab should be discontinued 4–8 weeks prior to the surgical procedure [7].

6.2.2   Cisplatin

It has been the most well proven effective agent with concurrent radiotherapy. The recommended dose is 40 mg/m^2 weekly or 100 mg/m^2 every 3 weeks. It causes inhibition of DNA synthesis and, to a lesser degree, inhibition of RNA and protein; it has not been shown to be cell-cycle specific [8]. Dose-related and cumulative renal insufficiency is the major dose-limiting adverse events associated with cisplatin. Ototoxicity has been observed even with a single dose of cisplatin 50 mg/m^2. It is manifested by tinnitus and or hearing loss in the high frequency range. Myelosuppression occurs in 25–30% of patients treated with cisplatin. Nadirs in circulating platelets and leukocytes occur between days 18 and 23 with most patients recovering by day 39. Most common side effect is marked nausea and vomiting which occur in almost all patients treated with cisplatin. Diarrhea and anorexia have also been reported. Other infrequent toxicities that have been reported include cardiac abnormalities, hiccups, elevated serum amylase, rash, alopecia, malaise, and asthenia [9].

6.2.3 Carboplatin

Carboplatin is in the platinum-based antineoplastic family of medications and works by interfering with duplication of DNA. Myelosuppression is the major dose-limiting toxicity. Thrombocytopenia, neutropenia, leucopenia, and anemia are common. Peripheral neuropathies have been observed in 4% of patients receiving carboplatin with mild paresthesia being the most common. Nausea and vomiting are the most common GI events; both usually resolve within 24 h and respond to antiemetics [10]. Elevated alkaline phosphatase, total bilirubin, and SGOT have been reported. Alopecia has been reported in 3% of the patients taking carboplatin. The standard dose of carboplatin is area under the curve (AUC) 5. The dose of carboplatin is calculated as follows, using the Calvert formula based on creatinine clearance: Total dose (mg) = Target AUC (in mg/mL per min) × (Estimated GFR + 25).

6.2.4 Paclitaxel

Paclitaxel is a natural product obtained via a semi-synthetic process from Taxus baccata. The dose of paclitaxel is 135 mg/m^2, with maximum body surface area (BSA) of 2.0 m^2. Myelosuppression is the major dose-limiting toxicity [11]. Neutropenia is both dose- and schedule-dependent and typically resolves rapidly. Fever is common, and infectious episodes are seen in about 1/3 of the patients receiving paclitaxel. Thrombocytopenia is uncommon and the cases that occur are usually mild to moderate. While anemia is common, it is severe in only 16% of cases. Severe reactions are rare and mostly occur within the first hour of administration. The most common symptoms in severe reactions include dyspnea, flushing, chest pain, and tachycardia. The most common GI toxicities, which include nausea, vomiting, diarrhea, and mucositis, are usually mild or moderate. Almost all of the patients receiving paclitaxel experience alopecia, nonetheless nail changes are infrequent.

6.3 Dose Constraints

Normal-Tissue Dose-Volume Analysis Criteria and Score Statistics based on recent studies are summarized in Tables 6.2, 6.3, 6.4, and 6.5.

Table 6.2 NRG ONCOLOGY/RTOG 0921/RTOG 0148/TIME-C [12] postoperative pelvic radiotherapy

Structure	Per protocol	Variation acceptable	Deviation unacceptable
Small bowel	30% receives <40 Gy	30% receives >40 to <45 Gy	>30% receives >45 Gy and ≥0.03 cc receives >65 Gy
Rectum	60% receives ≤40 Gy	60% receives 40 to <45 Gy	>60% receives >45 Gy and ≥0.03 cc receives >65 Gy
Bladder	35% receives ≤45 Gy	35% receives 45 to <50 Gy	>35% receives >50 Gy and ≥0.03 cc receives >65 Gy
Femoral heads	15% receives <35 Gy	>15% to ≤50% receives >35 Gy	>50% receives >35 Gy and ≥0.03 cc receives >65 Gy

Rx prescription, *Gy* Gray, *PTV* planning target volume

Table 6.3 EMBRACE-2 study protocol: Image guided intensity modulated external beam radio-chemotherapy and MRI based adaptive brachytherapy in locally advanced cervical cancer

		Hard dose constraints	Soft dose constraints
Targets	PTV45	V95% > 95% Dmax < 107%	
Help contour	CTV-HR + 10 mm		Dmax < 103%
OARS	Bowel	Dmax < 105% (47.3 Gy)	When no lymph node boost • V40 Gy < 100 cm³ • V30 Gy < 350 cm³ When lymph node boost or paraaortic irradiation • V40 Gy < 250 cm³ • V30 Gy < 500 cm³ Dmax <57.5 Gy
	Sigmoid	Dmax < 105% (47.3 Gy)	Dmax < 57.5 Gy
	Bladder	Dmax < 105% (47.3 Gy)	V40 Gy < 75% V30 Gy < 85% Dmax < 57.5 Gy
	Rectum	Dmax < 105% (47.3 Gy)	V40 Gy < 85% V30 Gy < 95% Dmax < 57.5 Gy
	Spinal cord	Dmax < 48 Gy	
	Femoral heads	Dmax < 50 Gy	
	Kidney		Dmean < 10 Gy
		Dmean < 15 Gy	
	Body	Dmax < 107%	
	Vagina PIBS—2 cm		When vagina not involved: Dras 2 cm < 5 Gy
Optional	Ovaries	<5–8 Gy	
	Duodenum	V55 < 15 cm³	

Table 6.4 RTOG 0126: a phase III randomized study of high dose 3D-CRT/IMRT vs. standard dose 3D-CRT/IMRT in patients treated for localized prostate cancer

Volume	Constraint
GTV (prostate)	100% to 79.2 Gy
PTV2 (GTV + 0.5 cm)	98% to 79.2 Gy
CTV (prostate/SV)	100% to 50.4 Gy
PTV1 (CTV + 0.5 cm)	98% to 50.4 Gy
Rectum	<50% to 60 Gy
	<35% to 65 Gy
	<25% to 70 Gy
	<15% to 75 Gy
	Dmax 84.7 Gy
Bladder	<50% to 65 Gy
	<35% to 70 Gy
	<25% to 75 Gy
	<15% to 80 Gy
	Dmax 84.7 Gy
Femoral head	Dmax 50 Gy
Penile bulb	Mean < 52.5 Gy

Table 6.5 Hypofractionation studies—prostate cancer

Trial	Total dose (cGy)	Fraction size (cGy)	Bladder goal Dose (cGy)	<Vol%	Rectum goal Dose (cGy)	<Vol%
Italian	6200	310	5425	50	5425	30
			3875	70	3875	50
PROFIT	6000	300	3700	50	3700	50
			4600	70	4600	70
CHHIP	6000	300	6000	5	6000	3
			4860	25	5700	15
			4080	50	5280	30
					4860	50
					4080	60
MD Anderson	7200	240	6500	20	6500	20
RTOG 0415	7000	250	7900	15	7400	15
			7400	25	6900	25
			6900	35	6400	35
			6400	50	5900	50

6.4   The Pathophysiology of Pelvic Radiation Disease

Radiation therapy is an important part of the multidisciplinary treatment of pelvic malignancies [13]. In patients with pelvic malignancies during radiotherapy, the surrounding healthy intestinal tissue such as the distal large bowel is also affected [14]. Although radiotherapy is a particular part of the treatment, gastrointestinal symptoms associated with radiation exposed tissues occur in almost half of the patients [15]. Pelvic radiation disease (PRD) includes the side effects that occur in patients who underwent radiation treatment for a pelvic tumor [14, 15]. Radiation toxicity is described as acute when it occurs during radiotherapy or within 3 months. If the symptoms occur after 3 months, it is described as chronic. In patients with PRD the most common symptoms are diarrhea, urgency, rectal bleeding, and fecal incontinence [16]. The target cell theory is the traditional explanation of radiation enteropathy which describes early pathology due to epithelial injury as well as fibroblast and endothelial cell damage could be detected for late-onset harm [17]. However, this theory is considered insufficient and in recent years other possible factors were regarded. The current approach for the pathophysiology of pelvic radiation disease is thought to be associated with the result of multiple interactions between epithelial damage, gut microvasculature, enteric nervous system, and gut microbiota [18].

It has been suggested that one of the main causes of the pathophysiology of pelvic radiation disease is oxidative injury [19, 20]. The cells which are exposed to radiation are damaged with oxidative stress injury. Although oxidative stress is harmful for all parts of the cell, the sub-cellular target is the nuclear DNA [15, 18]. After being exposed to ionizing radiation, the functions of nuclear DNA are impaired and as a result DNA transcription is deformed. These deformations include inter- and intra-strand cross-linkages, breaks, and mutations. In addition to the damage of radiation to the nucleus, the plasma membrane is also affected by radiation. The structure of the membrane is disturbed by the destruction of the rigid phospholipid bilayer structure which changes the electric gradient and also disrupts the integrity of the cell. Moreover, free radicals damage the cell in an indirect manner [21].

After DNA damage from radiation, the cell attempts to save itself using several repair mechanisms to fix the strand breaks and replication errors. However, the cell can only sustain these protection mechanisms under low levels of radiation. If the radiation dose becomes higher, the apoptotic mechanism starts and mitosis can be inhibited [17]. Another important point in pelvic radiation disease is the timing of receiving concomitant chemotherapy. In the case of concomitant chemotherapy, the protective repair system cannot work sufficiently. Chemotherapeutic agents may help to accumulate cells in the more radiosensitive stages of the cell cycle. Thus, the timing of chemotherapy during radiotherapy is considered to be essential for decreasing the harmful effects of pelvic radiation disease [22].

The degree of the damaging effect of radiotherapy differs based on the turnover capacity of the tissue. Thus, it can be said that damaging effects of radiation is the highest in tissues with high turnover capacity. As mentioned before, the repairing capacity of cells is important to decrease the effects of radiation; however, stage of the cell cycle is another important component of pelvic radiation disease. Thus, some kinds of cells such as crypt epithelium of the bowel are highly radiosensitive at the cell cycling phase of G_2M [23]. After damaging these cells by radiation the mucosal barrier breaks down and inflammation occurs. This issue is particularly important for the clinical outcomes of radiotherapy [14, 19, 20].

6.4.1   Gastrointestinal Toxicity

Acute small bowel toxicity was described as diarrhea, cramping, and abdominal pain starting from the third or fourth week of pelvis radiotherapy. These symptoms were usually treated with both dietary changes and medical approach. The rate of these symptoms was ranging from 3% to 20% mostly related to the radiotherapy planning technique [24, 25]. In the more advanced planning techniques such as stereotactic radiotherapy, grade 1 and 2 acute toxicity ranges from 10% to 31% and grade 2 0–7% [26].

Late toxicities can occur at least 6 months or years after the radiation treatment and usually presented with intermittent diarrhea, dysmotility, food intolerance, nutrient malabsorption, or fecal incontinence, and rarely fistula, obstruction, and hemorrhage (Fig. 6.5) [25]. Dosimetric studies revealed more normal organ dose delivery including small bowel and rectum with IMRT, compared to previous 3D conformal and 2D planning techniques. The rate has been diminished from 34%–50% to 6%–11% with the use of IMRT fields [27]. Another clinical study consisting of 293 men, whom received 76 Gy RT for prostate cancer, has showed that acute GI toxicity was significantly greater with 3D-CRT compared to IMRT. This result has not been affected by the duration of hormonal treatment (20% for 3D-CRT and 8% for IMRT) as well as the interval to the development of late GI toxicity was significantly longer in the IMRT group [28]. In contrast, androgen deprivation therapy has been detrimental effect to increase late grade 2 or greater rectal toxicity when used concurrently with three-dimensional conformal radiotherapy (3D-CRT) [28]. Intensity-modulated radiotherapy (IMRT) has been accepted as routine approach for pelvic radiotherapy with a potential to reduce toxicity by limiting the radiation dose received by the bowel and bladder [29].

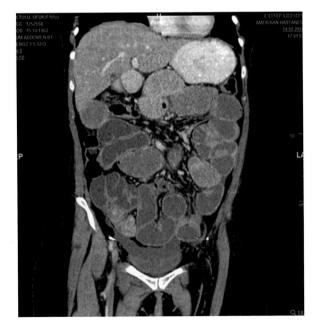

Fig. 6.5 A patient has been operated with advanced endometrium cancer, and received 45 Gy postoperative radiotherapy. After 9 months from the treatment, the patient admitted to emergency service with vomiting. Whole abdomen tomography revealed bowel obstruction due to surgery and radiotherapy fibrosis

The treatment approaches for acute proctitis were topical hydrocortisone, steroid, or sucralfate enemas, whereas the approach for chronic proctitis starts with more intensive approach such as argon laser, hyperbaric oxygen, vitamin A, and metronidazole [25, 30]. Also colonoscopy is considered to be important for excluding other reasons of rectal bleeding. However if the colonoscopy is not mandatory, it should be postponed 1 year after radiation in terms of being aware of no issues with poor wound healing, bleeding, or ulceration secondary to biopsy performed at the time of colonoscopy [30]. While the symptoms and rectal bleeding persist, laser treatment and interrectal administration of formaldehyde can be an option [31]. Also formaldehyde had also reported as safe without any complications and well tolerated [31]. Rarely, colostomy is needed if conservative management does not work. Another rare problem is anal incontinence during radiotherapy [32]. In the literature, even, it has been reported that only 2.2% of patients developed anal incontinence after radiotherapy, it has been reported that 67% of patients who received radiotherapy exhibited abnormal manometric parameters of anorectal functioning [33]. The total pelvis dose should not be >40–45 Gy in terms of avoiding severe pelvic complications. Irradiation of paraaortic lymph-nodes can cause increased pelvic complications [34]. Willett et al. found that 28 patients who received external-beam abdominal or pelvic irradiation developed inflammatory bowel disease [35]. They also reported that eight of 28 patients needed hospitalization or surgical intervention. Although occurrence of malignancies related to radiation is not common, this issue should be also kept in mind [30].

6.4.2 Genitourinary Toxicity

Low-grade urinary symptoms, including dysuria, urinary frequency, nocturia, and hesitancy, are relatively common during pelvic radiotherapy [36]. About half of patients treated with definitive external beam radiotherapy experience grade 1–2 genitourinary toxicity [37, 38]. In the ProtecT trial, men treated with definitive RT for their prostate cancer had an increase in nocturia from 19% at baseline to 59% as well as day time urinary frequency increased from 32% at baseline to 55% at 6 months after treatment. Even urinary voiding and nocturia were worse in the radiotherapy group at 6 months but then mostly recovered and were similar to the other groups after 12 months. Effects on quality of life mirrored the reported changes in function. No significant differences were observed among the groups in measures of anxiety, depression, or general health-related or cancer-related quality of life [39]. Similar effects were seen in women treated with pelvic radiotherapy [40]. Grade 3–4 urinary toxicity rates were reported as 12.3%, and the grade 3–4 chronic genitourinary toxicity incidence decreased to 2.7% [41]. It has been reported that radiotherapy to the cervix and prostate caused 2.5% ureteral stricture [42, 43]. Flank pain and urinary tract abnormalities were found to be the most common symptoms. Almost half of the patients could need diversion of the urinary stream and ileal conduits. Need for a nephrectomy is an uncommon condition [44]. The incidence of late urinary morbidity was reported up to 10% [44]. Patients who had gynecologic malignancies and who received radiation therapy have a tendency to develop urinary tract infections [45]. The dose of radiotherapy was considered to be important for the development of urinary tract infections [45, 46].

In a review of three RTOG trials using definitive radiotherapy with or without HT, 2922 patients were accrued with a median follow-up of 10.3 years for surviving patients. The RTOG scoring scheme was used to assess GI, GU, and other toxicities. Toxicity reported was grade 3 or higher late toxicity. Maximum grade 3+ late GU toxicity was 9%, 5%, and 6% for RT only, RT + STH, and RT + LTH, respectively. Additionally, the GU toxicity occurs over a longer period of time [47].

Non-infective cystitis is usually more severe and can cause intense pain, irritative voiding symptoms, and hematuria. Hemorrhagic cystitis is the most advanced clinical situations of radiation cystitis [44]. Montana et al. analyzed 527 patients of carcinoma cervix treated with radiotherapy and the mean bladder dose for the group of patients with cystitis was higher, 6661 ± 1309 cGy, than that for the patients without cystitis, 6298 ± 1305 cGy, $P = 0.19$. The risk of cystitis increased as a function of bladder dose ranging from 3% for patients receiving ≤ 5000 cGy to the bladder to 12% for patients receiving ≥ 8001 cGy to the bladder [48].

6.4.3 Neurologic Toxicity

The incidence of this first complication ranges from 0.8% to 3.0%, the radiotherapy-induced impairment of the lumbosacral plexus in cervical cancer patients treated with irradiation is very rare [49]. Lumbosacral plexopathy has been reported to develop occasionally in patients treated for pelvic tumors with doses of 60–67.5 Gy [50]. The differential diagnosis is important in patients who had plexopathy with recurrent tumors. Thomas et al. reported that indolent leg weakness has seen early in radiation-induced plexopathy while pain was found to be the most common symptom in patients with tumor plexopathy [50]. Muscular weakness, numbness, and paresthesia are common in both radiation-induced plexopathy and tumor plexopathy groups. In such cases, CT is particularly important in the detection of pelvic masses or bone destruction caused by the tumor. Symptomatic treatment involved steroids, analgesics including narcotics, neurological drugs such as galantamine hydrobromide preparations and alendronic acid preparations. The patient has been receiving physiotherapy. Unfortunately, the neurologic deficit is irreversible, and there is no any effective therapy unlike radiation myelopathy [49, 50].

6.4.4 Bone Toxicity

Insufficiency fracture due to pelvic radiotherapy is a kind of stress fracture, which is caused by normal stress placed on weakened bone where bone demineralization and decreased bone elastic resistance result from osteoporosis (Fig. 6.6) [51]. Although they are rarely life-threatening, these fractures need attention as they directly affect the quality of life of patient. In the analysis of 235 patients with

Fig. 6.6 Sacral
insufficiency fracture, no
clinical symptom, only
diagnosed with T2 MR
imaging

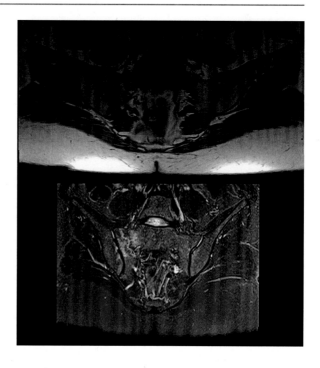

non-metastatic cervical cancer who were treated with definitive chemoradiation or postoperative radiotherapy, the 5-year detection rate of PIF was reported as 9.5%. The median radiation dose was 55 Gy (range 45–60 Gy) [52]. The median time to development of PIF was 12.5 months (range 5–30 months). The sites of fracture were sacroiliac joints, pubic rami, iliac bones, and femoral neck. The pain requiring medications was recorded in $11n$ of 16 patients. The significant risk factors of PIF were old age, body mass index <23, bone mineral density <−3.5 SD, more over radiation dose and concurrent chemotherapy had no impact on bone complications [52]. Grigsby et al. analyzed 1313 patients with gynecologic tumors treated with radiation therapy and reported that 207 of them received pelvic irradiation to the inguinal areas, including the hips. The cumulative actuarial incidence of fracture was 11% at 5 years and 15% at 10 years. In contrast to the previous report, most of the fractures were reported to occur in patients who were exposed 45–63 Gy doses [53]. Some risk factors such as cigarette smoking and osteoporosis were identified as risk factors for fracture.

Similarly prostate cancer patients who were treated for pelvic fields have the similar insufficiency fracture. In a paper by Igdem et al., of the 134 male patients, eight patients were identified with symptomatic IF after a median follow-up period of 68 months (range 12–116 months). The 5-year cumulative incidence of symptomatic IF was 6.8%. All patients are presented with lower back pain. Insufficiency fracture developed at a median time of 20 months after the end of radiotherapy and was managed conservatively without any need for hospitalization. No predisposing factors for development of IF could be identified [54].

More importantly, pelvic IF and metastatic disease had to be ruled out in order to prevent unnecessary treatment, especially in a patient cohort with high-risk features for distant spread. Also distinguishing insufficiency fractures from metastases on PET/CT could be challenging problem. Furthermore, radiation-induced toxicity results in significant decrease in the quality of life (Fig. 6.3).

6.4.5   Sexual Function

Patients undergoing radiotherapy for their pelvic cancer suffer from a considerable amount of late effects influencing negatively on sexual functioning. The literature has conflicting results about this quality of health metrics. Quick et al. analyzed early stage endometrium cancer patients who were treated either with adjuvant vaginal brachytherapy (VB) (n: 16) or only surgery group (n: 53). Of the sexually active patients, 33% of the VB patients and 42% of the surgery-alone patients felt their vagina was dry during sexual activity ($P = 0.804$) and 17% versus 20% felt their vagina was short ($P = 0.884$). Seventeen percent of patients in the VB group felt their vagina was tight compared to 29% in the surgery-alone group ($P = 0.891$) and 0% versus 14% of patients reported pain during intercourse ($P = 0.808$). As a result, there was no statistically significant difference in sexual/vaginal functioning, sexual worry, or sexual enjoyment between the two groups [55]. On contrast to this result, Bruner et al. investigated 90 patients treated with intracavitary irradiation for either carcinoma of the cervix (42 patients) or endometrial carcinoma (48 patients), 78 of whom also received external pelvic irradiation (44.5-Gy mean dose). They reported that vaginal length decreased in majority of the patients. Twenty two percent of women who participated in this study reported that their sexual frequency and sexual satisfaction decreased significantly [56]. Grigsby et al. reported that there were significant problems including decreased frequency of sexual intercourse, desire, orgasm, and enjoyment of intercourse in patients who had gynecologic tumors and who received radiotherapy. There were also some evidence which showed impairment in reproductivity in patients who received pelvic radiotherapy [57, 58]. The major improvement in the sexual outcome results, in the newer analyses, could be related to the radiotherapy techniques such as IMRT, 3DCRt, and 3D brachytherapy which could increase the knowledge about the normal tissue sparing and this has a positive impact on the modern series.

6.4.6   Vaginal Toxicity

Pathological alterations in the vaginal mucosa following radiotherapy involve mucosal atrophy, epithelial thinning, and loss of the squamous layer. Furthermore hyalinization and colonization can appear in connective tissue. These changes cause tissue damage, probable ulceration, and fistula formation. Histologic abnormalities are common in the 6 months following radiotherapy. It is quite important to distinguish this atypical formation from recurrent malignancies. In clinical settings vaginal stenosis and shortening can be seen several months after radiotherapy. However this duration may be long as 15 years after treatment [59]). The incidence of vaginal toxicity has been mostly obtained from patients who were treated for cervical cancer with radiotherapy. It has been reported that the risk of severe vaginal shortening was higher in patients who were older than 50 years old.

Rectovaginal fistula is a very serious anorectal complication with a significant impact on quality of life. In recent years, new options of surgical treatment have been re-introduced with improved treatment results, especially when dealing with low fistulas. Rectovaginal-vesicovaginal fistulas were reported to appear within 2 years following radiotherapy [60]. Diagnosis is made with vaginal scopy as well as CT or MRI. Zelga et al. reported 50 patients whom developed fistula after pelvic radiotherapy with a median age of 60 years (range 40–84 years). Cervical cancer was the most common cause of radiotherapy and median time of fistula development after radiotherapy was 20 months (range 5–240 months). Majority of the patients (96%) were reported to have fecal diversion, except two patients whom underwent rectal resection. Factors that correlated with fistula healing were a distance from the anal verge above 7 and creation of loop ileostomy, whereas a prolonged course of radiotherapy of more than 6 weeks ($P = 0.047$) correlated negatively [60]. Perez et al. reported that 25 patients developed vaginal toxicity among 205 patients who were treated with radiotherapy for VAIN or vaginal carcinoma. These complications included rectovaginal fistulas, vesicovaginal fistulas, bladder neck contractures or urethral strictures, rectal strictures, and proctitis [61]. In a retrospective study 193 patients with vaginal SCC who were treated with radiotherapy were investigated. It has been revealed that 17% of patients exposed to severe vaginal toxicity had complications at 10 years [62]. Although the vagina is regarded to be a radio-resistant organ, the tolerant dose of radiotherapy is still not clearly described. In a retrospective study, it has been reported that a radiation dose >70 Gy was significantly related to development of vaginal toxicity [63, 64]. In a literature review, acute endovaginal toxicity reported in <20.6% (vaginal inflammation, vaginal irritation, dryness, discharge, soreness, swelling, and fungal infection). G1-G2 late toxicity occurred in <27.7%. Finally, G3–G4 late vaginal occurred in <2%. The most common late side effects consisted of vaginal discharge, dryness, itching, bleeding, fibrosis, telangiectasias, stenosis, short or narrow vagina, and dyspareunia [63].

Hofsjo et al. investigated 34 patients with cervical cancer survivors who were treated with radiotherapy in terms of morphology of the vaginal epithelium and its correlation to serum levels of sex steroid hormones and sexual function [59]. The vaginal epithelium volume was reduced compared to control women. Longer distance between the dermal papillae ($P < 0.001$) and a shorter distance from basal layer to epithelial surface ($P < 0.05$) were measured in this group. Mucosal atrophy was observed in 91% of the survivors despite no difference in serum estradiol between cancer survivors and control women. The epithelial thickness was parallel to serum levels of estradiol. The cervical cancer survivors claimed more physical sexual symptoms. The relative risk factors were insufficient vaginal lubrication (RR 12.6), vaginal inelasticity (RR 6.5), reduced genital swelling when sexually aroused (RR 5.9), and for reduction of vaginal length during inter-course (RR 3.9) [59].

6.4.7 Testicular Function

Testicular radiation affects both germ cells and spermatogenesis as well as Leydig cells and testosterone production. The germinal epithelium is very sensitive even spermatogonia changes were seen following as low doses as 0.2 Gy. The significant effect on FSH levels or sperm counts, starts at a level between 0.2 and 0.7 Gy. This effect is transient dose-dependent and causes increase in FSH and reduction in sperm concentration. This effect a return to normal values within 12–24 months. No radiation dose threshold has been defined above which permanent azoospermia is inevitable; however, doses of 1.2 Gy and above are likely to be associated with a reduced risk of recovery of spermatogenesis [65]. Leydig cells which are related testosterone function are more radiosensitive than testicular germ cells. Usually, planned insertion of a sperm to provide a pregnancy was advised to be planned at least 12 months after radiotherapy.

Following radiation, vascular changes leading to cavernous artery insufficiency are primarily implicated in male erectile dysfunction [66]. In the evaluation of 16 men with a mean age of 61 years presenting with erectile dysfunction after radiation underwent arterial hemodynamics tests at a mean duration postradiation of 11 months, 85% had abnormal veno-occlusive parameters. Of the patients who could undergo cavernosography, 80% had venous leak, most commonly from the crura [66]. Following RT, sexual functions have been affected almost ranging from 50 to 75% after either external radiotherapy or brachytherapy [67].

Phosphodiesterase inhibitors such as sildenafil and tadalafil have been shown to effectively enhance sexual function. The RTOG performed a double-blinded cross-over trial randomizing patients receiving radiation and androgen deprivation therapy to sildenafil or placebo therapy for 12 weeks, and then crossed over. The study consists of 115 patients and sildenafil effect was significant ($P = 0.009$) with an erectile response of 0.17 compared to placebo with a response of 0.21 for patients receiving ≤120 days of ADT. However, only 21% of patients had a medication-specific response and they could benefit from sildenafil treatment [68]. Besides sildenafil, treatment option could be served as vacuum erection devices, intracavernosal injections with prostaglandins, and penile implants.

Potential risk factors during planning included large radiation field size, penile doses, and 70 Gy or more dose prescribed to the penile bulb.

6.4.8 Cutaneous Toxicity

Skin reactions for conventional fractionated radiotherapy are usually seen starting from second or third week (Fig. 6.7) [69]. The most significant acute morbidity of radiotherapy is reported to be the development of mucocutaneous reactions in the

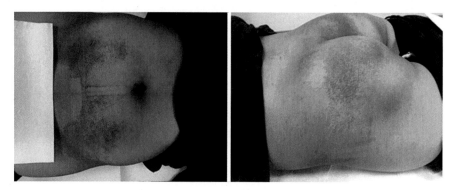

Fig. 6.7 A patient was treated with AP-PA pelvic fields for locally advanced cervical cancer. At the fifth week of the treatment, skin reactions were observed

vulva, perineum, and other inguinal areas. It has been assumed that the severity of the reaction was significantly associated with the radiation fractionation and comorbid usage of chemotherapy. Sometimes these acute reactions can cause interruption of treatment. Treatment of acute reactions includes topical agents, sitz baths, antifungal agents, and narcotic pain medications. The late complications of radiotherapy are telengiectasis and atrophy of the skin and mucosa of the vulva, dryness of the mucosa of the vagina and vulva, and narrowing of the vaginal introitus [70].

The progress of radiation-induced fibrosis is also facilitated by inflammation, which starts parallel to the start of radiotherapy and continues for months to years [71]. Cytokines such as TNF-a, IL-6, and IL-1 create an inflammatory response. TGF-β and platelet-derived growth factor regulate fibroblast activity and promote the production of extracellular matrix proteins. Fibroblasts are responsible for the development of late skin fibrotic changes like atrophy, contraction, and fibrosis [71]. In clinical practice, skin hygiene by washing with mild soaps and lukewarm water maintains skin barrier, and the risk for acute radiodermatitis decreases. The patients have to be informed for wearing loose fitting clothes, avoiding sun exposure and metallic topical products, and using water-based lipid-free moisturizers. Topical corticosteroids have been used to prevent radiodermatitis as well as itching due to inflammation [69, 71] (Fig. 6.2).

6.5　Management of Pelvic Radiation Disease

6.5.1　Prevention

Prevention is the first stage of the management of pelvic radiation disease. Preventing adverse effects of radiation is a multidisciplinary topic. Firstly, the patient should be assessed in terms of comorbid clinical conditions such as diabetes, hypertension, smoking, etc. The collaboration of medical oncologists, radiation oncologists, and surgeons is essential for preventing the side effects of radiation [19, 20].

There have been some important factors for prevention of side effects of radiation. The factors which are associated with host should be considered carefully.

Some co-morbid medical conditions such as hypertension, irritable bowel disease, and diabetes mellitus make patients tend to be effected by radiation much more. Before radiotherapy, comorbid disease such as diabetes or hypertension or some lifestyle characteristics such as smoking should be controlled. Smoking cessation is an important issue for decreasing the side effects of radiation. Smoking is considered to be an independent risk factor for development of side effects of radiotherapy [19]. Additionally, body mass index is another independent factor; a patient whose body mass index is >30 is reported to be a candidate for side effects of pelvic radiotherapy. Moreover, previous abdominal surgery and genetic predispositions are host related risk factors for the development of side effects of pelvic radiotherapy [14, 19, 20].

There are also some factors that are not associated with the host. Resistance of tumor against radiotherapy is an important factor for development of radiation related side effects. When resistance occurs, higher doses of radiotherapy should be considered for the tumor management. It has been well established that higher doses of radiotherapy are beneficial for overcoming the resistance; however, it is also strongly associated with higher collateral damage to surrounding healthy tissue in the radiotherapy beam [72]. Administering radiotherapy with higher doses and in larger fields is also associated with radiation related tissue damage. Larger doses of radiotherapy are considered to be associated with chronic complications. These observations are not new; for example, it has been demonstrated that when patients with uterine cervix carcinoma were treated with >1000 cGy/min over 2–3 min, this resulted in irreparable tissue damage in the 1970s. Thus, dose-volume histograms are routinely used to decrease the toxicity of radiotherapy [73]. Administration of radiotherapy to patients is performed in two ways: the beam radiation or brachytherapy. In this treatment approach, an external photon generator is used and exposes the patient to X-rays, electron beams, and gamma rays in a four-beam approach. This condition results a significant exposure to surrounding tissues [20]. However, large field sizes of treatment can cause damage to the surrounding tissue and lead to acute side effects such as diarrhea. Three dimensional conformal radiotherapy attempts to minimize the exposure to surrounding tissues. Radiation exposure can be avoided by calculating the tumor margin with computed tomography or magnetic resonance imaging. Surgical clips can be used to avoid more exposure; however, it is less useful compared to imaging modalities. Another important issue is the postoperative radiotherapy intervention. Postoperative radiotherapy was reported to be more toxic compared to preoperative radiotherapy. In postoperative radiotherapy cases, it is more likely to affect the pelvis with radiation. Studies demonstrated that postoperative radiotherapy-induced side effects on bowel was significantly higher compared to those who received radiotherapy preoperatively [74]. Prophylactic surgical techniques, image guiding, and supine position during radiotherapy were reported to decrease radiation associated side effects [20].

Managing patients with pelvic radiation disease is an ongoing subject of the oncology field. It has been considered that this situation is untreatable until understanding the etiology and pathogenesis. Currently, several medications, dietary supplements, and supportive measures are placed in guidelines. Pelvic radiation disease can affect various systems including urological, gastrointestinal, gynecological, dermatological, lymphatic, nervous, vascular structures, and sexual organs. Thus, management of patients should be individualized. The classification of patients in acute and chronic phases is essential for the management of the disease. Moreover, the psychological effects of pelvic radiation disease should be never neglected and be taken into account during the management [75]. There can be serious sexual problems such as ejaculation problems, erectile dysfunction, and vaginal stenosis [75]. Bowel is always kept in the mind as an affected system during pelvic radiation disease. Thus, a holistic approach including physical, psychological, and social factors should be implemented during management of pelvic radiation disease [76].

6.5.2 Management of Acute Phase

The main idea behind the acute phase management is supporting and solving the symptoms. Antikinetic medications such as fybogel, codeine, and loperamide should be considered to increase fluid absorption in the bowel and reduce peristaltism. Anti-cholinergic, antispasmodics, antiemetics, and analgesics are commonly used for resolving the related symptoms. In severe diarrhea cases, electronic imbalance must be followed up and supplementations must be admitted if necessary [14].

6.5.3 Management of Chronic Phase

Radiation can damage intestinal villi and inadequate enzyme production can cause malabsorption. In such situations, patients can misdiagnose with irritable bowel syndrome. Dietary interventions should be considered [77]. If the symptoms persist, medication should be considered, such as anti-inflammatory agents. Malabsorption of bile acids was reported to be the cause of diarrheal symptoms in 35–72% of patients with chronic pelvic radiation disease [73]. The most affected part of the small bowel is the terminal ileum in pelvic radiation disease [19]. Cholestyramine, colestipol, and colesevelam bind bile salts and have been administered to patients with pelvic radiation disease [73]. Evidence demonstrated that patients who were suffering from pelvic radiation disease responded well to the former agents.

6.5.3.1 Medical Treatments
Medical treatment is the first-line approach for the management of radiation-induced pelvic radiation disease. Recently, aminosalicylates, sucralfate, antibiotics, probiotics, steroids, and hyperbaric oxygen therapy have been recommended for the medical treatment of pelvic radiation disease [14].

6.5.3.2 Sucralfate
Sucralfate is an alkaline aluminum hydroxide of sulfated sucrose. It protects the mucosa by forming a viscous superficial coating and to stimulate mucosal healing by its angiogenic action [78].

Prospective studies have demonstrated that topical sucralfate treatment is effective in the treatment of PRD associated symptoms such as reducing the volume of rectal bleeding [79, 80]. Majority of patients who were suffering from these symptoms benefited as 73–100% in 4 and 6 weeks periods. However, patients who survived much more experienced recurrence range between 10% and 20% [80]. Oral sucralfate was reported to be ineffective for improving the symptoms. Regarding available evidence, topical administration of sucralfate should be considered as one of the first-line treatments of radiation-induced rectal bleeding [79–81]. Sucralfate can be used twice daily as a retention enema or can be used as two 1 g sucralfate tablets mixed with 4.5 mL of water in an enema applicator [81].

6.5.3.3 Metronidazole

Metronidazole is a bactericidal agent that kills anaerobic and microaerophilic bacteria and it has an immunomodulator effect. Thus it can be said that metronidazole has dual action reducing the risk of rectal bleeding and supporting the management of PRD [15].

There has been evidence which showed that metronidazole was effective in treating chronic rectal bleeding and diarrhea [82]. In a randomized study, metronidazole was found to be superior to mesalazine (3 × 1 g/day orally) and betamethasone enema (once a day during 4 weeks) or only the combination of mesalazine and betamethasone for the treatment of radiation-induced rectal bleeding, diarrhea, and ulcerations. Sahakitrungruang et al. enrolled in a RCT including 50 patients with chronic radiation-induced PRD; patients were randomized to daily colonic irrigation plus metronidazole (3 × 500 mg/day orally) and ciprofloxacin (2 × 500 mg/day orally) for a week, or to receive 4% formalin by using proctoscopy. After 8 weeks, it was found that there had been a significant improvement in rectal bleeding, urgency, diarrhea in patients treated with metronidazole [81]. Regarding the evidence based results, metronidazole can be administered orally (3 × 400 mg/day) from 1 week up to 12 weeks. Although it has been considered as a safe drug, skin rash, nausea, and vomiting are commonly seen as side effects [15, 81].

6.5.3.4 Probiotics

As mentioned previously, radiation damages the intestinal mucosa and causes problems in motility. These changes affect the natural bacterial colonies in the bowel [82]. Ionizing radiation disturbs the homeostasis of intestinal microflora which directly influences bowel functions. These changes in microflora create some associated problems. For example, enteric bacteria produce host's health system by synthesizing essential molecules such as vitamin K and folate. Furthermore, these commensal bacteria support the immune system indirectly [83]. During long-term radiotherapy, patients can need broad-spectrum antibiotics such as co-amoxiclav, ciprofloxacin, tetracycline, and rifaximin. Concerning the usage of probiotics in patients with pelvic radiation disease, there has been evidence which showed beneficial effects of heralding lactobacilli probiotics [83]. However, other probiotic studies failed to demonstrate the reduction of diarrheal symptoms. Unfortunately, there is no evidence for the prevention of pelvic radiation disease with probiotics or antibiotics [82].

6.5.3.5 Aminosalicylates

Aminosalicylates are compounds that contain 5-aminosalicylic acid (5ASA). It is a strong inhibitor of the synthesis and release of proinflammatory mediators (e.g., nitric oxide, leukotrienes, thromboxanes, and platelet activating factor). Aminosalicylates also inhibit the acute inflammatory and immune response [84]. They are marketed currently as pro-drugs (sulfasalazine) and the active compound (mesalazine). They are mainly effective for the improvement of early-onset PRD.

There is solely one randomized, controlled trial which showed that mesalazine significantly improved symptoms of PRD including diarrhea, abdominal pain, and flatulence [85]. However, current evidence does not support the use of mesalazine for the treatment of acute or chronic PRD. It has been suggested that mesalazine can be used for rectal bleeding as a second-line therapy [31].

6.5.3.6 Corticosteroids

Corticosteroids affect many metabolic and physiological systems in the human body. The main action of mechanism of corticosteroids is inhibiting the inflammation by blocking cytokine release and production, inhibiting histamine release and activation of macrophages, and finally by stabilizing cell membranes [86]. Thus, using corticosteroids has been considered rational at the early phase of PRD.

Unfortunately, corticosteroids have not been definitely shown to provide substantial benefits for treating pelvic radiation disease [14]. The studies that investigated the treatment effects of corticosteroids on patients with PRD were small sample sized, not randomized or had short follow-up time. However, enema forms of corticosteroids were reported to be effective for rectal bleeding in short time treatment periods [15, 86].

6.5.3.7 Endoscopic Approaches

While considering several endoscopic techniques, only argon plasma coagulation (APC) and formalin application have been reported to be effective for treating severe rectal bleeding. Other techniques, such as radiofrequency ablation (RFA), cryoablation, and band ligation should not be considered for treatment [14].

6.5.3.8 Argon Plasma Coagulation

The other main treatment modality of pelvic radiation disease is endoscopic approaches. Argon plasma coagulation (APC) treatment is a noncontact thermal coagulation technique on a probe that can be passed through the scope during endoscopy. A high voltage filament then ionizes the gas which heats the mucosa and results in coagulation of tissues damaged by PRD and aims to prevent them from bleeding. This technique allows reduced rectal bleeding in 80–90% of patients [19]. However, the use of this technique can be said to be limited to rectal bleeding. Furthermore, there can be serious side effects of APC therapy. Similar to other medical approaches, further studies are needed to support effectiveness of APC therapy in patients with pelvic radiation disease [15, 19].

6.5.3.9 Formalin

Formalin is an aldehyde which is used to preserve or fix tissues by cross-linkage of primary amino groups in proteins with other nearby nitrogen atoms in proteins or DNA through a CH2 bond. It is highly irritant and direct application to radiation-damaged tissues leads to local chemical cauterization [15]. Regarding this effect, formalin has been advised to be used in treatment for refractory severe rectal bleeding cases.

Formalin can be seen as an alternative to thermal coagulation therapy with argon plasma in patients with severe rectal bleeding. Besides this effect, the evidence showing the effectiveness of formalin in the treatment of PRD is said to be insufficient. During application side effects including anorectal pain, fecal incontinence, severe diarrhea, fever, and severe formalin-induced colitis should be taken into account [86].

6.5.3.10 Other Medications

Angiotensin I-converting enzyme inhibitors (ACEi) and the cholesterol lowering statins have been demonstrated to reduce gastrointestinal symptoms associated with radiation-induced side effects during pelvic radiotherapy [87]. Statins were found to have anti-thrombotic and anti-fibrotic properties in human cells exposed to radiation [19]. The actions of mechanism of statins were suggested to be inhibition of 3-hydroxymethylglutaryl coenzyme reductase. ACEi causes blood pressure homeostasis. These medications were shown to have protective effects on bowel tissue which was exposed to radiation. In a clinical study, only statin treatment or statin treatment combined with ACEi was reported to reduce gastrointestinal symptoms related to radiotherapy [87]. However, these findings need confirmation with further prospective studies.

6.5.3.11 Hyperbaric Oxygen Treatment

Hyperbaric oxygen (HBO) therapy is considered to be an alternative choice for the management of pelvic radiation disease. However, the results of studies which researched the effects of HBO therapy in pelvic radiation disease are inconsistent. HBO therapy was reported to have hypoxia decreasing properties by inducing angiogenesis in patients whose bowel was affected by radiotherapy [16]. In a randomized controlled trial, HBO treatment was shown to reduce the risk of pelvic radiation disease [88]. However, further studies are needed to confirm the beneficial effects of HBO treatment on the symptoms of pelvic radiation disease [20].

6.6 Rx: Sample Prescriptions

6.6.1 Diarrhea

- Evaluation of symptoms: diarrhea, determining watery diarrhea versus loose/soft stool, frequency, flatus/gas cramping, urgency or rectal/hemorrhoidal pain, and whether urination triggers bowel movement.
- Monitor weight loss, fluid loss (tenting and dry mucous membranes), and electrolyte imbalance (especially potassium should be replaced).

Initiation: A high fiber diet and increase the liquid intake initially. Also, increase foods high in pectin (i.e., oatmeal, bananas, and applesauce) which help bind stool. You can start psyllium tablets and probiotics.

Stool <4 times/day: Imodium is more accessible, and maximum dose is 16 mg (8 tablet/day).

Stool >4 times/day: Lomotil may be much cheaper with more side effects and can be used up to 8 tablets/day (4 × 2 tbl). Lomotil or imodium is usually prescribed after each loose bowel movement. However, when required on a daily basis, 1–2 tablets prescribed in the morning may reduce the need for subsequent tablets.

- Consider IV fluid support.
- Obtain stool culture to rule out *C. difficile*.

If there is refractory diarrhea, opium or Sandostatin (octreotide)—50–200 mcg SQ bid—tid could be preferred and hospitalization is recommended.
Chronic gastroenteritis:

- Chronic diarrhea and/or weight loss secondary to previous abdominal or pelvic irradiation may persist or develop after one to several years
- Multidisciplinary approach
- Psylliums, probiotics, and fiber rich diet are recommended
- Diarrhea may exist alone or may be associated with malabsorption. Fecal fat assays may be helpful to determine if malabsorption or maldigestion is present
- Classic radiation enteritis, a combination of imodium and lactulose
- Check vitamin B12 level
- No improvement, consider 2-week trial courses of pancreatic enzyme products and finally prednisone. Fecal incontinence: Physical therapy could increase the strength of perianal muscle

6.6.2 Chronic Radiation Proctitis, or Rectal Bleeding

- For chronic proctitis or rectal bleeding, initiate therapy with steroid suppositories (cortos sup) and sulfasalazine sup
- Consider the use of argon plasma coagulation
- A 3 month course of Trental and vitamin E (extend to 6 months if improvement), and then proceed to hyperbaric oxygen if needed

Hydrocortisone retention enema—1 pr q hs, retain for 1 h

- Supplied as single dose units, 100 mg hydrocortisone/60 cc
- Formalin—apply directly to involved area—most studies use a 4% solution
- Pancrelipase—1–2 po with meals, one with snacks
- Prednisone—10–40 mg po, q day, tablets 1, 2.5, 5, 10, 20, 50 mg

- Cholestyramine—one packet or one scoopful mixed per directions
- Pentoxifylline—400 mg po tid with meals, tablets 400 mg Note: do not use if history of cerebral or retinal bleeding
- Vitamin E (tocopherol)—1000 IU po, qd
- Hyoscine butylbromide, 3 times 1–2 tablet daily
- Chronic proctitis
- Symptoms related to trauma could be eased with stool softener
- Biopsy has to be prevented
- Argon laser could be administered
- hyperbaric O2
- Vaseline/lidocaine (1:1) combination, topical application
- 5 mg hydrocortisone acetate and 27 mg polidocanol supp (cortos supp), 3 × 1 or 3 × 2 and mesalazine, daily 3 × 1

6.6.3 Nausea/Vomiting

- Lorazepam—anticipatory—1–2 mg po 45 min prior to XRT, adjunct to antinausea medications 0.5–1 mg po tid—tablets 0.5, 1, 2 mg
- (Prochlorperazine) 10 mg po q 6—oral—5–10 mg po q 6–8 h
- Dexamethasone—2–4 mg po q 8 h
- Granisetron—1 mg po bid
- Promethazine—12.5–25 mg po/im/pr q 4–6 h
- Ondansetron—8 mg po q 8 h
- Metoklopramid HCl 10 mg

6.6.4 Genitourinary

- Symptoms: cystitis—urgency, frequency, dysuria, and nocturia. Bladder infection may occur during the first week
- Non-infectious cystitis is mild and intermittent initially, beginning in the third to fifth week
- Rule out infection and glucosuria
- Urgency/frequency or dysuria with a good stream and no hesitancy but small volume suggests bladder spasms and/or XRT cystitis—treat with analgesics or antispasmodics

Urgency or dysuria with hesitancy and intermittent stream suggests obstruction which should be treated with a urinary obstruction modifier, adding analgesics if needed.

- XRT cystitis from bladder spasms as both can cause dysuria from the tip of the penis to the suprapubic region.

Bladder spasms: Tolterodine (2 × 1–2 mg), oxybutynin (2–3 × 5 mg) or flavoxate (3–4 × 1 tbl), trospium chloride (3 × 15–30 mg).

- Methenamine effervescent 70 g: Gram negative and gram positive antibacterial
- Trimethoprim/sulfamethoxazole
- Ciprofloxacin—250–500 mg po q 12 h
- Levofloxacin—500 mg qd
- Nitrofurantoin
- Norfloxacin—400 mg po q 12 h

6.6.5 Hematuria and Chronic Radiation Cystitis

Late reacting cystitis, direct application (by the urologist) of dilute formalin, usually 4%, or use of argon plasma coagulation.

- A 3 month course of Trental and vitamin E (extend to 6 months if improvement), and then proceed to hyperbaric oxygen if needed.

Botox—active bladder

6.6.6 Perineal Reaction

- Hydrations are essential
- If the reaction is severe and early, consider candidal infection and treat with topical Nizoral cream or oral antifungals
- Pain management, consider the aquaphor/xylocaine mixture

Hydrocortisone 0.5% (OTC)—apply qid prn
Hydrocortisone 1%
2% Cream Ketoconazole—apply to affected area bid
Ketoconazole tablets—200 mg po qd × 10 days; 400 mg qd if
Metronidazole—375 mg, po bid—750 mg po qd × 7 days
Vaginal Moisturizer
Vaginal Hyaluronic supp

References

1. Viana R, Batourina E, Huang H, et al. The development of the bladder trigone, the center of the anti-reflux mechanism. Development. 2007;134:3763–9.
2. Sica GT, Teeger S. MR imaging of scrotal, testicular, and penile diseases. Magn Reson Imaging Clin N Am. 1996;4:545–63.
3. Roach M 3rd, Nam J, Gagliardi G, et al. Radiation dose-volume effects and the penile bulb. Int J Radiat Oncol Biol Phys. 2010;76:S130–4.

4. Sala EJ, Atri M. Magnetic resonance imaging of benign adnexal disease. Top Magn Reson Imaging. 2003;14:305–27.
5. Gay HA, Barthold HJ, O'Meara E, et al. Pelvic normal tissue contouring guidelines for radiation therapy: a radiation therapy oncology group consensus panel atlas. Int J Radiat Oncol Biol Phys. 2012;83:e353–62.
6. Ranieri G, Patruno R, Ruggieri E, et al. Vascular endothelial growth factor (VEGF) as a target of bevacizumab in cancer: from the biology to the clinic. Curr Med Chem. 2006;13:1845–57.
7. Jain RK, Duda DG, Clark JW, Loeffler JS. Lessons from phase III clinical trials on anti-VEGF therapy for cancer. Nat Clin Pract Oncol. 2006;3:24–40.
8. Dasari S, Tchounwou PB. Cisplatin in cancer therapy: molecular mechanisms of action. Eur J Pharmacol. 2014;740:364–78.
9. Rancoule C, Guy JB, Vallard A, et al. 50th anniversary of cisplatin. Bull Cancer. 2017;104:167–76.
10. Xue R, Cai X, Xu H, et al. The efficacy of concurrent weekly carboplatin with radiotherapy in the treatment of cervical cancer: a meta-analysis. Gynecol Oncol. 2018;150:412–9.
11. Zagouri F, Korakiti AM, Zakopoulou R, et al. Taxanes during pregnancy in cervical cancer: a systematic review and pooled analysis. Cancer Treat Rev. 2019;79:101885.
12. Viswanathan AN, Moughan J, Miller BE, et al. NRG Oncology/RTOG 0921: a phase 2 study of postoperative intensity-modulated radiotherapy with concurrent cisplatin and bevacizumab followed by carboplatin and paclitaxel for patients with endometrial cancer. Cancer. 2015;121:2156–63.
13. Siegel RL, Miller KD, Jemal A. Cancer statistics, 2015. CA Cancer J Clin. 2015;65:5–29.
14. Frazzoni L, La Marca M, Guido A, et al. Pelvic radiation disease: updates on treatment options. World J Clin Oncol. 2015;6:272–80.
15. Andreyev HJ, Wotherspoon A, Denham JW, Hauer-Jensen M. Defining pelvic-radiation disease for the survivorship era. Lancet Oncol. 2010;11:310–2.
16. Dearnaley DP, Khoo VS, Norman AR, et al. Comparison of radiation side-effects of conformal and conventional radiotherapy in prostate cancer: a randomised trial. Lancet. 1999;353:267–72.
17. Atwood KC, Norman A. On the interpretation of multi-hit survival curves. Proc Natl Acad Sci U S A. 1949;35:696–709.
18. Hauer-Jensen M, Denham JW, Andreyev HJ. Radiation enteropathy--pathogenesis, treatment and prevention. Nat Rev Gastroenterol Hepatol. 2014;11:470–9.
19. Morris KA, Haboubi NY. Pelvic radiation therapy: between delight and disaster. World J Gastrointest Surg. 2015;7:279–88.
20. Matta R, Chapple CR, Fisch M, et al. Pelvic complications after prostate Cancer radiation therapy and their management: an international collaborative narrative review. Eur Urol. 2019;75:464–76.
21. Yarnold J. Molecular aspects of cellular responses to radiotherapy. Radiother Oncol. 1997;44:1–7.
22. Metheetrairut C, Slack FJ. MicroRNAs in the ionizing radiation response and in radiotherapy. Curr Opin Genet Dev. 2013;23:12–9.
23. Pawlik TM, Keyomarsi K. Role of cell cycle in mediating sensitivity to radiotherapy. Int J Radiat Oncol Biol Phys. 2004;59:928–42.
24. Zelefsky MJ, Levin EJ, Hunt M, et al. Incidence of late rectal and urinary toxicities after three-dimensional conformal radiotherapy and intensity-modulated radiotherapy for localized prostate cancer. Int J Radiat Oncol Biol Phys. 2008;70:1124–9.
25. Nicholas S, Chen L, Choflet A, et al. Pelvic radiation and normal tissue toxicity. Semin Radiat Oncol. 2017;27:358–69.
26. McBride SM, Wong DS, Dombrowski JJ, et al. Hypofractionated stereotactic body radiotherapy in low-risk prostate adenocarcinoma: preliminary results of a multi-institutional phase 1 feasibility trial. Cancer. 2012;118:3681–90.
27. Chen MF, Tseng CJ, Tseng CC, et al. Clinical outcome in posthysterectomy cervical cancer patients treated with concurrent cisplatin and intensity-modulated pelvic radiotherapy: comparison with conventional radiotherapy. Int J Radiat Oncol Biol Phys. 2007;67:1438–44.

28. Sharma NK, Li T, Chen DY, et al. Intensity-modulated radiotherapy reduces gastrointestinal toxicity in patients treated with androgen deprivation therapy for prostate cancer. Int J Radiat Oncol Biol Phys. 2011;80:437–44.

29. Kwak YK, Lee SW, Kay CS, Park HH. Intensity-modulated radiotherapy reduces gastrointestinal toxicity in pelvic radiation therapy with moderate dose. PLoS One. 2017;12:e0183339.

30. Vanneste BG, Van De Voorde L, de Ridder RJ, et al. Chronic radiation proctitis: tricks to prevent and treat. Int J Color Dis. 2015;30:1293–303.

31. Denton AS, Andreyev HJ, Forbes A, Maher EJ. Systematic review for non-surgical interventions for the management of late radiation proctitis. Br J Cancer. 2002;87:134–43.

32. Pan YB, Maeda Y, Wilson A, et al. Late gastrointestinal toxicity after radiotherapy for anal cancer: a systematic literature review. Acta Oncol. 2018;57:1427–37.

33. Lindgren A, Dunberger G, Steineck G et al. Identifying female pelvic cancer survivors with low levels of physical activity after radiotherapy: women with fecal and urinary leakage need additional support. Support Care Cancer. 2019. https://doi.org/10.1007/s00520-019-05033-3.

34. Choi KH, Kim JY, Lee DS, et al. Clinical impact of boost irradiation to pelvic lymph node in uterine cervical cancer treated with definitive chemoradiotherapy. Medicine (Baltimore). 2018;97:e0517.

35. Willett CG, Ooi CJ, Zietman AL, et al. Acute and late toxicity of patients with inflammatory bowel disease undergoing irradiation for abdominal and pelvic neoplasms. Int J Radiat Oncol Biol Phys. 2000;46:995–8.

36. Viswanathan AN, Yorke ED, Marks LB, et al. Radiation dose-volume effects of the urinary bladder. Int J Radiat Oncol Biol Phys. 2010;76:S116–22.

37. Grun A, Kawgan-Kagan M, Kaul D, et al. Impact of bladder volume on acute genitourinary toxicity in intensity modulated radiotherapy for localized and locally advanced prostate cancer. Strahlenther Onkol. 2019;195:517–25.

38. Brand DH, Tree AC, Ostler P, et al. Intensity-modulated fractionated radiotherapy versus stereotactic body radiotherapy for prostate cancer (PACE-B): acute toxicity findings from an international, randomised, open-label, phase 3, non-inferiority trial. Lancet Oncol. 2019;20:1531.

39. Donovan JL, Hamdy FC, Lane JA, et al. Patient-reported outcomes after monitoring, surgery, or radiotherapy for prostate cancer. N Engl J Med. 2016;375:1425–37.

40. Portelance L, Chao KS, Grigsby PW, et al. Intensity-modulated radiation therapy (IMRT) reduces small bowel, rectum, and bladder doses in patients with cervical cancer receiving pelvic and Para-aortic irradiation. Int J Radiat Oncol Biol Phys. 2001;51:261–6.

41. Wang W, Hou X, Yan J, et al. Outcome and toxicity of radical radiotherapy or concurrent chemoradiotherapy for elderly cervical cancer women. BMC Cancer. 2017;17:510.

42. Kim S, Moore DF, Shih W, et al. Severe genitourinary toxicity following radiation therapy for prostate cancer--how long does it last? J Urol. 2013;189:116–21.

43. McIntyre JF, Eifel PJ, Levenback C, Oswald MJ. Ureteral stricture as a late complication of radiotherapy for stage IB carcinoma of the uterine cervix. Cancer. 1995;75:836–43.

44. Mallick S, Madan R, Julka PK, Rath GK. Radiation induced cystitis and proctitis - prediction, assessment and management. Asian Pac J Cancer Prev. 2015;16:5589–94.

45. Prasad KN, Pradhan S, Datta NR. Urinary tract infection in patients of gynecological malignancies undergoing external pelvic radiotherapy. Gynecol Oncol. 1995;57:380–2.

46. Levenback C, Eifel PJ, Burke TW, et al. Hemorrhagic cystitis following radiotherapy for stage Ib cancer of the cervix. Gynecol Oncol. 1994;55:206–10.

47. Lawton CA, Bae K, Pilepich M, et al. Long-term treatment sequelae after external beam irradiation with or without hormonal manipulation for adenocarcinoma of the prostate: analysis of radiation therapy oncology group studies 85-31, 86-10, and 92-02. Int J Radiat Oncol Biol Phys. 2008;70:437–41.

48. Montana GS, Fowler WC. Carcinoma of the cervix: analysis of bladder and rectal radiation dose and complications. Int J Radiat Oncol Biol Phys. 1989;16:95–100.

49. Georgiou A, Grigsby PW, Perez CA. Radiation induced lumbosacral plexopathy in gynecologic tumors: clinical findings and dosimetric analysis. Int J Radiat Oncol Biol Phys. 1993;26:479–82.
50. Klimek M, Kosobucki R, Luczyńska E, et al. Radiotherapy-induced lumbosacral plexopathy in a patient with cervical cancer: a case report and literature review. Contemp Oncol (Pozn). 2012;16:194–6.
51. Henry AP, Lachmann E, Tunkel RS, Nagler W. Pelvic insufficiency fractures after irradiation: diagnosis, management, and rehabilitation. Arch Phys Med Rehabil. 1996;77:414–6.
52. Park SH, Kim JC, Lee JE, Park IK. Pelvic insufficiency fracture after radiotherapy in patients with cervical cancer in the era of PET/CT. Radiation Oncol J. 2011;29:269–76.
53. Grigsby PW, Roberts HL, Perez CA. Femoral neck fracture following groin irradiation. Int J Radiat Oncol Biol Phys. 1995;32:63–7.
54. Igdem S, Alco G, Ercan T, et al. Insufficiency fractures after pelvic radiotherapy in patients with prostate cancer. Int J Radiat Oncol Biol Phys. 2010;77:818–23.
55. Quick AM, Seamon LG, Abdel-Rasoul M, et al. Sexual function after intracavitary vaginal brachytherapy for early-stage endometrial carcinoma. Int J Gynecol Cancer. 2012;22:703–8.
56. Bruner DW, Lanciano R, Keegan M, et al. Vaginal stenosis and sexual function following intracavitary radiation for the treatment of cervical and endometrial carcinoma. Int J Radiat Oncol Biol Phys. 1993;27:825–30.
57. Grigsby PW, Russell A, Bruner D, et al. Late injury of cancer therapy on the female reproductive tract. Int J Radiat Oncol Biol Phys. 1995;31:1281–99.
58. Jensen PT, Froeding LP. Pelvic radiotherapy and sexual function in women. Transl Androl Urol. 2015;4:186–205.
59. Hofsjo A, Bergmark K, Blomgren B, et al. Radiotherapy for cervical cancer - impact on the vaginal epithelium and sexual function. Acta Oncol. 2018;57:338–45.
60. Zelga P, Tchórzewski M, Zelga M, et al. Radiation-induced rectovaginal fistulas in locally advanced gynaecological malignancies-new patients, old problem? Langenbeck's Arch Surg. 2017;402:1079–88.
61. Perez CA, Camel HM, Galakatos AE, et al. Definitive irradiation in carcinoma of the vagina: long-term evaluation of results. Int J Radiat Oncol Biol Phys. 1988;15:1283–90.
62. Frank SJ, Jhingran A, Levenback C, Eifel PJ. Definitive radiation therapy for squamous cell carcinoma of the vagina. Int J Radiat Oncol Biol Phys. 2005;62:138–47.
63. Delishaj D, Barcellini A, D'Amico R, et al. Vaginal toxicity after high-dose-rate endovaginal brachytherapy: 20 years of results. J Contemp Brachytherapy. 2018;10:559–66.
64. Stryker JA. Radiotherapy for vaginal carcinoma: a 23-year review. Br J Radiol. 2000;73:1200–5.
65. Howell SJ, Shalet SM. Spermatogenesis after cancer treatment: damage and recovery. J Natl Cancer Inst Monogr. 2005;2005:12–7.
66. Mulhall J, Ahmed A, Parker M, Mohideen N. The hemodynamics of erectile dysfunction following external beam radiation for prostate cancer. J Sex Med. 2005;2:432–7.
67. Chen RC, Clark JA, Talcott JA. Individualizing quality-of-life outcomes reporting: how localized prostate cancer treatments affect patients with different levels of baseline urinary, bowel, and sexual function. J Clin Oncol. 2009;27:3916–22.
68. Watkins Bruner D, James JL, Bryan CJ, et al. Randomized, double-blinded, placebo-controlled crossover trial of treating erectile dysfunction with sildenafil after radiotherapy and short-term androgen deprivation therapy: results of RTOG 0215. J Sex Med. 2011;8:1228–38.
69. Fisher J, Scott C, Stevens R, et al. Randomized phase III study comparing best supportive care to Biafine as a prophylactic agent for radiation-induced skin toxicity for women undergoing breast irradiation: radiation therapy oncology group (RTOG) 97-13. Int J Radiat Oncol Biol Phys. 2000;48:1307–10.
70. Kouvaris JR, Kouloulias VE, Plataniotis GA, et al. Dermatitis during radiation for vulvar carcinoma: prevention and treatment with granulocyte-macrophage colony-stimulating factor impregnated gauze. Wound Repair Regen. 2001;9:187–93.

71. Wei J, Meng L, Hou X, et al. Radiation-induced skin reactions: mechanism and treatment. Cancer Manag Res. 2019;11:167–77.
72. Do NL, Nagle D, Poylin VY. Radiation proctitis: current strategies in management. Gastroenterol Res Pract. 2011;2011:917941.
73. Shadad AK, Sullivan FJ, Martin JD, Egan LJ. Gastrointestinal radiation injury: prevention and treatment. World J Gastroenterol. 2013;19:199–208.
74. Frykholm GJ, Glimelius B, Pahlman L. Preoperative or postoperative irradiation in adenocarcinoma of the rectum: final treatment results of a randomized trial and an evaluation of late secondary effects. Dis Colon Rectum. 1993;36:564–72.
75. Klee M, Thranov I, Machin D. Life after radiotherapy: the psychological and social effects experienced by women treated for advanced stages of cervical cancer. Gynecol Oncol. 2000;76:5–13.
76. Brand AH, Bull CA, Cakir B. Vaginal stenosis in patients treated with radiotherapy for carcinoma of the cervix. Int J Gynecol Cancer. 2006;16:288–93.
77. Stacey R, Green JT. Radiation-induced small bowel disease: latest developments and clinical guidance. Ther Adv Chronic Dis. 2014;5:15–29.
78. Szabo S, Vattay P, Scarbrough E, Folkman J. Role of vascular factors, including angiogenesis, in the mechanisms of action of sucralfate. Am J Med. 1991;91:158s–60s.
79. Kochhar R, Sriram PV, Sharma SC, et al. Natural history of late radiation proctosigmoiditis treated with topical sucralfate suspension. Dig Dis Sci. 1999;44:973–8.
80. Gul YA, Prasannan S, Jabar FM, et al. Pharmacotherapy for chronic hemorrhagic radiation proctitis. World J Surg. 2002;26:1499–502.
81. Cavcic J, Turcic J, Martinac P, et al. Metronidazole in the treatment of chronic radiation proctitis: clinical trial. Croat Med J. 2000;41:314–8.
82. Chitapanarux I, Chitapanarux T, Traisathit P, et al. Randomized controlled trial of live lactobacillus acidophilus plus bifidobacterium bifidum in prophylaxis of diarrhea during radiotherapy in cervical cancer patients. Radiat Oncol. 2010;5:31.
83. Fuccio L, Guido A. Probiotics supplementation for the prevention of gastrointestinal radiation-induced side effects: the time is now. Am J Gastroenterol. 2013;108:277.
84. Cole AT, Slater K, Sokal M, Hawkey CJ. In vivo rectal inflammatory mediator changes with radiotherapy to the pelvis. Gut. 1993;34:1210–4.
85. Seo EH, Kim TO, Kim TG, et al. The efficacy of the combination therapy with oral and topical mesalazine for patients with the first episode of radiation proctitis. Dig Dis Sci. 2011;56:2672–7.
86. Pikarsky AJ, Belin B, Efron J, et al. Complications following formalin installation in the treatment of radiation induced proctitis. Int J Color Dis. 2000;15:96–9.
87. Wedlake LJ, Silia F, Benton B, et al. Evaluating the efficacy of statins and ACE-inhibitors in reducing gastrointestinal toxicity in patients receiving radiotherapy for pelvic malignancies. Eur J Cancer. 2012;48:2117–24.
88. Clarke RE, Tenorio LM, Hussey JR, et al. Hyperbaric oxygen treatment of chronic refractory radiation proctitis: a randomized and controlled double-blind crossover trial with long-term follow-up. Int J Radiat Oncol Biol Phys. 2008;72:134–43.

Toxicity Management for Other Sites in Radiation Oncology

7

Cagdas Yavas and Melis Gultekin

7.1 Breast

7.1.1 Anatomy

The breasts are located on the anterior and also partly the lateral aspects of the chest. Each of them extends cranially to the second rib, caudally to the sixth costal cartilage, medially to the sternum, and laterally to the mid-axillary line. The nipple-areola complex is located between the 4th and 5th ribs. The inner structure of the mammary gland is composed of epithelial components that consist of lobules, where milk is made, which connect to ducts that lead out to the nipple. The functional unit of the breast is the ductal-lobular unit. These lobules and ducts are located and surrounded by fibrous and adipose tissue [1, 2].

The breast lies upon the deep pectoral fascia, that in turn overlies pectoralis major and serratus anterior, and caudally, external oblique muscle and its aponeurosis as the latter forms the anterior wall of the sheath of rectus abdominis muscle. The superior pectoral fascia, with the anterior layer, envelops the breast ventrally and a posterior layer dorsally.

The blood supply of the breast is derived from the internal thoracic artery (internal mammary artery), the intercostal artery, and the axillary arteries. The lymphatic drainage of the breast is diffuse and variable. The lymphatics of the breast spreads through two sets of lymphatic vessels: the superficial (subepithelial or subdermal)

C. Yavas
Selcuk University, Faculty of Medicine, Department of Radiation Oncology,
Konya, Turkey

M. Gultekin (✉)
Hacettepe University, Faculty of Medicine, Department of Radiation Oncology,
Ankara, Turkey
e-mail: melisgultekin@hacettepe.edu.tr

© Springer Nature Switzerland AG 2020
G. Ozyigit, U. Selek (eds.), *Prevention and Management of Acute and Late Toxicities in Radiation Oncology*, https://doi.org/10.1007/978-3-030-37798-4_7

and the deep lymphatics. The subepithelial plexus connects to subdermal lymphatic vessels by vertical lymphatics and from them to the deep plexus. The subepithelial and subdermal plexus of the breast are confluent with the subareolar plexus in which the fine lymphatics of the lactiferous ducts. From the deep lymphatics, the lymph flows towards the axillary and internal thoracic nodes [2].

The axilla is bounded medially with the chest wall, laterally by the latissimus dorsi muscle, cranially by the axillary vein, posteriorly by the subscapularis muscle, and caudally by the interdigitation of the serratus anterior and latissimus dorsi muscles. The axilla is divided into three levels, with respect to their anatomical relationship to the pectoralis minor muscle. Level I nodes are situated inferiorly or laterally to the lower border of the pectoralis minor muscle. The external mammary, axillary vein, and scapular lymph nodes form level I nodes. Level II nodes lie deep or behind the pectoralis minor and include the central lymph node group and the subclavicular nodes. Lastly, level III nodes are situated above the upper border of the pectoralis minor muscle and include the subclavicular and apical node groups. The internal thoracic lymph nodes lie along the internal thoracic vessels and are very small. They drain the inner aspect of the mammary gland and also the anterior chest wall, the anterior portion of the diaphragm, the upper portion of the rectus sheath and muscle, and the superior portion of the liver [1, 2].

7.1.2 Contouring

The total glandular breast tissue, whose borders are often not clearly visible, should be delineated (Fig. 7.1). The cranial border is highly variable depending on breast size and patient position, and defined as second rib insertion. The caudal border is defined as loss of apparent breast tissues on computed tomography (CT) scans. The lateral aspect can be more cranial then the medial aspect depending on breast shape and patient position. Laterally mid-axillary line should be included; however, latissimus dorsi muscle should be excluded. Medial border is highly variable depending on breast size and amount of ptosis. Clinical reference needs to be taken into account and should not cross midline. The anterior border is the skin overlying the breast tissue. In the posterior border pectoralis muscles, chest-wall muscles, and ribs should be excluded [3, 4].

7.1.3 Dose Constraints

Despite there being very good evidence for a radiation dose-volume effect in many organs, there appears to be a paucity of published data on dose-volume effect of radiation on breast tissue (Table 7.1) [5].

Skin reactions and the constitutional symptom of fatigue dominate the early toxicity profile [6, 7]. Over 90% of women who receive radiation for breast cancer will develop some skin changes during their course of treatment. Acute side effects of treatment are generally common in occurrence, self-limiting, and resolve within 4–6 weeks after the treatment is completed.

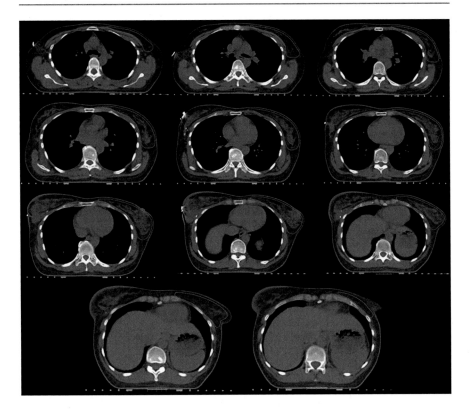

Fig. 7.1 Delineation of breast as normal structure

Table 7.1 Dose constraints

Organ	Emami			Quantec	SRS	SBRT	End point
	1/3	2/3	3/3				
Breast							
Skin	TD 5/5: 10 cm² (−) TD 50/5: 10 cm² (−)	TD 5/5: 30 cm² (−) TD 50/5: 30 cm² (−)	TD 5/5: 100 cm²: 50 Gy TD 50/5: 100 cm²: 65 Gy		23 Gy: <10 cc D_{max}: 26 Gy	30 Gy/3 fx (10 Gy/fx) D_{max}: 33 Gy (11 Gy/fx) 36.5 Gy/5 fx (7.3 Gy/fx) D_{max}: 39.5 Gy (7.9 Gy/fx)	Telangiectasia Ulceration

The risk of radiation dermatitis is influenced by many factors including total dose, dose per fraction, volume and surface area exposed to radiation, and the use of bolus material. Acute radiation toxicity is usually encountered with doses above 45 Gy. Total skin doses of ≥60 Gy are associated with moist desquamation that does not heal as well. For the treatment of breast cancer, 45–50.4 Gy with 1.8–2.0 Gy fractionations are commonly utilized for the whole breast irradiation (WBI). Cumulative doses of

60–66 Gy may be given to smaller boost volumes of the lumpectomy site or chest wall. With this standard dosing, breast radiation will result in 80–90% of patients developing some skin erythema and dry desquamation; in 30–50% of patients, the erythema is more severe and is associated with skin tenderness; in 5–10% of patients, patchy moist desquamation confined mostly to skin folds can be seen; and the confluent moist desquamation encountered in <5% of the patients [7, 8]. Among patients with early breast cancer undergoing adjuvant RT, evidence from literature data indicates that hypofractionated RT (40–42.5 Gy given in 3–4 weeks) is associated with a lower risk of acute toxic effects compared with conventionally fractionated RT [9].

The most common long-term sequelae of breast irradiation are fibrosis, which is encountered approximately 30% of the patients who underwent breast RT. Radiation-induced fibrosis typically presents 4–12 months after RT and progresses over several years. Late-radiation induced reactions include persistant breast edema, hyperpigmentation, chronic ulcerations and wounds, fibrosis, telangiectasias, and secondary skin cancers. Mukesh et al. reviewed the current literature and recorded dose-volume effects of breast irradiation [5]. The European Organization for Research and Treatment of Cancer (EORTC) "boost versus no boost" trial randomized 5318 patients with early breast cancer between boost (16 Gy) versus no boost treatment after WBI [10]. After 10 years of follow-up the incidence of moderate to severe fibrosis was 28.1% versus 13.2%, respectively ($p < 0.0001$). In this trial patients with microscopically incomplete tumor excision were also randomized to either a boost dose of 10 Gy or 26 Gy. The cumulative incidence of moderate to severe fibrosis for low-dose and high-dose schedules at 10 years was 24% and 54%, respectively. Yarnold et al. randomized 1410 patients with the diagnosis of breast cancer into one of three RT regimens after local tumor excision of early stage breast cancer; 50 Gy in 25 fractions vs. two dose levels of a test schedule giving 39 or 42.9 Gy in 13 fractions over 5 weeks [11]. Fraction sizes were 2.0, 3.0, and 3.3 Gy, respectively. The equivalent doses in 2 Gy fractions using an α/β ratio of 3.1 Gy for palpable breast induration were 46.7 Gy and 53.8 Gy for test arms 1 and 2, respectively. The risk of moderate to severe induration at 10 years for arms 1 and 2 was 27% and 51%, respectively.

The Hungarian PBI trial [12] and TARGIT trial [13] are two randomized trials supporting a strong qualitative indication on a volume-normal tissue complication relationship. They report superior cosmetic outcome and reduced normal tissue complication rate in the PBI arm when compared to the WBI. However, these are significant differences regarding the RT techniques and fractionation schedules between the two groups, therefore it is difficult to draw conclusions on the radiation volume effect on breast tissue. Accelerated partial breast irradiation (APBI) has also been implicated in post-radiation breast toxicity. The Christie group reported that patients treated with APBI had significantly higher rates of marked breast fibrosis (14% vs. 5%) and telangiectasia (33% vs. 12%) when compared to WBI group [14]. A dose–response relationship for late radiation effects including telangiectasia and breast fibrosis is well established and these dissimilar results can possibly be explained by calculating the 2 Gy equivalent dose (EQD2) for the PBI and WBI groups using an α/β ratio of 3.1 for fibrosis [11].

7.1.4 Pathophysiology

The most common acute side effects of breast irradiation are radiodermatitis, including irritation, pain, and itching, peeling, and moist desquamation. The moist desquamation is the most uncomfortable one, and may cause disruption of the treatment. Approximately 85% of patients who underwent breast irradiation treated with RT will experience a moderate-to-severe skin reaction. Acute radiation-induced skin reactions often lead to itching and pain, delays in treatment, and deteriorate aesthetic appearance and subsequently to a decrease in quality of life and are correlated with long-term cosmesis.

The exact pathophysiology of radiation-induced acute skin reactions of the breast tissue has not understood. The two main components of the skin are the outermost layers or epidermis and the deeper layers or dermis, each of which have unique structures and function and respond variably to radiation exposure. Acute radiation changes in the skin primarily reflect injury to the epidermis. Ionizing produces direct and indirect ionization events that leads to damage of cellular macromolecules, most importantly in the form of double-stranded DNA breaks. Through this DNA damaging mechanism, RT affects all cellular types within the epidermis and dermis and leads to the clinical syndrome of radiation dermatitis. Within the epidermis, radiation-induced DNA damage disrupts the normal proliferation and differentiation of basal keratinocytes. The destruction of a large proportion of basal keratinocytes results in the disruption of the self-renewing property of the epidermis. Repeated exposures do not allow time for basal skin cells to replenish in order to maintain optimal renewal of the epidermis [15].

The effects of ionizing radiation to dermis are probably more complex. Microvascular injury within the dermis also contributes to both the acute and chronic skin effects of radiation. Pro-inflammatory cytokines and chemokines, including interleukin (IL)-1, IL-6, IL-8, and tumor necrosis factor (TNF)-alpha, among others, have been demonstrated to play roles in immune cell activation, leukocyte transendothelial migration, and inflammatory edema. The immune response is exacerbated with the degranulation of mast cell and histamine release, which contribute the clinical radiation dermatitis syndrome. Radiation effects on dermal fibroblasts, mediated by transforming growth factor (TGF)-beta, are felt to be more important for late tissue fibrosis, rather than acute dermatitis [16].

Radiation-induced skin change usually occurs 10–14 days after initiation of RT and often will progressively worsen throughout the course of treatment. The first clinically apparent lesion is mild erythema (Fig. 7.2). Edema, dryness, burning, itching, tenderness, and hyperpigmentation can also be seen. Skin or nipple-areolar hyperpigmentation often occurs approximately 2–3 weeks after treatment initiation, particularly in patients with increased melanin content (Fig. 7.3). If there is any hair follicle in the radiation field, epilation is also being seen [15, 17]. As the dose increases desquamation, either dry or moist may be encountered. Dry desquamation usually seen at doses above 20 Gy and is characterized by peeling of dry, scaly skin and may not particularly add to patient symptomatology. However, moist desquamation is painful as a result of destruction and sloughing of dermal

Fig. 7.2 A breast cancer patient with mild grade 1 dermatitis

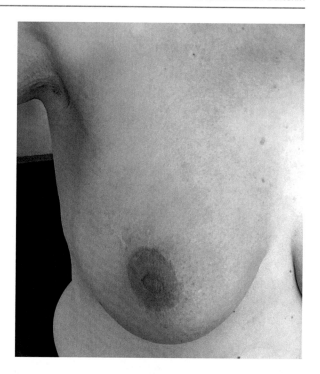

Fig. 7.3 A breast cancer patient with grade 2 dermatitis

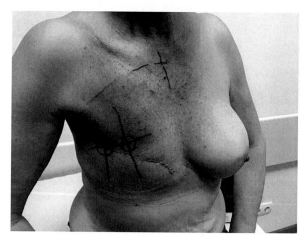

layer. Moreover, serous fluid drainage, or "weeping," may be seen. It is typically only experienced after cumulative doses of >30 Gy [18]. Moist desquamation usually initiates as small patches in skin folds and can progress to involve larger, confluent areas of irradiated skin. These symptoms are most pronounced in the axilla and inframammary fold and peak in intensity 1–2 weeks after the completion of the RT course. The acute dermatitis heals by the repopulation of epidermal keratinocytes and reversal of the immune response cascade. Re-epithelialization begins at approximately day 10 and competes with ongoing radiation damage to maintain homeostasis of the epidermal layer. Once radiation treatments are complete, the majority of symptoms usually resolve 2–4 weeks following the treatment. Hyperpigmentation may last for several months but does eventually resolve over time [18–21].

Breast edema is also an important acute side effect of breast RT. During the acute period after irradiation, inflammatory markers are induced and the expression of these proteins contributes to increased vascular permeability of breast tissue and it causes edema. Breast edema that manifests as skin and trabecular thickening appears generally in the first several weeks after completion of RT. Initially, there is engorgement of the dermal as well as of the intramammary lymphatics (trabecular thickening). This edema usually resolves over a period of weeks, months, or sometimes years [22].

Another complication of breast irradiation is fat necrosis. Some of the common causes of fat necrosis are RT, surgery, or trauma, particularly one associated with anticoagulation therapy. It is hypothesized that outpouring of blood into the parenchyma may result in swollen trabecular framework in the breast. This is usually associated with disruption of fat cells. This destruction may form intracellular vacuoles which are usually filled with necrotic material [23].

Radiation-induced fibrosis in breast tissue is one of the important late toxicities of breast RT. It can be the cause of aesthetic and functional problems, which give rise to a permanent scar. Skin thickening or fibrosis of the breast or chest wall is observed in about 1/3 of patients. However, moderate or severe fibrosis is found in less than 5% of patients. Clinically, this fibrosis involves a loss of suppleness of the skin, which shows an induration and feeling of firmness to the touch. The development of radiation-induced fibrosis is influenced by multiple factors, including RT dose and volume, fractionation schedule, previous or concurrent treatments, genetic susceptibility, and comorbidities. Although radiation-induced fibrosis originally was assumed to be a slow, irreversible process, contemporary studies suggest that it is not necessarily a fixed process as fibrosis or telangiectasia can appear months to years after the completion of RT (Fig. 7.4). Radiation-induced fibrosis of the breast is similar to inflammation, wound healing, and fibrosis of any origin. Typical histologic features include the presence of inflammatory infiltrates, particularly macrophages in the earlier stages of fibrosis, differentiation of fibroblasts into postmitotic fibrocytes, and changes in the vascular connective tissue with excessive production and deposition of extracellular matrix proteins and collagen [24, 25]. The pathophysiology of the radiation-induced fibrosis probably begins with the cytokine expression immediately after RT, and continues for months or years. Inflammatory mediators that have been implicated include TNF-alpha, IL-6, and IL-1. Fibrogenic cytokines that modulate the proliferation and differentiation of fibroblasts and the synthesis of extracellular matrix proteins and matrix metalloproteinases include TGF-β and platelet-derived growth factor (PDGF). Other growth factors, such as the connective tissue growth factor (CTGF), which is secreted by fibroblasts and endothelial cells, also promote fibrosis [26, 27].

Fig. 7.4 Telangiectasia developed after radiotherapy as late toxicity

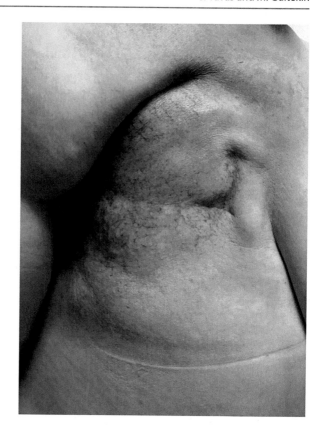

7.1.5 Treatment

For the prevention of radiation-related acute skin reaction, modern RT techniques including intensity-modulated RT (IMRT) and volumetric-modulated arc therapy (VMAT), advanced forms of RT that deliver radiation to the planned treatment volume while minimizing radiation to normal tissue outside the target, have been reported to reduce the occurrence of skin reactions [28]. Furthermore, hypofractionated RT has become increasingly popular for WBI. Shaitelman et al. demonstrated that rates of dermatitis, pruritus, hyperpigmentation, and pain are decreased with hypofractionated RT when compared to standard scheme [9].

The skin in the treatment field needs to be protected from irritation and friction during and for 2 to 4 weeks after RT. The patients should be advised to (i) maintain the RT field clean and dry, (ii) wash with lukewarm water and mild soap (synthetic soaps are preferable), (iii) use unscented, lanolin-free, water-based moisturizers two to three times per day, including non-treatment day on the weekend, (iv) to avoid skin irritants, such as perfumes and alcohol-based lotions, (v) wear loose-fitting clothes to avoid friction injuries, (vi) avoid corn starch or baby powder in skin folds, (vii) avoid sun exposure, (viii) avoid wet shaving within the treatment area; an electric razor is a safe alternative. It is important to instruct patients to gently clean and dry the skin in the RT field before each fraction [18, 29]. Randomized studies showed that patients who used soap and water had significant reductions in itching at the end of treatment and reduced erythema [30].

Patients are typically advised to avoid applying topical moisturizers, gels, emulsions, or dressings shortly before RT, as they can cause a bolus effect meaning that these agents increase the doses to the epidermis. Therefore the use of metallic-based formulations would increase the skin reaction when interacting with radiation, and furthermore, that the actual application could potentially create a bolus effect and increase skin dose. However, a randomized trial conducted in breast cancer patients, using aluminum-containing deodorants, nonaluminum-containing deodorants, or none, during conventionally fractionated RT did not find any significant difference among the three groups in the incidence or severity of radiation dermatitis [31].

Dry desquamation may be treated with hydrophilic (oil-in-water) moisturizers including dexpanthenol cream and aloe vera. Bepanthen®, or dexpanthenol cream, had been used extensively at the reporting institution for acute skin reactions. Patients applied the Bepanthen® cream twice daily beginning with the first day of treatment to half the field and none to the other half. Statistically significant reduction in desquamation with the use of the cream was observed. With further analysis, this effect on desquamation was mainly for "low-grade lesions." The authors concluded that there was no overall significant effect of the ointment [32]. Chamomile cream and almond ointment have also been studied in breast cancer patients in a similar fashion using the patient as her own control. Neither agent had a significant overall effect, but the almond ointment did reduce grade II toxicity [33].

The soft, absorbent, silicone foam bandages can be used for moist desquamation. This type of dressing is not traumatic to the wound and surrounding skin when removed. The bandage can be applied with or without topical agents. The dressing should be changed daily or more frequently, depending upon the severity of weeping. Macmillan et al. conducted a randomized controlled trial to evaluate the effect of a hydrogel or dry dressing on the time to healing of moist desquamation after RT to different body areas including the breast [34]. A total of 357 patients randomized before RT to receive simple dry dressings (Tricotex) or a hydrogel (Intrasite), with Tricotex as a secondary dressing. Patients were instructed to use their dressings from the onset of moist desquamation, if it occurred. The results of this study have not supported the routine use of hydrogels in the care of patients with moist desquamation and suggest that the healing times are prolonged, without any improvement in patient comfort.

Mid-potency topical corticosteroids may be useful to control itch or irritation. Evidence from several randomized trials and one meta-analysis indicates that the regular use of topical corticosteroids during the RT and for a few additional weeks after the completion of treatment may reduce the incidence of severe dermatitis (moist desquamation). Antihistamines are generally not effective in reducing pruritus related to radiation dermatitis [29, 30].

In a meta-analysis including 919 breast cancer patients it was shown that topical corticosteroids applied once or twice daily to the breast or chest wall from the first day of RT to up to 3 weeks after completion of RT reduced the risk of wet desquamation compared with placebo creams [35].

There is conflicting evidence with respect to use of aloe vera gel. In a randomized trial including breast cancer, more patients in the aloe vera gel group than in the aqueous cream group developed dry desquamation, dermatitis of grade 2 or higher, and greater pain [36]. A subsequent systematic review did not find evidence for efficacy of aloe vera in preventing or minimizing radiation dermatitis in cancer patients [37]. Furthermore in a randomized trial, it was found that the use of either an aloe cream or placebo cream during RT increased the incidence and severity of radiation dermatitis compared with a dry powder regimen [38]. The use of other agents and dressings including silver sulfadiazine (SSD), petroleum-based ointments, ascorbic acid, allantoin, almond oil, olive oil, dexpanthenol, calendula, barrier film, silver nylon dressings, and silicone-based film-forming gel dressing also evaluated; however, there is no evidence with respect to the efficacy of any of these topical agents in preventing or reducing the severity of radiation dermatitis.

Many agents are used to relive radiation-induced acute skin toxicity. Washing with mild soap and water and use of topical corticosteroids and silver nylon dressings have proved effective in managing the severity of radiation-induced dermatitis. Several other agents, including calendula, catechins, b-sitosterol, HA, EGF, GM-CSF, statins, and SSD, may potentially be useful in managing acute radiation dermatitis, as respective studies have demonstrated positive results. However, additional, confirmatory studies are needed before asserting their clinical efficacy. There is limited number of randomized trials evaluating the role of aloe vera, trolamine (triethanolamine), chamomile, ascorbic acid, pantothenic acid, sucralfate, or hyaluronic acid for the prevention of radiation dermatitis; however, most of the evidence does not support the use of them [39].

The treatment of radiation-induced late skin toxicity of the breast is conflicting. Pentoxifylline and vitamin E combinations up to >3 years may be effective for the treatment of radiation-induced fibrosis [40]. However, the optimal dose and duration of therapy and the role of tocopherol have not been determined. It is also unclear whether this therapy should be continued indefinitely to maintain benefit. Physical therapies including active and passive range of motion exercises may be advised. For the treatment of radiation-induced fibrosis there is limited evidence with respect to the use of hyperbaric oxygen. There are a few reports of successful treatment of RT-induced telangiectasias and hyperpigmentation with laser therapy [40, 41].

7.1.6 Rx: Prescription Samples

Radiation-induced acute dermatitis

- Bepanthen® (dexpanthenol cream): twice daily
- Mometasone furoate 0.1% or hydrocortisone 1% cream twice daily, after RT session.
- Silver sulfadiazine cream: SSD 1% cream three times a day, 3 days a week, for 5 weeks during RT and 1 week thereafter

7.2   Skin

7.2.1   Anatomy

The skin is the largest organ of the body covering the body's entire external surface, and accounts for approximately 15–20% of the total body weight in adults. It is composed of three layers from outermost level to inner level: (i) the epidermis, (ii) the dermis, (iii) subcutaneous tissue [42].

The superficial epidermis, which is the outermost part of the skin, is a stratified epithelium largely composed of keratinocytes that are formed by division of cells in the basal layer, and give rise to several distinguishable layers as they move outwards and progressively differentiate. Keratinocytes are specific constellation of cells that synthesize keratin, a long, threadlike protein with a protective role for the skin. In addition to keratinocytes there are also some other cell populations, including melanocytes, which donate pigment to the keratinocytes. The epidermis is a continually renewing layer and gives rise to derivative structures, such as pilo-sebaceous apparatuses, nails, and sweat glands. The eccrine sweat glands, also derived from epidermis and opening directly to the surface of the skin, present in every region of the body in densities of 100–600/cm^2. Total thickness of the epidermis is usually about 0.5–1 mm [42–44].

Between epidermis and the dermis there is a porous basement membrane zone that allows the exchange of cells and fluid and holds the two layers together. Basal keratinocytes are the most important components of structures of the dermal-epidermal junction; dermal fibroblasts are also involved in a lesser extent. The dermal-epidermal junction has many important roles including supporting the epidermis, establishing cell polarity and direction of growth. It directs the organization of the cytoskeleton in basal cells, provides developmental signals, and functions as a semipermeable barrier between layers [44].

The dermis is the middle layer and composed of the fibrillar structural protein known as collagen. The dermis is connected to the epidermis at the level of the basement membrane and consists of two layers of connective tissue, the papillary and reticular layers which merge together without clear demarcation. The upper layer, papillary layer, is thinner, composed of loose connective tissue and contacts epidermis. The reticular layer is the deeper layer and it is thicker, less cellular than papillary layer. The reticular layer is composed of dense connective tissue/bundles of collagen fibers. The dermis houses the sweat glands, hair, hair follicles, muscles, sensory neurons, and blood vessels. Although no vessels pass through the dermal-epidermal junction, the dermis has a very rich blood supply. The dermis has very important functions including protecting of the body from mechanical injury, aiding thermoregulation. In addition, the dermis includes receptors of sensory stimuli. The main component of the dermis is collagen which is an important structural protein for the entire body. Collagen is found in many structures including tendons, ligaments, the lining of bones, and the dermis. It is a major stress-resistant material of the skin. On the other hand, elastic fibers play an important role during maintaining elasticity; however, it has a relatively little capacity to resist deformation and tearing of the skin. Collagen represents 70% of the skin's dry weight [44].

Beneath the dermis there is a subcutaneous tissue, is also called as hypodermis, or panniculus, which contains small lobes of fat cells known as lipocytes. It is the deepest layer of skin and contains adipose lobules along with some skin append- ages like the hair follicles, sensory neurons, and blood vessels. According to the anatomical site of the body, the thickness of the panniculus varies considerably. Considered an endocrine organ, the subcutaneous tissue provides the body with buoyancy and functions as a storehouse of energy. In the panniculus there is also hormone conversion takes place, converting androstenedione into estrone by aro- matase. Lipocytes produce leptin, a hormone that regulates body weight by way of the hypothalamus [44].

The thickness of all three layers of the skin changes depending on body region, and geographical area, and categorized based on the thickness of the epidermal and dermal layers. The thinnest layer of the epidermis is located in the eyelids, measur- ing less than 0.1 mm. On the other hand, the palms and soles of the feet have the thickest epidermal layer, measuring approximately 1.5 mm. The dermis is thickest on the back, where it is 30–40 times as thick as the overlying epidermis [43, 44]. The three layers of the skin form an important barrier to the external environment, allow the transmission of sensory information, and serve a significant role in main- taining homeostasis. The dynamic epidermis continually produces a protective outer layer of corneocytes as cells undergo the process of keratinization and termi- nal differentiation. Collagen and elastic filaments of the dermal layer provide the underlying tensile strength of the skin, whereas the layer of subcutaneous fat pro- vides a store of energy for the body. The high rate of cell proliferation in the epider- mis and in epithelial tissue in general and the fact that this tissue is most frequently exposed to physical and chemical damage result in the exceedingly high rate of skin cancers found in humans as compared with other types of cancer [42, 43].

7.2.2 Contouring

There has been no available contouring atlas/guideline for skin yet.

7.2.3 Dose Constraints

Skin cells are relatively radiosensitive, since they originate from a rapidly repro- ducing differentiated stem cell. The basal keratinocytes, hair follicle stem cells, and melanocytes are highly radiosensitive to ionizing radiation. Radiation skin injury can be classified as acute or late injuries (Table 7.2). Acute injury occurs within hours to weeks after radiation exposure, whereas late injury presents months to years after radiation exposure. Acute skin toxicity is frequent during RT and can lead to temporary arrest of the treatment. Chronic toxicity can occur and conduct to cosmetic problems. Radiation-induced skin reactions depend on many treatment

Table 7.2 Scoring systems for acute radiation dermatitis [18, 45–47]

Classification scale	Scores	Clinical description
RTOG	0	No change
	1	Erythema; dry desquamation, epilation
	2	Bright erythema, moist desquamation, edema
	3	Confluent moist desquamation, pitting edema
	4	Ulceration, hemorrhage, necrosis
NCI CTCAE	0	No change
	1	Faint erythema or dry desquamation
	2	Moderate to brisk erythema; patchy, moist desquamation, mostly confined to skin folds and creases; moderate edema
	3	Moist desquamation in areas other than skin folds and creases; bleeding induced by minor trauma or abrasion
	4	Life-threatening consequences; skin necrosis or ulceration of full-thickness dermis; spontaneous bleeding from involved site; skin graft indicated
Radiation dermatitis severity	0.0	None
	0.5	Patchy or faint erythema; faint hyperpigmentation
	1.0	Faint, diffuse erythema; diffuse hyperpigmentation; mild epilation
	1.5	Definite erythema; extreme darkening/hyperpigmentation
	2.0	Definite erythema/hyperpigmentation with fine dry desquamation and mild edema
	2.5	Definite erythema/hyperpigmentation with branny/scaly desquamation
	3.0	Deep red erythema with diffuse dry desquamation; peeling in sheets
	3.5	Violaceous erythema with early moist desquamation; peeling in sheets; patchy crusting
	4.0	Violaceous erythema with diffuse moist desquamation; patchy crusting; ulceration; necrosis

and patient-related factors including total dose, fraction dose, use of bolus material, type of beam and energy, and under-nutrition, older age, obesity, smoking, skin diseases, autoimmune diseases, failure of DNA reparation. Acute reactions are primarily effected by dose per fraction and are increased when the dose per fraction increases. Chronic and acute toxicities are more often when total dose increases. Under 45 Gy, the risk of severe skin toxicity is low, and begins above 50 Gy [18, 48].

Radiation-induced acute skin reactions include erythema, dry desquamation, hyperpigmentation, and moist desquamation. Acute skin reactions are a reflection of inflammatory response to ionizing radiation, and there is a dose-dependent loss of cells from the epidermis, dermis, and microvascular endothelium. When the doses are above the tolerance limits, a devastating side effect of ionizing radiation, necrosis, may be encountered. Acute changes include erythema and pain and occur within 90 days. Even with modern RT techniques, approximately 85% of patients will experience a moderate to severe acute skin reaction in exposed areas. It has been demonstrated that the fields treated with a conventional 2 Gy daily fractionation do not cause any changes in the basal cell density until total doses of 20–25 Gy are delivered. Higher radiation doses cause a significant reduction in the number of mitotic cells and an increase in degenerate cells [18, 48, 49]. If the total RT dose to the skin does not exceed 30 Gy, the erythema phase is followed during the 4th or 5th week by a dry desquamation phase, characterized by pruritus, scaling, and an increase in melanin pigmentation in the basal layer. If the total radiation dose to the skin is ≥50 Gy the erythema phase is followed by a moist desquamation phase. This stage usually begins in the 4th week and is often accompanied by considerable discomfort [50].

For the radiation-induced late skin reactions two different end points were chosen as necrosis and telangiectasia. The recommended tolerance doses of the skin necrosis are as follows: for a 100 cm^2 field, the TD 3/5 was 51 Gy, TD 5/5 was 55 Gy, and TD 50/5 was 70 Gy. For a 30 cm^2 field, the TD 3/5 was 57 Gy. For a 10 cm^2 field, the TD 3/5 was 69 Gy. For the endpoint of telangiectasia with an area of approximately 100 cm^2, the TD 10/5 was 50 Gy, TD 30/5 was 59 Gy, and the TD 50/5 was 65 Gy [51, 52]. According to the stereotactic body RT (SBRT) dose recommendations of the American Association of Physicists in Medicine (AAPM) report 101, 23 Gy should be received <10 cc of the skin; and D_{max} should be <26 Gy for a single fraction stereotactic radiosurgery (SRS). For the fractionated SBRT, D_{max} point dose is suggested as 33 Gy (11 Gy/fraction), and threshold dose should be 30 Gy (10 Gy/fraction) [53].

7.2.4 Pathophysiology

The exact pathophysiology of radiation-induced acute skin reactions has not been fully understood; however, the underlying mechanisms of the radiation-induced skin reactions are inflammatory response and oxidative stress. The two main components of the skin are the outermost layers or epidermis and the deeper layers or dermis, each of which have unique structures and function and respond variably to radiation exposure. Acute radiation changes in the skin primarily reflect injury to the epidermis. Basal keratinocytes, stem cells in the hair follicles, and melanocytes are highly radiosensitive. Ionizing radiation produces direct and indirect effects that lead to damage of cellular macromolecules, most importantly in the form of double-stranded DNA breaks. Through this DNA damaging mechanism, RT affects all cellular types within the epidermis and dermis and leads to the clinical syndrome of radiation dermatitis. The destruction of a large proportion of basal keratinocytes results in the disruption of the self-renewing property of the epidermis. Ionizing radiation causes an acute reaction that causes changes in skin pigmentation through the migration of melanosomes, interrupted hair growth, and damage to the deeper dermis, while sparing the upper epidermal layer.

Damage to the dermis disrupts the normal process of skin cell repopulation, initially resulting in erythema due to dermal vessel dilation and histamine-like substance release (Fig. 7.5) [49, 54–56]. Repeated exposures do not allow time for basal skin cells to replenish in order to maintain optimal renewal of the epidermis.

Fig. 7.5 A patient with grade 2 radiation dermatitis

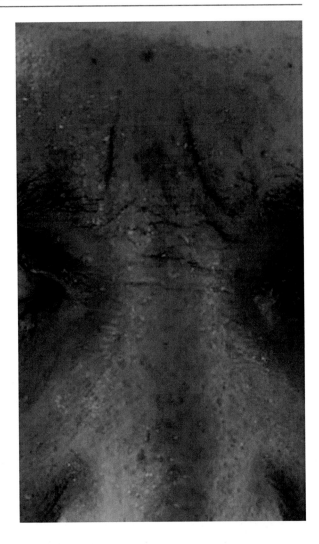

Ionizing radiation incites signaling between the epidermis and dermis through resident skin cells. The hallmark of radiation-induced skin injury is the transendothelial migration of leukocytes and other immune cells from circulation to irradiated skin. The resident and circulating immune cells in the skin are stimulated by keratinocytes, Langerhans cells, and fibroblasts. Numerous cytokines and chemokines are produced in response to these activation signals, which act on the endothelial cells of local vessels, causing the up-regulation of adhesion molecules including intercellular adhesion molecule-1 (ICAM1), vascular cell adhesion molecule-1 (VCAM1). These factors can create a local inflammatory response of eosinophils and neutrophils leading to self-perpetuating tissue damage and loss of protective barriers [49, 55]. At higher doses of RT, greater damage occurs and the skin attempts to compensate by increasing its rate of mitosis in the basal keratinocyte cell layer. However, as

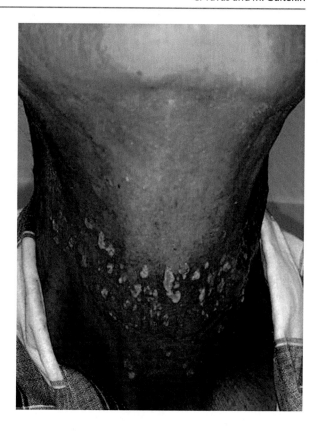

the turnover of novel cells is faster than the shedding of the old cells, this leads to thickened, scaly skin (dry desquamation). At even higher RT doses, the basal layer is unable to recover and an exudate is released; this is referred to as moist desquamation (Fig. 7.6). These varying degrees of damage compromise the integrity of the physical barrier produced by the skin and its immune function, resulting in increased risk of infection [55]. Damage to the vascular endothelium induces hypoxia and upregulates transforming growth factor (TGF)-β, which is a cytokine that plays a central role in mediating radiation-induced fibrosis. Fibrosis and tissue hypoxia resulting from vascular damage result in the generation of reactive oxygen species (ROS) [55, 57].

The acute phase of the skin reactions usually occurs within 90 days. A transient early erythema can be seen within a few hours after RT exposure and subsides after 24–48 h. Due to an inflammatory response, temporary erythema and histamine-like substances that cause dermal edema and skin erythema are released because of the increases permeability and dilation of capillaries. Generalized erythema, sometimes undetectable without special instrumentation, may occur hours after radiation exposure, and fade within hours to days. A second phase of more sustained erythema is apparent 10–14 days after dosing, and is characterized by a blanchable reactive pink hue, without other epidermal changes, most likely mediated by cytokines. The main erythematous reaction occurs 3–6 weeks after the RT begins and reflects a varying severity of loss of epidermal basal cells. Acute radiation skin toxicity has been correlated with increased formation of various cytokines and chemokines as discussed above [54].

The development of radiation-induced fibrosis is also mediated by inflammation, which begins immediately after RT and continues for months to years. Available data suggest that chronic radiation dermatitis is caused by imbalance of pro-inflammatory and pro-fibrotic cytokines, which starts after irradiation and lasts for months or even many years. These include tumor necrosis factor-alpha (TNF-α), interleukins 6 and 1 (IL-6 and IL-1), TGF-β, platelet-derived growth factor (PDGF), and connective tissue growth factor [49]. TNF-a, IL-6, and IL-1 are involved in the inflammatory response, while TGF-β and PDGF regulate fibroblast activity and promote the production of extracellular matrix proteins. Fibroblasts are the key cells in the development of late radiation-induced fibrotic changes. Permanently atypical fibroblasts can cause skin atrophy, contraction, and fibrosis. The TGF-β is a regulatory protein that controls wound healing, proliferation, and differentiation of multiple cell types and synthesis of extracellular matrix proteins in the normal tissue inflammatory response. Its main function on connective tissues in vivo is to promote growth. The proliferation of endothelial cell is also stimulated, but the growth of epithelial cell is inhibited [49, 58–60].

Radiation-induced alterations of the vascular system, particularly damage to endothelial cells, appear to contribute significantly to late toxicity. The concomitant radiation-induced endothelium damage results in improper vascularization of irradiated skin and restricts blood perfusion. It may exacerbate the fibrosis and deteriorate healing process. This phenomenon, together with secretion of PDGF, can also play a role in pathogenesis of telangiectasia. Moreover, persistent inflammation and secretion of pro-inflammatory cytokines lead to leukocyte infiltration, which may cause other manifestations of chronic radiation dermatitis, such as skin atrophy or necrosis [61–63].

7.2.5 Treatment

Before discussing the treatment methods of radiation-related skin reactions, the preventive strategies should be overviewed. Firstly, the modern RT techniques including intensity-modulated radiation therapy (IMRT) and volumetric-modulated arc radiation therapy (VMAT), advanced forms of RT that deliver radiation to the planned treatment volume while minimizing radiation to normal tissue outside the target, have been reported to reduce the occurrence of skin reactions [28]. The use of proper RT techniques helps to avoid unnecessary irradiation of healthy skin. Secondly the skin in the treatment area needs to be protected from irritation and friction during the treatment, and for 2–4 weeks after the radiation treatment has finished [29]. Thirdly, the patients should be advised to (i) maintain the irradiated area clean and dry, (ii) wash with lukewarm water and mild soap (synthetic soaps are preferable), (iii) use unscented, lanolin-free, water-based moisturizers two to three times per day, including non-treatment day on the weekend, (iv) to avoid skin irritants, such as perfumes and alcohol-based lotions, (v) wear loose-fitting clothes to avoid friction injuries, (vi) avoid corn starch or baby powder in skin folds, (vii) avoid sun exposure, (viii) avoid wet shaving within the treatment area; an electric razor is a safe alternative. It is important to instruct patients to gently clean and dry the skin in the radiation field before each irradiation session [18, 29].

From the clinical perspective, the reduction in the incidence of chronic radiation-induced skin reactions is expected especially for soft tissue sarcomas and breast or head and neck cancer patients due to the high dose received by skin and predictable long survival. The most important prevention method of chronic radiation dermatitis is, as in the case of acute reactions, the use of proper RT techniques to avoid unnecessary irradiation of healthy skin. It was shown that the application of IMRT leads to the reduction of late radiation complications, for example, breast induration and telangiectasia. IMRT allowed reducing acute wound healing complication rates in patients with lower extremity sarcomas. However, the results may vary depending on treatment site and localization of target volumes, thus preparing a few treatment plans in different techniques and comparing them is recommended [61, 64, 65].

Another approach for skin sparing may be the avoidance of putting bolus when there is no necessity to ensure the full dose to targets near or at the skin. The trends in modern RT allow using altered fractionation schedules, such as hypofractionation. It was shown that late skin reactions are related to the dose per fraction. Larger daily doses received by skin may increase the risk of chronic radiation dermatitis, so it is important to apply skin-sparing techniques of irradiation, but only when it is possible to obtain satisfactory dose coverage of target volumes [9].

Historically, there was a concern with respect to washing with soap and water could cause mechanical trauma and worsen of radiation dermatitis resulted in recommendations against washing in the radiation treatment fields. Three trials challenge this practice and compared washing versus no washing during RT [66–68]. There were less patients with a maximum toxicity grade of ≥ 2 in one trial [66] (36% versus no washing 56%, $p = 0.04$) when washing was permitted, and the other trials reported a trend in favor of washing [67, 68]. Given the important psychosocial benefit of allowing patients to maintain their normal hygienic routine, the practice of allowing washing with water and mild soap is generally accepted as standard clinical practice. The patients should be advised to follow gentle washing practices with a mild shampoo [69].

The irradiated skin should be dry and clean. There are many trials comparing the use of antiperspirant versus no antiperspirant during RT [69]. Given the physical properties of RT, there was a concern of bolus effect on the skin and enhanced acute toxicities from antiperspirants, especially metallic-based preparations. The use of deodorants, and in particular metallic deodorants, during RT has been debated due to concerns that the deposition of aluminum salts may influence the superficial radiation dose or cause a bolus effect. Several authors challenged this belief and examined non-metallic-based antiperspirant. The trial by Théberge et al. was the only study that used a non-inferiority design [70]. Watson et al. examined the use of aluminum-based antiperspirant [71]. There was no evidence to suggest that the use of antiperspirants resulted in increased toxicities. Using unscented, lanolin-free, water-based moisturizers two to three times per day, including non-treatment day on the weekend is recommended [69].

Patients are typically advised to avoid applying topical moisturizers, gels, emulsions, or dressings shortly before RT, as they can cause a bolus effect by increasing the radiation dose delivered to the epidermis [72].

Topical steroids may be used for the prevention of severe radiation dermatitis and the reduction of discomfort and itching [69]. There are many studies comparing the topical steroids with placebo, emollients, or dexpanthenol (a pro-vitamin B5 preparation). Shukla et al. investigated the role of topical steroid (beclomethasone dipropionate spray) used as prophylaxis with the purpose of reducing risk of the wet desquamation of skin in irradiated field [73]. Their results demonstrated that the use of topical steroid (beclomethasone dipropionate spray) for skin during radiotherapy significantly reduces the risk of wet desquamation of the skin. Miller et al. reported significant reduction in the mean grade of discomfort or burning (1.5 versus 2.1; $p = 0.02$) and itching (1.5 versus 2.2; $p = 0.002$) [74]. A meta-analysis including 10 randomized trials (919 participants with breast cancer) found that topical corticosteroids applied once or twice daily to the breast or chest wall from the first day of RT to up to 3 weeks after completion of RT reduced the risk of wet desquamation compared with placebo creams [75]. Evidence from several randomized trials and one meta-analysis indicates that the regular use of topical corticosteroids during the RT and for a few additional weeks after the completion of treatment may reduce the incidence of severe dermatitis (moist desquamation) [69, 73, 74]. Low- to medium-potency topical corticosteroids including mometasone furoate 0.1% or hydrocortisone 1% cream can be applied to the treatment field once or twice daily, after each RT session.

There is limited evidence regarding the use of aloe vera, trolamine (triethanolamine), sucralfate, silver sulfadiazine (SSD), petroleum-based ointments, ascorbic acid, allantoin, almond oil, olive oil, dexpanthenol, calendula, barrier film, silver nylon dressings, and silicone-based film-forming gel dressing or hyaluronic acid for the prevention of radiation dermatitis. The use of prophylactic trolamine was investigated in a randomized trial conducted on patients with advanced squamous cell carcinoma of the head and neck [76]. The patients were assigned to three groups as prophylactic trolamine group, interventional trolamine group, and institutional preference product group. Grade ≥ 2 dermatitis was reported in 79, 77, and 79 percent of the three groups, respectively. In another study, Wells et al. investigated whether sucralfate or aqueous cream reduced acute skin toxicity during radiotherapy when compared with no treatment to the head and neck, breast or anorectal area. After 5 weeks, the severity of erythema, desquamation, itch, pain, and discomfort, as reported by patients, was similar in the three groups [77]. Moreover a randomized trial Hemati et al. evaluated the effectiveness of topical silver sulfadiazine (SSD) in preventing acute radiation dermatitis in women receiving RT for breast cancer. The intervention group received SSD cream 1%, three times a day, 3 days a week, for 5 weeks during RT and one week thereafter [78]. Their results demonstrated that patients in the SSD group experienced a less severe dermatitis than patients in the control group. Due to the conflicting results of the limited literature data, the use of aloe vera, trolamine (triethanolamine), sucralfate, SSD, petroleum-based ointments, ascorbic acid, allantoin, almond oil, olive oil, dexpanthenol, calendula, barrier film, silver nylon dressings, and silicone-based film-forming gel dressing or hyaluronic acid for the prevention of radiation dermatitis is not recommended.

Radiation-induced early skin reactions including erythema and dry desquamation are best treated symptomatically. The affected area is washed gently with plain water alone or combined with a mild, low pH cleansing agent that does not exacerbate the existing dermatitis. Washing may also reduce the bacterial load and thereby reduce potential superantigen-induced inflammation. Patients should wear well-fitting, nonbinding clothing and avoid unnecessary topical irritants and friction. The severity of radiation dermatitis varies between people and radiation doses in the following grades: (i) grade 1, faint redness and skin peeling, (ii) grade 2, moderate redness and swelling, skin thinning in the skin folds, (iii) grade 3, skin thinning more than 1.5 cm across, not just on the skin folds, plus severe swelling, and (iv) grade 4, death of skin cells and deep skin ulcers (Table 7.2) [18, 45, 46].

Patients with grade 1 acute dermatitis with faint erythema and dry desquamation usually do not require any therapeutic intervention. General skin care should be advised. For the dry desquamation hydrophilic (oil-in-water) moisturizers may be used. Mid-potency topical corticosteroids such as clocortolone pivalate cream or fluocinolone acetonide ointment may be useful to control itch or irritation. Antihistamines are generally not effective in reducing pruritus related to radiation dermatitis [61, 69].

The use of special dressings does not seem to be effective in patients with grade 1 dermatitis; however, there is insufficient evidence against them. Special dressings including hydrocolloid dressing, gentian violet have been investigated in different studies [79–82]. Mak et al. [80] and Macmillan et al. [81] observed a detrimental effect for hydrogel although only the later was statistically significant, while Gollins et al. [81] showed a significant benefit. The methodological limitations of these trials result in the role of hydrocolloid dressings for established radiation-induced moist desquamation remaining unclear.

Patients with grade 2 and 3 dermatitis present with moist desquamation involving the skin folds or other skin areas. Treatment involves measures aimed at preventing secondary skin infection and the use of dressings over the areas of skin sloughing [69]. If infection occurs, standard therapy for bacterial infections should be initiated with topical and/or systemic antibiotics. The specialized dressings for moist desquamation, bleeding, exudates, or drainage should be considered. The use of dressings in the management of moist desquamation is based upon the observation that a moist environment promotes the rate of re-epithelialization and increases the speed of wound healing. There are many types of dressings; however, there is little evidence to aid in the choice among the various types of dressings. Silicone foam bandages with/without topical agents may be used. This type of dressing is atraumatic to the wound and surrounding skin when removed. The dressing should be changed daily or more frequently, depending upon the severity of weeping. Non-adherent, hydrogel, or hydrocolloid dressings also seem to be reasonable. A few randomized trials have compared different dressings or dressings versus other topical agents with inconclusive results [69, 81, 82]. Grade 3 radiodermatitis with moist desquamation may require interruption of RT, depending upon the body location and the patient's discomfort.

Grade 4 dermatitis is rarely encountered. Patients presenting with full-thickness skin necrosis and ulceration should be treated on a case-by-case basis. They may require discontinuation of RT. Treatment may include surgical debridement, full-thickness skin graft, or myocutaneous or pedicle flaps. For infected or at-risk wounds, systemic or topical antibacterial agents should be considered [83].

Available literature data on the management of chronic radiation dermatitis are unsatisfactory. Most of the interventions are based only on clinical practice and extrapolation of management used in similar conditions. In a phase II trial Delanian et al. investigated a combination of pentoxifylline (800 mg/day) and vitamin E (1000 IU/day) for at least 6 months was administered orally to subjects who displayed late fibrosis (0.5–30 years post-treatment) [84]. Treatment was well tolerated. All assessable injuries exhibited continuous clinical regression and functional improvement. There are some small, randomized trials suggest that prolonged treatment with pentoxifylline in combination with vitamin E for up to >3 years may be helpful for the treatment of subcutaneous radiation-induced fibrosis [69, 85]. These data suggest that the combination of pentoxifylline plus tocopherol can reverse superficial radiation-induced fibrosis in some patients; however, the optimal dose and duration of therapy and the role of tocopherol are unknown. In patients with radiation fibrosis adequate analgesic medication is important as well, since radiation-induced fibrosis can be painful.

Hyperbaric oxygen has been evaluated as a treatment for radiation-induced fibrosis; however, there is currently insufficient evidence to show efficacy [86]. There are a few reports of successful treatment of radiation therapy-induced telangiectasias and hyperpigmentation with laser therapy [87, 88].

7.2.6   Rx: Sample Prescriptions

Radiation-induced acute dermatitis prevention:

- Bepanthen® (dexpanthenol cream): twice daily
- Mometasone furoate 0.1% or hydrocortisone 1% cream twice daily, after RT session.
- Silver sulfadiazine cream (SSD) 1% cream three times a day, 3 days a week, for 5 weeks during RT and 1 week thereafter

Radiation-induced acute dermatitis treatment:

- Hydrophilic (oil-in-water) moisturizers: Hydrolipid cream (e.g., XClair®) (gently apply a thin layer of product using clean hands 2–4 times daily to the skin in the treatment area)
- Cloderm® Clocortolone pivalate cream
- Synalar® Fluocinolone acetonide ointment
- Cordran® Flurandrenolide ointment
- Westcort® Hydrocortisone valerate ointment

Radiation-induced fibrosis

- Pentoxifylline (800 mg/day) and vitamin E (1000 IU/day) for at least 6 months
- NSAID (non-steroidal anti-inflammatory drugs)

7.3 Bones

7.3.1 Anatomy

There are total 206 bones (excluding sesamoid bones) in the adult human skeleton. It can be classified into two divisions: (i) axial skeleton and (ii) appendicular skeleton [89].

Axial skeleton consists of 80 bones and forms the axis of human body, and consists of skull, vertebral column, and thoracic cage. The skull is formed by 22 bones. Additionally, seven bones including the hyoid bone and the ear ossicles, three small bones found in each middle ear, are located in the head skeleton. The vertebral column composed of 24 bones, each called a vertebra, in addition to the sacrum and coccyx. The 12 pairs of ribs, and the sternum, the flattened bone of the anterior chest are located in the thoracic cage.

In an adult there are 126 bones in the appendicular skeleton. It includes all bones of the upper and lower limbs, in addition the bones that attach each limb to the axial skeleton. The bones of the appendicular skeleton are covered in later section on bones of the upper extremities and the lower extremities.

There are four types of bones: (i) long bones, (ii) short bones, (iii) flat bones, and (iv) irregular bones. The clavicles, humerus, radius, ulnae, metacarpals, femurs, tibiae, fibulae, metatarsals, and phalanges are the long bones in the body. Short bones include the sesamoid bones, patellae, and carpal and tarsal bones. The skull, mandible, scapulae, sternum, and ribs are the flat bones. Irregular bones include the vertebrae, sacrum, coccyx, and hyoid bone.

The long bones are formed by combination of endochondral and membranous bone formation. On the other hand, the flat bones form by membranous bone formation. The long bones include a hollow shaft, or diaphysis; flared, cone-shaped metaphyses below the growth plates; and rounded epiphyses above the growth plates. A dense cortical bone is the primary structure of the diaphysis. The epiphysis and diaphysis include a trabecular meshwork bone surrounded by a relatively thin shell of dense cortical bone. In the adult human being the skeleton is composed of 80% cortical bone and 20% trabecular bone. Different bones and skeletal sites within bones have different ratios of cortical to trabecular bone. The cortical to trabecular bone ratio for vertebra is 25:75, and for femoral head it is 50:50.

Cortical bone is dense and solid and surrounds the marrow space. The trabecular bone composed of a honeycomb like network of trabecular plates and rods interspersed in the bone marrow compartment. Cortical bone has two surfaces: an outer periosteal surface and inner endosteal surface. Periosteal surface activity is very crucial for appositional growth and fracture repair. Bones increase in diameter with aging due to exceeding bone formation to bone resorption on the periosteal surface. On the other hand, with aging, bone resorption typically exceeds bone formation on the endosteal surface, so the marrow space normally expands. Cortical bone and trabecular bone are normally formed in a lamellar pattern, in which collagen fibrils are laid down in alternating orientations [89, 90].

7.3.2   Contouring

There has been no available contouring atlas/guideline for all parts of the bony structures yet; however, some special parts of the bony structures that have an importance during irradiation of different site of the tumors have been defined. Femoral head is important during the irradiation of the pelvic tumors. For the delineation of femoral head, the ball of the femur, trochanters, and proximal shaft to the level of the bottom of ischial tuberosities should be included (Fig. 7.7) [91].

7.3.3   Dose Constraints

Emami et al. proposed dose constraints for humoral and femoral head, mandible and temporomandibular joint (TMJ), and rib cage [51]. For the femoral head the selected end points were necrosis and femoral neck fracture. The incidence of femoral necrosis and femoral neck fracture has been encountered with different doses ranging from 20 Gy to 70 Gy. The estimated TD 5/5 and TD 50/5 are 52 Gy and 65 Gy, respectively (Table 7.3). According to the stereotactic body RT (SBRT) dose recommendations of the American Association of Physicists in Medicine (AAPM) report 101, 14 Gy should be received <10 cc of the head of the femur for a single fraction stereotactic radiosurgery (SRS). For the fractionated SBRT, threshold doses for the 3 fraction and 5 fraction schedules are suggested as 28.8 Gy (9.6 Gy/fraction) and 30 Gy (6 Gy/fraction), respectively [53].

For the mandible and TMJ, the selected endpoint is osteoradionecrosis. It may be affected by several factors including the tumor location, dental status, RT technique, and total treatment dose [51, 53, 92–94]. There is imprecise data with respect to TMJ toxicity and it was thought that necrosis was a more viable endpoint for determining a TD 5/5 and TD 50/5. TD 5/5 for 1/3, 2/3, and 3/3 of the mandible are

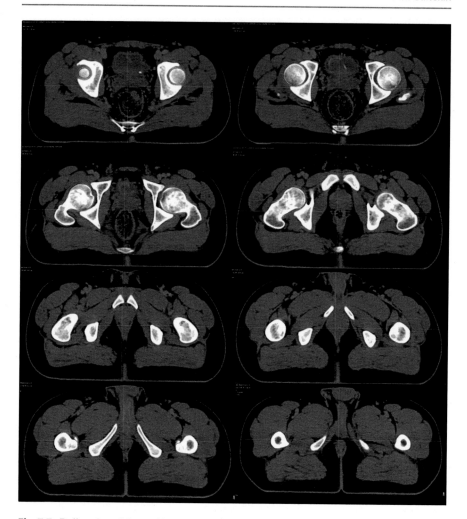

Fig. 7.7 Delineation of femoral heads as normal structures

defined as 65 Gy, 60 Gy, and 60 Gy, respectively. TD 50/5 can be projected as approximately 77 Gy for a small (1/3) volume with 72 Gy for the 2/3 and full volume [51]. The risk of fracture in upper femora is estimated as 5% with 45–50 doses using conventional fractionation. Osteonecrosis is rarely encountered with <60 Gy doses [95].

The endpoint chosen for the rib cage is pathologic fracture. Recommendations by Emami et al. for the 1/3 of the rib cage are 50 Gy, and 65 Gy for TD 5/5, and TD 50/5, respectively. Moreover, their recommendations for TD 2/5 were 48 Gy, TD 8/5 was 58 Gy, and TD 20/5 was 65 Gy [51]. Many factors including dental hygiene and volume of the mandible that is irradiated have an important role with respect to the induction of osteonecrosis of the mandible. Cooper et al. demonstrated that with doses <65 Gy, there is no increased risk of osteonecrosis;

Table 7.3 Dose constraints

Organ	Emami			Quantec	SRS	SBRT	End point
	1/3	2/3	3/3				
Bones							
Femoral head	(−) (−)	(−) (−)	TD 5/5: 52 Gy TD 50/5: 65 Gy	45–50 Gy: 5% (fracture risk)	14 Gy <10 cc	21.9 Gy/3 fx (7.3 Gy/fx) 30 Gy/5 fx (6 Gy/fx)	Necrosis and fracture
Rib	TD 5/5: 50 Gy TD 50/5: 65 Gy	(−) (−)	(−) (−)		22 Gy <1 cc		Pain or fracture
Temporomandibular joint mandible	TD 5/5: 65 Gy TD 50/5: 77 Gy	TD 5/5: 60 Gy TD 50/5: 72 Gy	TD 5/5: 60 Gy TD 50/5: 72 Gy		D_{max}: 30 Gy	28.8 Gy/3 fx (9.6 Gy/fx) 35 Gy/5 fx (7 Gy/fx)	

however, doses ≥75 Gy the risk is about 80% [96]. The risk of trismus has been reported as 5–38% using therapeutic dose levels [97].

7.3.4   Pathophysiology

The most commonly encountered radiation-induced bone toxicities are: (i) radiation-induced bone fractions including pelvic and femoral insufficiency fractures, radiation-induced rib fracture, vertebral fractures, (ii) radiation-induced osteonecrosis including mandibular osteoradionecrosis and osteoradionecrosis of the femoral head, and (iii) radiation-induced growth abnormalities in pediatric patients.

7.3.4.1 Radiation-Induced Bone Fractures

Radiation-induced bone injury has become increasingly rare complication of the RT with the use of megavoltage radiation and improved planning and radiation delivery techniques. The skeletal tissue is known as a relatively radioresistant tissue [98].

There has been limited data regarding the impact of focal RT on normal bone tissue. There are many factors contributing the radiation-induced bone toxicity including chemotherapy use, steroid use, reduced mobility, and even direct tumor infiltration of the bone [98–101]. The α/β ratio of the bone is suggested as 1.8–2.8 Gy, implying that the bone is a relatively slow or late responding tissue with the capacity for sublethal DNA damage repair [102].

Evidence from literature data illustrates that the bone is actually an acute responding tissue to ionizing radiation [98, 102]. Within the days after RT exposure, acute reactive changes including decreased osteoblast numbers, diminished collagen production, and increased osteoclast activity have been determined. An increased risk of local fracture has been encountered with RT to the pelvis, vertebrae, and ribs in cancer patients. Acute cortical bone loss has been shown in the ribcage within 4 months of thoracic SBRT [103–105].

The multipotent mesenchymal and hematopoietic stem cells are progenitors for cells that lead to bone formation and resorption. Depletion of one population of these osteoprogenitor cells can disrupt the other in different ways including altered cell signaling or damaged vascularity within the marrow [98, 106, 107]. Osteoclasts are derived from hematopoietic lineage precursors [106], and the osteoblast/osteocyte is derived from mesenchymal origin [108]. Recent studies examining the effects of irradiation on the bone have mainly focused on the osteogenic potential and colony-forming ability of multipotent mesenchymal cells after RT exposure [98, 107]. It has been observed that the number of osteoblast is diminished in the irradiated bone because of reactive oxygen species mediated DNA damage that leads to apoptosis. Moreover, in the irradiated volume of the bone an increase in adiposity could indicate a preferential shift of multipotent mesenchymal cells toward adipocytes at the expense of osteoblasts [107, 109]. Radiation-induced osteoblast injury impairs matrix production and lowers bone mineral density which eventually increases bone fragility. The prolonged and/or transient reduction in bone formation via effects on multipotent mesenchymal cells and osteoblasts can serve to decline new bone formation and compromise the microstructure and mechanical properties of the bone [98, 106, 107, 109].

The damage to ionizing radiation to hematopoietic stem cells lineage precursors, which produce osteoclast, is well-documented. It is also well known that the number of the osteoclasts decrease after the exposure to RT. Due to this reduced turnover, decreased bone formation and resorption shrinking of the bone may be seen. Disproportional activation promotes excessive resorption, lowers bone mass, and diminishes bone quality and strength. Substantial bone loss occurring as an early response due to elevated osteoclast activity, coupled with prolonged periods of reduced turnover and subsequent embrittlement of the bone, could contribute to the etiology of radiation-induced insufficiency fractures, as are detailed below in multiple skeletal locations [98, 110–112].

The radiation tolerance of the femoral head and neck is substantially lower than the radiation tolerance of long bones. The femoral neck fraction is increasingly rare as routine pelvic fields include blocking of the femoral neck and most of the femoral heads. If the inguinal nodes must be treated, the femoral head and neck will unavoidably receive a substantial radiation dose, and care must be taken not to exceed the radiation tolerance of these structures. The pathophysiology of the femoral neck fraction is same with other bone fractions, due to the microvasculature alterations of the mature bone, which causes decreased blood supply to the periosteum which compromises osteoblastic function and can result in an insufficiency fracture. Insufficiency fractures of bone occur as a result of physiological stress on bones with deficient elastic resistance.

7.3.4.2 Radiation-Induced Osteoradionecrosis

Osteoradionecrosis is a complication of RT due to vascular obliteration and decreased vascular supply of the irradiated tissues. There are many different proposed mechanisms of osteoradionecrosis development. The most widely accepted pathophysiologies for the development of osteoradionecrosis are as follows:

According to Marx, osteoradionecrosis should be considered as a non-healing wound of the bone due to metabolic and tissue homeostatic disturbances. It is the result of hypoxic, hypovascular, and hypocellular tissue, followed by tissue breakdown that causes to a non-healing wound. There is no interstitial infection, only superficial contamination [113].

According to Bras et al., the major factor for leading ischemic necrosis of the mandible is radiation-induced obliteration of the inferior alveolar artery [114].

Several authors proposed that, the initial event in the development of osteoradionecrosis is damage to osteoclasts as a result of radiation which occurs earlier compared with vascular alterations. This theory is supported by the similar disease process of medication-related osteonecrosis of the jaw [108].

Delanian et al. proposed that osteoradionecrosis occurs due to a radiation-induced fibroatrophic mechanism, including free radical formation, endothelial dysfunction, inflammation, microvascular thrombosis, fibrosis and remodeling, and finally bone and tissue necrosis [115].

Lastly Store et al. demonstrated that bacteria may play a fundamental role in the pathogenesis of osteoradionecrosis, stating that teeth present in the field of irradiation might represent the port of entry for microorganisms [115].

Recent evidence in cellular and molecular biology more accurately evaluate the progression of microscopically observed osteoradionecrosis and support the radiation-induced fibrosis theory. Combining all the above theories, it can be concluded that three phases have been observed during the development of osteoradionecrosis [116]:

- The pre-fibrotic phase: The endothelial cells are mainly observed, with an accompanying acute inflammatory response.
- The constitutive organized phase: There is an abnormal fibroblastic activity, and the extracellular matrix loses organization.
- The late fibroatrophic phase: In order to attempt to remodel the tissue with formation of fragile healed tissues that are at an increased risk of reactivated inflammation when the tissue sustains local injury, this could possibly lead to tissue necrosis.

7.3.4.3 Radiation-Induced Growth Abnormalities in Pediatric Patients

The primary skeletal toxicity following irradiation of pediatric patient is growth retardation. Growth abnormality associated with ionizing irradiation may be clinically seen as loss of stature and problems associated with asymmetric growth. The human skeleton grows from birth until late puberty. The growth of the long bones takes place in the epiphyseal (growth) plate. The epiphysis is the most sensitive portion of bone to radiation. Microscopic changes can be seen with doses as low as 3 Gy, with growth retardation occurring at 4 Gy; however, the doses above 15 Gy result in larger and more lasting deficits in stature [117]. The radiation-related changes in the epiphysis may be reversible at low doses. The growth plate may be widened 1–2 months after irradiation, often returning to normal by 6 months.

At doses greater than 12 Gy, there is increasing cellular damage to chondrocytes, with chondroblasts receiving maximum radiation effects. Delayed changes, occurring ≥6 months after RT, include bone marrow atrophy and cartilage degeneration. Late radiation changes are due to underlying vascular fibrosis and direct cellular damage. In the epiphysis, marked growth retardation occurs.

Apparent joint space widening has been described 8–10 months after therapy. Metaphyseal changes include bowing, with little or no change in bone length. Irregularity and fraying of the metaphysis resembling rickets may be present. Abnormal tubulation with premature fusion of the physis may occur. Growth retardation due to RT is most marked in the rapidly growing long bones and spine irradiated before epiphyseal closure. The spine is of particular importance in RT planning. Scoliosis results from both asymmetric vertebral growth changes and from secondary changes in the overlying soft tissues [117, 118].

7.3.5 Treatment

7.3.5.1 Radiation-Induced Bone Fractures

Radiation-induced bone toxicity as a late effect of RT, and the bone fractures are the worst adverse effects of RT on bone tissue and these fractures are generally named as "insufficiency or stress fractures," which are generally the subgroup of fractures that result from normal or physiologic stress applied to weakened bone.

Radiation-induced long bone fracture which is a rare complication of RT is most commonly seen following the higher doses used in the management of extremity sarcoma. Contemporary publications on limb-sparing treatment of soft tissue sarcoma of the extremities report a post-RT fracture incidence ranging from 4% to 8.6% [119]. For the treatment of radiation-induced long bone fracture, surgery is recommended. Therefore, the patient should be consulted orthopedic surgeon immediately.

The neck of the femur has a substantially lower radiation tolerance than other parts of the femur and long bones. This complication is increasingly rare as routine pelvic fields include blocking of the femoral neck and most of the femoral heads. The best strategy for femoral head and neck fractures is prevention. However, when the radiation-induced femoral neck fracture is encountered the surgical treatment should be done. Surgical repair of femoral head/neck fractures following RT may require special mechanical reinforcement due to the poor quality of bone following irradiation.

Pelvic RT is commonly used in many types of the tumors including cervical cancer, endometrial cancer, bladder cancer, and rectal cancer. Previous studies have demonstrated that pelvic RT results in demineralization of bone matrix, with a pelvic fracture rate of 2–89% reported among women undergoing RT for gynecologic malignancies [120]. Almost any part of the bony pelvis can fracture following pelvic RT, and fractures have been observed following RT for almost all pelvic disease sites. Particularly the patients who are at greater risk for osteoporosis such as older patients should be screened with respect to the osteoporosis and if necessary appropriate therapy should be advised. When insufficiency fractures do occur, they almost always resolve with conservative therapy including analgesics and physical therapy. Bisphosphonates may be used to promote healing and decrease the risk of subsequent fractures. Bisphosphonate, which induces apoptosis in osteoclasts and inhibits bone resorption, has been widely used for osteoporosis. Several reports have described that bisphosphonate is useful for bone loss associated with bone metastasis and is also effective for treating and preventing pelvic fracture after RT. However, it should be kept in mind that bisphosphonate has an antiangiogenic effect similar to that of RT and suppresses bone turnover. Therefore, it may confound osteonecrosis and induce pathologic fractures [120–122]. Again the patient should be evaluated and managed with orthopedic surgeon [117].

Pierce et al. showed that the incidence of rib fractures following breast irradiation ranged from 0% to almost 20%, though when restricting the review to studies using "modern techniques," the incidence was 1–3% [123]. In other contemporary series, the incidence of rib fracture following breast-conserving therapy is well below 1% [124]. Risk factors for chest wall toxicity after SBRT have been reported, but few studies evaluate predictive factors specifically for rib fracture. Among these risk factors patient-related factors such as gender, age, race, tobacco use, hypertension, and peripheral vascular disease have not been associated with risk of such chest wall toxicity; the impact of obesity and diabetes remains controversial [98, 125]. Further investigation into the effects of SBRT on rib cortical thickness and bone mineral density would allow better quantification of the relationship between RT dose and the risk for significant changes in bone structure that could lead to rib fracture. The recurrent tumor should be ruled out before further interventions. The vast majority of rib fractures will heal without intervention. Analgesics may be given as needed [123].

Vertebral compression fractures (VCF) are the most common osteoporotic fracture [98, 126]. Although the majority of cases are asymptomatic, approximately one-third of cases can lead to significant pain, reduced mobility, and decreased quality of life [127, 128]. RT has been associated with an increased risk of VCFs in cancer patients. The pathophysiology of post-RT VCFs is not well understood. With the increased use of SBRT, the occurrence of VCFs after SBRT has become an important issue. In some series, SBRT-associated VCFs incidence has been reported as high as 39%, with the majority of reports indicating a VCF rate of 10–20% and most fractures occurring within 3–4 months of treatment [98]. Most symptomatic patients were fully resolved after conservative treatment using analgesics and rest; however, but some patients need narcotics or hospitalization because of severe pain and disability. The patient should be evaluated and managed with orthopedic surgeon.

7.3.5.2 Radiation-Induced Osteoradionecrosis

The management of osteoradionecrosis is a rather complex issue. The tumor recurrence should be ruled out before any intervention. With conservative measures that are commonly employed, including improvement of oral hygiene, irrigation, and antibiotic therapy, complete osteoradionecrosis resolution is estimated to occur in 8–33% of patients after 1 year [116]. Conservative debridement and antibiotics is usually effective for mild osteoradionecrosis. Saline irrigation and antibiotic medications during the infectious period are the conservative therapies commonly employed, especially in early stage disease. Bacterial identification and sensitivity testing can be used before administration of antibiotics. Penicillin with metronidazole or clindamycin is empirically prescribed until bacterial identification has been completed [116, 129]. However, when bone and soft tissue necrosis are extensive, resection of the mandible with immediate microvascular reconstruction may provide better results. The surgical approaches for treatment of osteoradionecrosis of the jaws include wound debridement, sequestrectomy, decortication, and resection [130].

Hyperbaric oxygen is used at many centers to prevent and/or treat osteoradionecrosis. Hyperbaric oxygen is thought to act by stimulating monocyte and fibroblast function, thereby increasing vascular density and improving circulation [131]. The available data regarding the efficacy of hyperbaric oxygen are limited and conflicting. In a randomized trial hyperbaric oxygen was tested for prevention. In this trial, irradiated patients needing teeth extractions were randomized to perioperative penicillin versus perioperative penicillin plus hyperbaric oxygen therapy. The incidence of osteoradionecrosis in patients treated with hyperbaric oxygen was found as 5%; however, it was 30% for the patients who did not receive hyperbaric oxygen [132]. Hyperbaric oxygen is time consuming and is expensive treatment option. The most common side effect is reversible myopia.

The other agents used in the treatment of osteoradionecrosis is pentoxifylline and vitamin E. Pentoxifylline is a methylxanthine derivative that has multiple effects and may be advantageous for management of osteoradionecrosis. Pentoxifylline induces vascular dilation and increased erythrocyte flexibility resulting in enhanced blood flow. It also has an anti-tumor necrosis factor α activity and is believed to reduce the cytokine cascade driving the osteoradionecrosis disease process [133]. A single institution phase II study using pentoxifylline and vitamin E in patients with refractory osteoradionecrosis resulted in all 54 patients experiencing a complete recovery in a median of 9 months [134]. This finding needs to be confirmed in a randomized trial.

There is no standardized protocol established for the prevention of osteoradionecrosis following tooth removal. The use of perioperative antibiotics, hyperbaric oxygen, and strict adherence to surgical principles, such as primary closure and alveoloplasty, have all been implemented by several authors with varying rates of success.

7.3.5.3 Radiation-Induced Growth Abnormalities in Pediatric Patients

Radiation-induced growth retardation is one of the most devastating side effects of ionizing RT in pediatric patients. Growth abnormalities can be broadly grouped into loss of stature and problems associated with asymmetric growth. The

radiation-induced growth abnormalities are primarily treated with surgical intervention. To avoid this invasive therapy, careful field design is essential in minimizing
the extent of the abnormalities. Although there has been no human data, preclinical
studies have promising results with respect to the use of radioprotectants such as
amifostine to minimize growth abnormalities [117, 135, 136].

7.3.6   Rx: Prescription Samples

Radiation-induced bone fractures:

- Bisphosphonates
- Acetaminophen 325 mg, taken every 4 h.
- Narcotics

  Osteoradionecrosis

- Chlorhexidine gluconate 0.12% (dispense 1 bottle rinse with 20 ml for 30 s
  3 times/day).
- Penicillin V potassium 500 mg (dispense 28 tablets, take 1 tablet 4 times/day).
- Amoxicillin 500 mg (dispense 28 tablets, take 1 tablets 4 times/day)
- Clindamycin 150 mg or 300 mg (dispense 150–300 mg (dispense 28 capsules,
  take 1 capsule every 6 h).
- Acetaminophen 325 mg, taken every 4 h.

7.4   Extremities

7.4.1   Anatomy

The upper extremity or limb is a functional unit of the upper body. It is composed
of three sections, the upper arm, forearm, and hand. The upper extremity extends
from the shoulder joint to the fingers and contains 30 bones. Moreover, it contains of many nerves, blood vessels, and muscles. The nerves of the arm are supplied by the brachial plexus, which is one of the two major nerve plexus of the
human body [137].

The lower extremity is designed for weight-bearing, balance, and mobility. The
bones and muscles of the lower limb are larger and stronger than those of the upper
limb, which is necessary for the functions of weight-bearing and balance. The lower
extremity comprises the twenty-six bones of the feet, seven tarsal bones, and the leg
bones including the femur, fibula, and tibia. Femur is the longest and strongest bone
in the body. Its rounded head, located on the proximal, medial aspect of the femur,
fits beautifully in the acetabulum to form the hip joint. The tibia and fibula are the
bones of the leg. The tibia is larger and is located medial to the fibula. The tibia is
the weight-bearing bone and is part of the knee joint [138].

7.4.2 Contouring

There has been no available contouring atlas/guideline for all parts of both the upper and lower extremities yet; however, some special parts of the bony structures that have an importance during irradiation of different site of the tumors have been defined. Femoral head is important during the irradiation of the pelvic tumors. For the delineation of femoral head, the ball of the femur, trochanters, and proximal shaft to the level of the bottom of ischial tuberosities should be included [91].

7.4.3 Dose Constraints

Radiation effects on bones vary as a consequence of dose, energy, and fractionation. The pathological effects of radiation differ from the immature (growing) to the mature (adult) skeleton. In an immature skeleton, radiation affects chondrogenesis and resorption of calcified cartilage [139]. On the other hand, in an adult skeleton, the effects of radiation occur mainly on osteoblasts, with consequent reduction in bone formation [140, 141].

In the immature bones chondrocytes in the epiphyseal growth cartilage are the most radiosensitive areas. Microscopic changes in growth cartilage chondrocytes may appear following doses <3 Gy, and growth may slow down after just 4 Gy. Usually, histological recovery occurs up to 12 Gy, but higher levels of exposure may cause more serious cellular damage [142]. In adults microscopic changes in growth cartilage chondrocytes may appear following doses. The threshold for these alterations is estimated at around 30 Gy, and cellular death occurs with a dose of 5 Gy. Alteration to bone ranges from slight osteopenia to osteonecrosis. One year after irradiation, the bone appears osteopenic in radiographic views [140].

Emami et al. proposed the selected end points for the femoral head as necrosis, and femoral neck fracture (Table 7.4). The incidence of femoral necrosis and femoral neck fracture has been encountered with different doses ranging from 20 Gy to 70 Gy. The estimated TD 5/5 and TD 50/5 are 52 Gy and 65 Gy, respectively [51]. According to the stereotactic body RT (SBRT) dose recommendations of the American Association

Table 7.4 Dose constraints

Organ	Emami			Quantec	SRS	SBRT	End point
	1/3	2/3	3/3				
Extremities							
Muscle	TD 1/5: 50 Gy						Myositis
Brachial plexus	TD 5/5: 62 Gy	TD 5/5: 61 Gy	TD 5/5: 60 Gy	60–66 Gy	14 Gy <3 cc	20.4 Gy/3 fx (6.8 Gy/fx)	
	TD 50/5: 77 Gy	TD 50/5: 76 Gy	TD 50/5: 75 Gy		D_{max}: 17.5 Gy	27 Gy/5 fx (5.4 Gy/fx)	Clinically apparent nerve damage/ neuropathy

of Physicists in Medicine (AAPM) report 101, 14 Gy should be received <10 cc of the head of the femur for a single fraction stereotactic radiosurgery (SRS). For the fractionated SBRT, threshold doses for the 3 fraction and 5 fraction schedules are suggested as 28.8 Gy (9.6 Gy/fraction), and 30 Gy (6 Gy/fraction), respectively [53].

For the muscles the end point was chosen as clinical myositis. Most of the clinical evidences come from tangential breast irradiation. Emami et al. recommended TD 1/5 for the muscle as 50 Gy [51]. In a study conducted on 29 patients with the diagnosis of Ewing sarcoma, Jentzsch et al. reported the results of 22 patients who were alive after ≥2 years [143]. The treatment protocol consisted of 50 Gy external beam RT in addition to cyclophosphamide along with various combinations of vincristine, actinomycin D, or doxorubicin. Patients were categorized into four groups based on whether the functional limitations were mild (group 1), moderate (group 2), severe (group 3), or requiring amputation (group 4). Of the 22 patients, 59% were in group 1, 23% were in group 2, 14% were group 3, and one patient (4%) was considered group 4. An important determinant of radiation-related muscle injury is the dose-fractionation schedule. Among 145 patients treated at the NCI for soft tissue sarcoma of the extremities, muscle morbidity was higher for those who received total radiation doses greater than 63 Gy [144].

7.4.4 Pathophysiology

Pathophysiology of the radiation-induced bone fractures and osteonecrosis is discussed under the "bone" section. Therefore, in this section three topics will be discussed regarding the pathophysiology of radiation-induced extremity toxicity: (i) radiation-induced muscle toxicity, (ii) radiation-induced joint toxicity, and (iii) radiation-induced artery, vein, and nerve toxicity (Table 7.5).

7.4.4.1 Radiation-Induced Muscle Toxicity
Radiation-induced muscle injury can be seen by two clinical scenarios as myositis, which is also the chosen endpoint by Emami et al., and muscle fibrosis as a late side

Table 7.5 The RTOG/EORTC late radiation morbidity scoring criteria

| Organ | Chronic toxicity | | | |
	Grade 1	Grade 2	Grade 3	Grade 4
Bone	Asymptomatic No growth retardation Reduced bone density	Moderate pain or tenderness Growth retardation Irregular bone sclerosis	Severe pain or tenderness Complete arrest of bone growth Dense bone sclerosis	Necrosis/ spontaneous fracture
Joint	Mild joint stiffness Slight limitation of movement	Moderate stiffness Intermittent or moderate joint pain Moderate limitation of movement	Severe joint stiffness Pain with severe limitation of movement	Necrosis/complete fixation

effect. Although radiation-induced muscle injury is observed in experimental animal studies, it is infrequently reported in the clinical literature. Skeletal muscle has been considered relatively resistant to radiation injury and damage induced by conventional external beam RT is rarely observed [145]. The cellular response to acute muscle injury has been studied in animals and in humans. Edema, myofilament disruption, and endothelial swelling are seen at 24 h after single doses of 11–13 Gy in rabbits [146]. Amino acid release occurs four to 6 h after doses of 15 Gy in rats suggesting protein breakdown [147]. Phillips et al. [148] studied human muscle response after irradiation, and observed muscle degeneration and vacuolization associated with a loss of capillaries 2–4 months after doses of 20 Gy. An increase in collagen deposition over time was also evident but eventually decreased at 1 year at which time capillary recovery was also observed. Few microscopic changes were noted at any time points after doses of less than 15 Gy [145, 148].

The pathophysiology underlying late radiation-induced muscle injury is believed to originate from vascular damage and consequent ischemia along with the inflammation which accompanies the vascular damage. Radiation primarily affects small arteries, arterioles, and capillaries. The endothelial cells are the most radiosensitive elements and exhibit swelling and necrosis acutely, followed by intimal proliferation and subintimal deposition of collagen. The ischemia and inflammation in turn lead to the development of muscle fibrosis, a nonspecific repair reaction resulting in marked alteration of the muscle parenchyma. Radiation-induced fibrosis is similar to inflammation, wound healing, and fibrosis of any origin. Typical histologic features include the presence of inflammatory infiltrates, particularly macrophages in the earlier stages of fibrosis, differentiation of fibroblasts into postmitotic fibrocytes, and changes in the vascular connective tissue with excessive production and deposition of extracellular matrix proteins and collagen. Fibrosis, which is a form of normal tissue healing process, is thus a marker of repair efforts from the initial vascular injury and is usually is irreversible, resulting in chronic pain, deformity, and impaired mobility in severe cases [144, 145].

7.4.4.2 Radiation-Induced Joint Toxicity

There is limited data regarding the radiation effects on adult articular (joint) cartilage, though joint damage has been reported following cancer treatment or occupational exposures. Ionizing radiation can cause a severe acute and persistent reduction in the structural integrity of exposed skeletal tissue. Although there are some reports demonstrating the extent and nature of bone and growth plate cartilage damage following exposure, radiation effects on articular cartilage within the joint structure are undefined and relatively unstudied. Progressive degeneration and arthritis have been reported in various joints exposed to radiation. Specifically, cartilage thinning, pain, swelling, and ultimately erosion of subchondral bone have been described from hips following pelvic RT and from joints within the hand following occupational exposures [149–151].

The articular cartilage matrix consists primarily of proteoglycan polymers and type-II collagen which determine the mechanical properties of the tissue. Reducing proteoglycan polymers content in cartilage matrix can lower compressive stiffness.

Progressive destruction and loss of matrix contribute to arthropathies such as osteo-arthritis [149, 152]. In preclinical studies it was proposed that ionizing radiation may decrease proteoglycan polymers and increase matrix degradation in the articular cartilage, which lowers compressive stiffness [149]. Recent preclinical evidence published in preliminary form has shown that radiation can induce an acute reduction in the surface mechanical properties of mouse and pig articular cartilage, specifically lowering compressive stiffness [153]. However the exact pathophysiology of the radiation-related joint dysfunction has not been studied in human beings.

7.4.4.3 Radiation-Induced Artery, Vein, and Nerve Toxicity

Radiation-induced arteritis of large vessels and brachial plexus neuropathy are uncommon delayed complications of local RT. Vascular injury due to radiation is rare sequelae of RT but has been detected in many major vessels, including the aortic, renal, iliac, carotid, and subclavian-axillary arteries [154]. The pathophysiology of arteriopathy has not been clearly defined yet; however, although experimental and histopathologic studies have shown several changes in the arteries. These changes include fibrosis of the internal elastic membrane, injury to the vasa vasorum and ischemic necrosis of the vessel wall, periarterial fibrosis, and hyalinization and thickening of the vessel wall with fibrin deposition [154–156].

Radiation-induced nerve injury most frequently presents with paresthesia, and is associated with pain and/or weakness in the ipsilateral extremity. Weakness tends to be slowly progressive. The onset of symptoms can be seen within 6 months of completing radiation. Radiation-induced peripheral neuropathy is a chronic handicap, frightening because progressive and usually irreversible, usually appearing several years after RT. The incidence of radiation-induced peripheral neuropathy is rare but increasing with improved long-term cancer survival. The pathophysiological mechanisms have not been understood yet fully; however, nerve compression by indirect extensive radiation-induced fibrosis of tissue around peripheral nerves is thought to play a central role. Moreover the direct injury to nerves through axonal damage and demyelination because of injury to blood vessels by ischemia following capillary network failure may cause the neuropathy. Pathologic studies have shown loss of myelin, fibrosis, and thickening of the neurolemma sheath, and obliteration of the vasonevum [157, 158].

7.4.5 Treatment

Approximately one-third of patients undergoing RT to a bone metastasis will experience an acute increase in focal bone pain. This pain is transitory, but if severe, it may necessitate treatment with an opioid or a short course of an oral glucocorticoid. The treatment of the radiation-induced bone fractions and osteonecrosis was discussed under the "bone" section. Therefore in this section three topics will be discussed regarding the treatment of radiation-induced extremity toxicity: (i) radiation-induced muscle toxicity, (ii) radiation-induced joint toxicity, and (iii) radiation-induced artery, vein, and nerve toxicity.

7.4.5.1 Radiation-Induced Muscle Toxicity

As with inflammation-related pain of other causes, in the management of radiation-induced myositis, non-steroidal anti-inflammatory drugs (NSAIDS) are a reasonable initial intervention for active radiation myositis. The value of corticosteroids for radiation myositis is anecdotal and extrapolated from the utility of prednisone in other subacute radiation-related inflammatory conditions such as radiation pneumonitis. Nonetheless, if non-steroidal anti-inflammatory agents fail, a 1–3 week course of prednisone at 30–60 mg/day may be initiated. Should such measures not provide adequate results or if there is laboratory or radiographic evidence of severe tissue breakdown, more aggressive approaches such as hyperbaric oxygen therapy may be considered. Hyperbaric oxygen therapy is of benefit in the treatment of extensive muscle tissue breakdown due to various causes including radiation injury. To further reduce the chances of developing long-term disability secondary to muscle fibrosis, early physical therapy and rehabilitation are advised [145].

7.4.5.2 Radiation-Induced Joint Toxicity

There is little evidence regarding the optimal management of the radiation-related joint dysfunction. Exercises and physical therapy may be considered. In order to prevent radiation-induced joint dysfunction and stiffness, patients also can be consulted appropriate exercise programs during the RT. In case of pain analgesics may be used. If there is associated moderate-to-severe joint pain with swelling, NSAIDs such as aspirin, ibuprofen (Advil, Motrin), or naproxen sodium (Aleve) can be prescribed in order to provide relief. For the patients whose joint is particularly painful and debilitating may require surgery.

7.4.5.3 Radiation-Induced Artery, Vein, and Nerve Toxicity

Radiation-induced neuropathic pain is a rare but devastating complication following cancer treatment. It is often progressive, refractory to conservative treatment, and sometimes irreversible. An acute, transient brachial plexopathy can occur after RT that involves a nerve [159]. Mimicking the syndrome known as acute brachial plexitis (brachial neuritis), this disorder is characterized by pain, paresthesia, and weakness in the shoulder, arm, and hand. The syndrome is usually self-limited but may cause persistent pain or dysfunction. Newer methods of RT appear to have substantially reduced the incidence of this condition.

The first treatment option may be non-opioid analgesic agents including aspirin, acetaminophen, NSAID, COX-2 inhibitors. If there is no response tramadol, opioids, antidepressants (tricyclics and serotonin-norepinephrine reuptake inhibitors), antiepileptic drugs (gabapentin, pregabalin, and other anticonvulsants), and N-methyl-D-aspartate (NMDA) receptor antagonists may be suggested. For many patients, an approach using combinations of drugs that target different metabolic pathways may result in improved analgesia and fewer side effects because lower doses of each drug can be used. In case of intractable pain, intravenous lidocaine may be used [160].

7.4.6   Rx: Sample Prescriptions

Radiation-induced myositis

- Acetaminophen 325 mg, taken every 4 h
- COX-2 inhibitors (Celecoxib: Celebrex® 200 mg, bid)
- Prednisone at 30–60 mg/day (1–3 weeks)

  Radiation-induced neuropathic pain

- Acetaminophen 325 mg, taken every 4 h
- COX-2 inhibitors (Celecoxib: Celebrex® 200 mg, bid)
- Pregabalin 450 mg/day
- High-dose transdermal fentanyl (350 µg/h)
- Lidocaine 5 mg/kg (IV)
- Nortriptyline (12.5 mg once daily at bedtime; may increase as tolerated up to 35 mg/day)

7.5   Ovaries

7.5.1   Anatomy

Ovaries are located in each side of the uterus close to the lateral pelvic sidewalls in women. They are connected by the mesovarium to the broad ligament of the uterus which covers the fallopian tubes, ovaries, ovarian and uterine arteries, and ligaments. It has no visceral peritoneum and is surrounded by germinal epithelium.

The primary arterial blood supply to the ovaries is ovarian arteries, which are branch of the abdominal aorta just below the level of the renal arteries and run through the suspensory (infundibulopelvic) ligaments of the ovaries. These ligaments attach each ovary to the pelvic sidewall. The ovarian (utero-ovarian) ligaments attach each ovary to the lateral surface of the uterus and do not contain any vessels. The right ovarian vein directly drains into the vena cava inferior while the left ovarian vein drains into the left renal vein. The primary ovarian lymphatic drainage toward the para-aortic nodes parallels the course of the ovarian veins and the secondary one mainly drains into the iliac lymphatic system [161].

Ovaries have gametogenic and endocrine functions where germ cells and steroid hormones are produced, respectively. Oogonia are formed during fetal life which originates from primordial germ cells and proliferate rapidly by active mitosis. The cortex of the ovaries consists of connective tissue which contains ovarian follicles. Follicles develop from the germinal epithelium which surrounding the free surface of the ovaries. As the fetal period progresses, primary oocytes and primordial follicles are formed and mitosis is terminated. Further development of primary oocytes is prevented until puberty. The number of primordial follicles decreases gradually until menopause and menopause occurs when there is no follicle left in the ovarian cortex due to involution, atresia, and ovulation.

Hypothalamic gonadotropin-releasing hormone (GnRH) controls follicular maturation and ovarian luteinization by stimulating the release of pituitary gonadotropins, follicle-stimulating hormone (FSH), and luteinizing hormone (LH). GnRH rises to initiate puberty in late childhood and primary follicles are formed. Follicle cells are now called granulosa cells. Granulosa cells surround the growing ovarian follicles and support oocyte function during maturation. Granulosa cells stimulated by follicle-stimulating hormone (FSH) and secrete estrogen. Increased estrogen stimulates luteinizing hormone (LH) release. LH plays a key role for oocyte maturation and ovulation. After ovulation, the corpus luteum produces progesterone, estradiol, and 17-hydroxyprogesterone, causing endometrial changes. If there is no chorionic gonadotropin released from the conceptus, the corpus luteum is disappeared and progesterone and estrogen levels were decreased and the endometrium is shed as a menstruation.

Ovarian hormones have also significant roles on integrity of the bone and cardiovascular system, maturation and maintenance of breast and vagina, and libido.

7.5.2 Contouring

There has been no available contouring atlas/guideline for ovaries yet. We showed CT images of 37 years of women with cervical cancer who had ovarian transposition before RT. Bilateral transposed ovaries are separately countered slice by slice considering clips localization (Fig. 7.8).

7.5.3 Dose Constraints

Premature ovarian failure (POF) is observed in 70–85% of patients who underwent abdomino-pelvic RT depending on age and dose [162]. Pre-pubertal girls are more resistant to gonadotoxic effects of radiotherapy (RT) and chemotherapy, most probably because of the greater number of primordial follicles which are more resistant to vascular damage and cortical fibrosis. However, as age progresses, the germ cell pool cannot be renewed and the number of primordial follicles decreases gradually. Consequently, the risk of ovarian failure increases with age [162]. After total body irradiation (TBI), POF is observed in 100% of patients after puberty and 50% of patients before age 10 [163].

The severity of ovarian damage also depends on the RT field, total dose, and fraction dose. When RT field in close proximity to or includes the ovaries, the risk of POF is very high and causing infertility [164].

Ovaries are extremely sensitive to very low RT doses, and 50% of patients develop permanent infertility or premature menopause after <2 Gy radiation

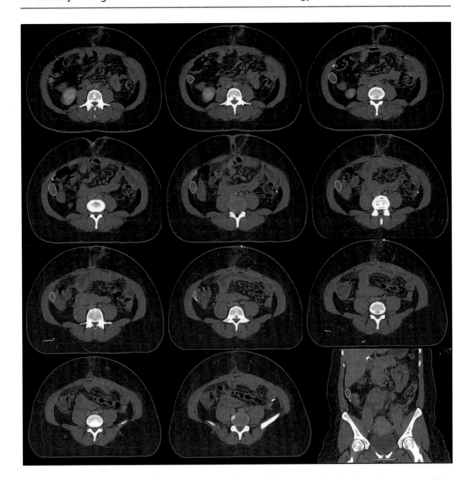

Fig. 7.8 CT images of 37 years of women with cervical cancer who had ovarian transposition before RT. Bilateral transposed ovaries are separately countered slice by slice considering clips localization

exposure [165]. A RT dose of 2.5–3 Gy may inhibit ovarian function, 5–15 Gy results in temporary sex hormone disorder and infertility, and 20–30 Gy leads to irreversible damage to the ovaries [166]. Fractionated RT reduces the risk of ovarian damage [167]. In 1980, Ash et al. analyzed the effect of fractionated RT on ovarian function in reproductive age women [168]. They showed that >8 Gy doses cause 100% permanent sterility, while the effect of low doses varies depending on age. Doses of >10 Gy to the ovaries are a significant risk factor for delayed/absent menarche or secondary amenorrhea in the first 5 years after treatment [162]. If ovarian dose is limited to ≤3 Gy, early menopause observed in only 11% of patients; however, 60% of patients became menopausal if the ovarian dose exceeds 3 Gy [169]. In 2005, Wallace et al. defined effective sterilizing dose, which leads to earlier and permanent ovarian failure in 97.5% of patients; 20.3 Gy at birth, 18.4 Gy at age <10 years, 16.5 Gy at age 20 years, and 14.3 Gy at age 30 years [170]. However, there is no clear threshold dose for the risk of POF in clinical practice. It depends on numerous other factors including age, genetic characteristics of the patients, comorbidities, and other treatment modalities [171].

In 2016, Du et al. found that limiting the ovarian RT dose to V7.5 <26% in intensity-modulated RT (IMRT) can prevent the disruption of ovarian function [172]. In a recent study, published by Yin et al. showed that better preserving ovarian function in transposed ovaries, RT dose should be limited to D_{max} <9.985 Gy, D_{mean} <5.32 Gy and V5.5 <29.65% in IMRT [173].

7.5.4 Pathophysiology

RT and chemotherapy (e.g., alkylating agents) alone or in combination may cause temporary or permanent changes in reproductive capacity and endocrine and sexual functions [174]. This condition is characterized by the depletion of oocytes which is called "female primary gonadal failure" or POF, resulting in early menopause which is defined by high serum FSH concentration.

Particularly in patients who receive RT to the lower abdomen, pelvis, spine, or total body, the number of oocytes or in other words ovarian reserve is reduced [175]. The damage of the ovaries leads to both sterilization and suppression of estrogen production which is caused by loss of the primordial follicles. Thus, affected individuals present with delayed puberty, decreased secondary sexual characteristics, amenorrhea, and menopausal symptoms.

Radiation-induced ovarian damage causes DNA double-strand breaks (DSBs) in the ovarian tissue, either directly or due to scattered radiation and leads to treatment-induced apoptosis, mitochondrial DNA damage, blood vessel damage, neovascularization, and cortical fibrosis. The primary target of radiation damage is granulosa cells [176, 177]. Thus, hormone production and follicle count decrease, and atresia develops in residual follicles.

7.5.5 Treatment

Patients with a high risk of POF should be evaluated for fertility preservation before gonadotoxic treatment (TBI, chemotherapy, RT, etc.). Ovaries should be prevented as much as possible when treatment planning. Using newer RT techniques can limit dose to the ovaries in order to prevent infertility and POF. Laparoscopic ovarian transposition (oophoropexy) should be performed before RT to preserve gonadal function in premenopausal patients less than 40 years of age with low risk of ovarian involvement. Prior to this procedure, the radiation oncologist and the surgeon should be in good collaboration and the ovaries should be moved at least 3 cm away from the border of the RT field. In addition, marking this region with the clips is important in terms of contouring the ovaries and determining the doses taken during the RT. The ovarian preservation rate after this procedure reaches as high as 80–88% and the success rates are higher with transposition of both ovaries [178, 179].

Embryo and oocyte cryopreservation can also be performed in suitable patients before RT with similar efficacy. Oocytes cryopreservation in post-pubertal women includes stimulation of ovaries with exogenous gonadotropins and collection of mature oocytes for future fertilization. However, only few oocytes can be collected with this method [180]. Again, embryo cryopreservation encompasses hormonal stimulation of the ovaries and collection of oocytes. Additionally, collected oocytes simultaneously brought together with sperm to create embryos for future implantation. However, this technique is not suitable for pediatric and adolescent cases. In addition, ovarian stimulation and in vitro fertilization process may lead to delay in starting cancer treatment [181]. Another one of the most important drawbacks is the risk of the specimen carrying cancer cells, especially in patients with hematologic or gonadal malignancies.

Ovarian tissue cryopreservation method in which ovarian tissue (the ovarian cortex) is removed by laparoscopic ovarian cortical tissue biopsy or oophorectomy and then stored together with primordial follicles is the only fertility preservation method suitable for both pre- and post-pubertal women [182]. However, this method is still considered to be experimental. In addition, hormone replacement therapy (HRT) containing estrogen and progesterone should be considered to decrease menopausal symptoms, unless contraindicated [183].

7.6   Testes

7.6.1   Anatomy

The testes are oval-shaped paired organs that are located in the scrotum. They are superiorly suspended by the spermatic cord, which include vessels, nerves, and ducts. Tunica vaginalis and tunica albuginea cover the testis externally and internally, respectively. Tunica albuginea also divides the testicular parenchyma into lobules. A lobule of the testis consists of one or more seminiferous tubules, where sperm develops.

The arterial supply of the testes is derived mainly from the testicular arteries and to a lesser extent from the artery of the vas deferens and the cremasteric artery. Venous drainage is provided by the pampiniform plexus which converge to form the testicular vein above the testis. Testicular veins drain directly into the inferior vena cava on the right, and the renal vein on the left. The lymphatic drainage of the testes follows the same route of the testicular vessels and drain to the pre-aortic and para-aortic lymph nodes.

The testis is a male reproductive organ that is responsible for producing the primary male sex hormone (testosterone) and production of sperm. Follicle-stimulating hormone (FSH) and luteinizing hormone (LH) released from the anterior pituitary stimulate the production of sperm and secretion of testosterone, respectively.

Leydig cells are primary androgen-secreting cells, providing 75% of testosterone produced in men [184]. Testosterone plays a role in the development of spermatogenesis and secondary sex characteristics. Sertoli cells found in the epithelial tissue are supporting cells that surround the germ cells. They have an important role in spermatogenesis. Spermatogenesis or formation of spermatozoa from immature germ cells occurs in the germinal epithelium of the seminiferous tubules. This process begins at puberty. Spermatogonia, the least differentiated germ cells, divide by mitosis to form spermatocytes. These cells soon form spermatids with meiosis and undergo metamorphosis to become spermatozoa. These cells are transported to the lumen of the epididymis for maturation.

7.6.2 Contouring

There has been no available contouring atlas/guideline for testis yet. We showed delineation of testes as critical organs in computed tomography (CT) and magnetic resonance imaging (MRI) slices of 33 years of men with rectal cancer (Fig. 7.9).

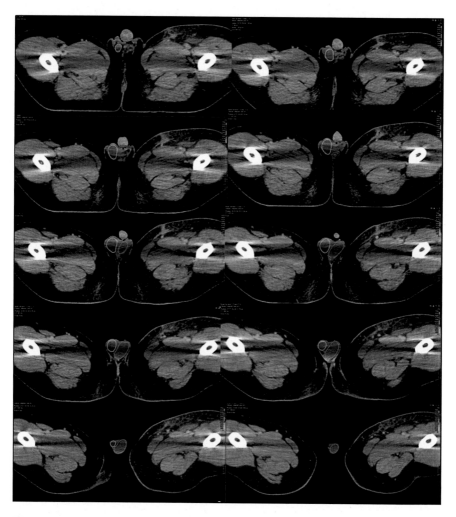

Fig. 7.9 Delineation of testes as critical organs in computed tomography (CT) and magnetic resonance imaging (MRI) slices of 33 years of men with rectal cancer

7.6.3   Dose Constraints

Germ cell integrity, Leydig and Sertoli cell functions, and neuromuscular control of ejaculation are highly sensitive to cancer treatment. Leydig cells and spermatogonia have different sensitivities to cytotoxic treatments. Spermatogonia are extremely sensitive to even very low radiation doses regardless of age and this may cause infertility. However, testosterone production often continues because Leydig cells are relatively radioresistant to radiation. Germinal epithelium can be damaged at very low doses compared to Leydig cells (<1 Gy vs. 20–30 Gy) [185].

Even radiation doses of 15 cGy may cause a decrease in sperm count and temporary sterility [186]. Doses <0.8 Gy can cause oligospermia, 0.8–2 Gy temporary azoospermia, and 2–3 Gy permanent azoospermia [187, 188]. This decrease may develop 3–6 weeks after RT and recovery may take 1–3 years depending on the RT dose.

Spermatocytes cannot perform the division required for maturation at doses of 2–3 Gy. Spermatids are more resistant than spermatocytes and higher radiation dose of 4–6 Gy is required for damage [189]. There is an increased risk of permanent sterility at higher doses. At low radiation doses (<2 Gy), sperm count decreases 60–80 days after exposure due to completion of maturation period of spermatogonia [190]. Azoospermia develops more rapidly due to concurrent spermatid damage at higher doses (>4 Gy).

Several studies have shown that multiple small RT fractions are more toxic than a large single fraction for spermatogenesis. This is called "reverse fractionation effect." This is due to excessive radiosensitivity of the testicular germinal epithelium, low number of stem cells, and rapid cell turnover [190].

Infertility may develop as a result of radiation exposure of the testes from scattered radiation or radiation leakage under testicular shield. In a study by Sklar et al., germ cell dysfunction was observed in 55% of ALL cases who were treated with 12 Gy RT to the abdomen [191]. Transient elevation of FSH level and oligospermia were observed in patients who underwent 20 Gy RT to the abdomen with the diagnosis of HL. There is no effect at lower doses. The dose of testes is insignificant in patients who underwent mantle or PA RT with the diagnosis of HL. However, testis doses vary between 3 and 10% in cases without testicular shield and <1% in cases with testicular shield depending on the distance between the testes and the inguinal region in patients treated with pelvic RT. With a well-designed testicular shield, testicular doses are <2 Gy, which can be further reduced with multileaf collimators (MLCs) and only temporary azoospermia may develop depending on the internal radiation scatter.

Direct testicular irradiation may cause chemical changes in Leydig cell functions. Unlike females, young males (pre-pubertal and peri-pubertal vs. post-pubertal and adult) are more radiosensitive and more prone to testicular damage [192]. Radiation doses that cause clinical effects on Leydig cell function are >20 Gy and >30 Gy in pre-pubertal and post-pubertal males, respectively [193]. Subclinical Leydig cell dysfunction is observed when 12 Gy is applied to the testes while significant dysfunction is observed when testis exposed to 24 Gy [194]. Shalet et al.

reported deterioration of gonadotropin secretion in 82% of cases due to testicular damage after 24 Gy in 12–16 fractions in patients treated with testicular recurrence of ALL [195].

7.6.4 Pathophysiology

Primary gonadal failure in males is characterized by low testosterone, elevated FSH and LH levels, absence of puberty signs until 14 years of age, or arrested pubertal development for more than 6 months [194]. Depending on the severity of gonadal injury, spermatogenesis and steroidogenesis may be affected differently in males.

Spermatogenic damage can be reversible or irreversible, depending on treatment modalities (RT, chemotherapy, etc.) and patient characteristics. Decrease in the number of proliferating germ cell pool plays a role in the etiology [196]. The damage to the production of sperm cell results in oligospermia (sperm concentration less than 20×10^6/ml measured in a semen sample) or azoospermia [188, 195]. Germ cell failure is characterized by elevated FSH, low inhibin B, reduced testicular volume and azoospermia.

RT effects on testes depend on patient age, RT dose, and RT field. In contrast to females, testosterone production may continue despite the germ cell failure. Therefore, normal spontaneous pubertal development, hormonal balance, libido or erection function are possible. After severe gonadal toxicity, both spermatogenesis and steroidogenesis may be impaired.

7.6.5 Treatment

Patients with a high risk of gonadal failure should be evaluated for fertility preservation before gonadotoxic treatment (TBI, chemotherapy, RT, etc.). Testes should be prevented as much as possible when treatment planning. Using testicular shield and newer RT techniques can reduce dose of the testes. Pre-pubertal testis is more sensitive to RT effect. In these cases, pubertal induction should be initiated with testosterone around the ages of 12–14 years [197].

Patients should be referred to the sperm bank for cryopreservation of spermatozoa before chemotherapy and pelvic RT in order to preserve fertility [198, 199]. It is the best option for fertility preservation. New technologies such as testicular sperm extraction method may be an option in cases that cannot provide semen samples due to their young age [200]. In vitro maturation of germ cells to sperm, testicular tissue cryopreservation, and autografting of biopsied tissue remain experimental [201].

Management strategies for management of acute and late radiation-induced toxicities for current chapter is summarized in Table 7.6.

Table 7.6 Management of acute and late radiation-induced toxicities breast, skin, bones, extremities, muscles, and nerves

Organ	Acute toxicity	Treatment	Chronic toxicity	Treatment
Breast	Radiation dermatitis	Skin emollients (not immediately before RT) Topical steroids (e.g., mometasone, betamethasone) for prevention Consider non-steroidal agents (e.g., silver sulfadiazine, calendula ointment, barrier films) Consider protective dressings for areas of moist desquamation Monitor for and treat secondary infections if necessary Provide reassurance, monitor symptoms for resolution	Fibrosis Telangiectasia and atrophy	Pentoxifylline Vitamin E Hyperbaric oxygen Pulsed dye laser (PDL)
Skin	Radiation dermatitis	Grade 1: hydrophilic (oil-in-water) moisturizers Corticosteroids Grade 2-3: Antimicrobial agents (in case of infection) Dressing Grade 4: Surgical debridement Full-thickness graft Flaps Antimicrobial agents (in case of infection)	Fibrosis Telangiectasia and atrophy Necrosis Ulceration	Pentoxifylline Vitamin E Hyperbaric oxygen Pulsed dye laser (PDL)
Bones			Fracture Osteoradionecrosis	Surgery Bisphosphonates Narcotics Antibiotics (Penicillin, metronidazole and clindamycin) Conservative debridement Hyperbaric oxygen Pentoxifylline Vitamin E Surgery

(continued)

Table 7.6 (continued)

Organ	Acute toxicity	Treatment	Chronic toxicity	Treatment
Extremities Muscles Nerves			Myositis Fibrosis Neuropathic pain	Analgesics (NSAID) Corticosteroid Hyperbaric oxygen therapy Non-opioid analgesic agents (e.g., aspirin, acetaminophen, non-steroidal anti-inflammatory drugs [NSAIDs], COX-2 Inhibitors) • Tramadol • Opioids • Alpha 2 adrenergic agonists • Antidepressants (tricyclics and serotonin-norepinephrine reuptake inhibitors) • Antiepileptic drugs (gabapentin, pregabalin, and other anticonvulsants) • Muscle relaxants • N-methyl-D-aspartate (NMDA) receptor antagonists • Topical analgesic agents

References

1. Jatoi I, Kaufman M, Petit JY. Atlas of breast surgery. New York: Springer; 2006.
2. Bistoni G, Farhadi J. Anatomy and physiology of the breast. Plast Reconstr Surg. 2015:477–85.
3. https://www.rtog.org/CoreLab/ContouringAtlases/BreastCancerAtlas.aspx.
4. Offersen BV, Boersma LJ, Kirkove C, Hol S, Aznar MC, Sola AB, Kirova YM, et al. ESTRO consensus guideline on target volume delineation for elective radiation therapy of early stage breast cancer, version 1.1. Radiother Oncol. 2016;118(1):205–8.
5. Mukesh M, Harris E, Jena R, Evans P, Coles C. Relationship between irradiated breast volume and late normal tissue complications: a systematic review. Radiother Oncol. 2012;104(1):1–10.

6. González Sanchis A, Brualla González L, Sánchez Carazo JL, Gordo Partearroyo JC, Esteve Martínez A, Vicedo González A, López Torrecilla JL. Evaluation of acute skin toxicity in breast radiotherapy with a new quantitative approach. Radiother Oncol. 2017;122(1):54–9.

7. White J, Joiner MC. Toxicity from radiation in breast cancer. Cancer Treat Res. 2006;128:65–109.

8. Podrock D, Kristjanson L. Skin reactions during radiotherapy for breast cancer: the use and impact of topical agents and dressings. Eur J Cancer Care. 1999;8:143–53.

9. Shaitelman SF, Schlembach PJ, Arzu I, Ballo M, Bloom ES, Buchholz D, Chronowski GM, et al. Acute and short-term toxic effects of conventionally fractionated vs hypofractionated whole-breast irradiation: a randomized clinical trial. JAMA Oncol. 2015;1(7):931–41.

10. Bartelink H, Horiot JC, Poortmans PM, et al. Impact of a higher radiation dose on local control and survival in breast-conserving therapy of early breast cancer: 10-year results of the randomized boost versus no boost EORTC 22881- 10882 trial. J Clin Oncol. 2007;25:3259–65.

11. Yarnold J, Ashton A, Bliss J, Homewood J, Harper C, Hanson J, Haviland J, Bentzen S, Owen R. Fractionation sensitivity and dose response of late adverse effects in the breast after radiotherapy for early breast cancer: long-term results of a randomised trial. Radiother Oncol. 2005;75(1):9–17.

12. Polgar C, Fodor J, Major T, et al. Breast-conserving treatment with partial or whole breast irradiation for low-risk invasive breast carcinoma – 5-year results of a randomized trial. Int J Radiat Oncol Biol Phys. 2007;69:694–702.

13. Vaidya JS, Joseph DJ, Tobias JS, et al. Targeted intraoperative radiotherapy versus whole breast radiotherapy for breast cancer (TARGIT-A trial): an international, prospective, randomised, non-inferiority phase 3 trial. Lancet. 2010;376:91–102.

14. Ribeiro GG, Magee B, Swindell R, Harris M, Banerjee SS. The Christie Hospital breast conservation trial: an update at 8 years from inception. Clin Oncol (R Coll Radiol). 1993;5:278–83.

15. Kole AJ, Kole L, Moran MS. Acute radiation dermatitis in breast cancer patients: challenges and solutions. Breast Cancer (Dove Med Press). 2017;9:313–23.

16. Koenig TR, Wolff D, Mettler FA, Wagner LK. Skin injuries from fluoroscopically guided procedures: part 1, characteristics of radiation injury. AJR Am J Roentgenol. 2001.

17. Brown KR, Rzucidlo E. Acute and chronic radiation injury. J Vasc Surg. 2011;253(1 Suppl):15S–21S.

18. Ryan JL. Ionizing radiation: the good, the bad, and the ugly. J Invest Dermatol. 2012;132(3 pt 2):985–93.

19. Pignol JP, Vu TT, Mitera G, Bosnic S, Verkooijen HM, Truong P. Prospective evaluation of severe skin toxicity and pain during postmastectomy radiation therapy. Int J Radiat Oncol Biol Phys. 2015;91(1):157–64.

20. Fisher J, Scott C, Stevens R, et al. Randomized phase III study comparing Best Supportive Care to Biafine as a prophylactic agent for radiation-induced skin toxicity for women undergoing breast irradiation: Radiation Therapy Oncology Group (RTOG) 97-13. Int J Radiat Oncol Biol Phys. 2000;48(5):1307–10.

21. Buchholz TA. Radiation therapy for early-stage breast cancer after breast-conserving surgery. N Engl J Med. 2009;360(1):63–70.

22. Yi A, Kim HH, Shin HJ, Huh MO, Ahn SD, Seo BK. Radiation-induced complications after breast cancer radiation therapy: a pictorial review of multimodality imaging findings. Korean J Radiol. 2009;10(5):496–507.

23. Boyages J, Bilous M, Barraclough B, Langlands AO. Fat necrosis of the breast following lumpectomy and radiation therapy for early breast cancer. Radiother Oncol. 1988;13(1): 69–74.

24. Williams NR, Williams S, Kanapathy M, et al. Radiation-induced fibrosis in breast cancer: a protocol for an observational cross-sectional pilot study for personalised risk estimation and objective assessment. Int J Surg Protoc. 2019;14:9–13.

25. Delanian S, Porcher R, Rudant J, Lefaix JL. Kinetics of response to long-term treatment combining pentoxifylline and tocopherol in patients with superficial radiation-induced fibrosis. J Clin Oncol. 2005.

26. Haase O, Rodemann HP. Fibrosis and cytokine mechanisms: relevant in hadron therapy? Radiother Oncol. 2004;73(Suppl 2):S144.
27. Bentzen SM. Preventing or reducing late side effects of radiation therapy: radiobiology meets molecular pathology. Nat Rev Cancer. 2006;6(9):702.
28. Pignol JP, Olivotto I, Rakovitch E, Gardner S, Sixel K, Beckham W, Vu TT, Truong P, Ackerman I, Paszat L. A multicenter randomized trial of breast intensity-modulated radiation therapy to reduce acute radiation dermatitis. J Clin Oncol. 2008;26(13):2085.
29. Salvo N, Barnes E, van Draanen J, Stacey E, Mitera G, Breen D, Giotis A, Czarnota G, Pang J, De Angelis C. Prophylaxis and management of acute radiation-induced skin reactions: a systematic review of the literature. Curr Oncol. 2010;17(4):94.
30. Chan RJ, Webster J, Chung B, Marquart L, Ahmed M, Garantziotis S. Prevention and treatment of acute radiation-induced skin reactions: a systematic review and meta-analysis of randomized controlled trials. BMC Cancer. 2014;14:53.
31. Lewis L, Carson S, Bydder S, Athifa M, Williams AM, Bremner A. Evaluating the effects of aluminum-containing and non-aluminum containing deodorants on axillary skin toxicity during radiation therapy for breast cancer: a 3-armed randomized controlled trial. Int J Radiat Oncol Biol Phys. 2014;90(4):765.
32. Lokkevik E, Slovlund E, Reitan J, et al. Skin treatment with bepanthen cream versus no cream during radiotherapy. Acta Onocol. 1996;35(8):1021–6.
33. Maiche AG, Grohn P, Maki-Hokkonen H. Effect of chamomile cream and almond ointment on acute radiation skin reaction. Acta Oncol. 1991;30(3):395–6.
34. Macmillan MS, Wells M, MacBride S, Raab GM, Munro A, MacDougall H. Randomized comparison of dry dressings versus hydrogel in management of radiation-induced moist desquamation. Int J Radiat Oncol Biol Phys. 2007;68(3):864–72. Epub 2007 Mar 23.
35. Haruna F, Lipsett A, Marignol L. Management of acute radiation dermatitis in breast cancer patients: a systematic review and meta-analysis. Anticancer Res. 2017;37(10):5343.
36. Heggie S, Bryant GP, Tripcony L, et al. A Phase III study on the efficacy of topical aloe vera gel on irradiated breast tissue. Cancer Nurs. 2002;25:442.
37. Richardson J, Smith JE, McIntyre M, et al. Aloe vera for preventing radiation-induced skin reactions: a systematic literature review. Clin Oncol (R Coll Radiol). 2005;17:478.
38. Hoopfer D, Holloway C, Gabos Z, et al. Three-arm randomized phase III trial: quality aloe and placebo cream versus powder as skin treatment during breast cancer radiation therapy. Clin Breast Cancer. 2015;15:181.
39. Rosenthal A, Israilevich R, Moy R. Management of acute radiation dermatitis: a review of the literature and proposal for treatment algorithm. J Am Acad Dermatol. 2019;81(2):558.
40. Magnusson M, Höglund P, Johansson K, Jönsson C, Killander F, Malmström P, Weddig A, Kjellén E. Pentoxifylline and vitamin E treatment for prevention of radiation-induced side-effects in women with breast cancer: a phase two, double-blind, placebo-controlled randomised clinical trial (Ptx-5). Eur J Cancer. 2009;45(14):2488.
41. Rossi AM, Nehal KS, Lee EH. Radiation-induced breast telangiectasias treated with the pulsed dye laser. J Clin Aesthet Dermatol. 2014;7(12):34.
42. Kanitakis J. Anatomy, histology and immunohistochemistry of normal human skin. Eur J Dermatol. 2002;12(4):390–401.
43. Montagna W, Kligman AM, Carlisle KS. Atlas of normal human skin. New York: Springer; 1992.
44. James WD, Berger TG, Elston DM. Andrews' diseases of the skin: clinical dermatology. 10th ed. Philadelphia: Elsevier Saunders; 2006.
45. Common Terminology Criteria for Adverse Events (CTCAE), Version 5.0, November 2017, National Institutes of Health, National Cancer Institute. Available at: https://ctep.cancer.gov/protocoldevelopment/electronic_applications/docs/CTCAE_v5_Quick_Reference_8.5x11.pdf. Accessed 27 Mar 2018.
46. Pommier P, Gomez F, Sunyach MP, et al. Phase III randomized trial of Calendula officinalis compared with trolamine for the prevention of acute dermatitis during irradiation for breast cancer. J Clin Oncol. 2004;22:1447.

47. Ryan JL, Ling M, Williams JP, et al. Curcumin intervention and plasma biomarkers for radiation dermatitis in breast cancer patients. J Invest Dermatol. 2011;131:S90.
48. Bray FN, Simmons BJ, Wolfson AH, Nouri K. Acute and chronic cutaneous reactions to ionizing radiation therapy. Dermatol Ther (Heidelb). 2016;26(2):185–206.
49. Wei J, Meng L, Hou X, Qu C, Wang B, Xin Y, Jiang X. Radiation-induced skin reactions: mechanism and treatment. Cancer Manag Res. 2019;11:167–77.
50. Mendelsohn FA, Divino CM, Reis ED, Kerstein MD. Wound care after radiation therapy. Adv Skin Wound Care. 2002;15(5):216.
51. Emami B, Lyman J, Brown A, Coia L, Goitein M, Munzenrider JE, Shank B, Solin LJ, Wesson M. Tolerance of normal tissue to therapeutic irradiation. Int J Radiat Oncol Biol Phys. 1991;21(1):109–22.
52. Turesson I, Notter G. The predictive value of skin telangiectasia for late radiation effects in different normal tissues. Int J Radiat Oncol Biol Phys. 1986;12:603–9.
53. Benedict SH, Yenice KM, Followill D, Galvin JM, Hinson W, Kavanagh B, Keall P. Stereotactic body radiation therapy: the report of AAPM Task Group 101. Med Phys. 2010;37(8):4078–101.
54. Hymes SR, Strom EA, Fife C. Radiation dermatitis: clinical presentation, pathophysiology, and treatment. J Am Acad Dermatol. 2006;54(1):28–46.
55. Singh M, Alavi A, Wong R, Akita S. Radiodermatitis: a review of our current understanding. Am J Clin Dermatol. 2016;17(3):277–92.
56. Morgan K. Radiotherapy-induced skin reactions: prevention and cure. Br J Nurs. 2014;23(16):S24, S26–32.
57. Kim JH, Kolozsvary AJJ, Jenrow KA, Brown S. Mechanisms of radiation-induced skin injury and implications for future clinical trials. Int J Radiat Biol. 2013;89(5):311–8.
58. Bentzen SM. Preventing or reducing late side effects of radiation therapy: radiobiology meets molecular pathology. Nat Rev Cancer. 2006;6(9):702–13.
59. Martin M, Lefaix J-L, Delanian S. TGF-β1 and radiation fibrosis: a master switch and a specific therapeutic target? Int J Radiat Oncol Biol Phys. 2000;47(2):277–90.
60. Tibbs MK. Wound healing following radiation therapy: a review. Radiother Oncol. 1997;42(2):99–106.
61. Spałek M. Chronic radiation-induced dermatitis: challenges and solutions. Clin Cosmet Investig Dermatol. 2016;9:473–82.
62. Denham JW, Hauer-Jensen M. The radiotherapeutic injury – a complex "wound". Radiother Oncol. 2002;63(2):129–45.
63. Quarmby S, Kumar P, Kumar S. Radiation-induced normal tissue injury: role of adhesion molecules in leukocyte–endothelial cell interactions. Int J Cancer. 1999;82(3):385–95.
64. Keller LMM, Sopka DM, Li T, et al. Five-year results of whole breast intensity modulated radiation therapy for the treatment of early stage breast cancer: the fox chase cancer center experience. Int J Radiat Oncol Biol Phys. 2012;84(4):881–7.
65. Mukesh MB, Qian W, Wilkinson JS, et al. Patient reported outcome measures (PROMs) following forward planned field-in field IMRT: results from the Cambridge Breast IMRT trial. Radiother Oncol. 2014;111(2):270–5.
66. Roy I, Fortin A, Larochelle M. The impact of skin washing with water and soap during breast irradiation: a randomized study. Radiother Oncol. 2001;58:333–9.
67. Westbury C, Hines F, Hawkes E, Ashley S, Brada M. Advice on hair and scalp care during cranial radiotherapy: a prospective randomized trial. Radiother Oncol. 2000;54:109–16.
68. Campbell IR, Illingworth MH. Can patients wash during radiotherapy to the breast or chest wall? A randomized controlled trial. Clin Oncol (R Coll Radiol). 1992;4:78–82.
69. Wong RK, Bensadoun RJ, Boers-Doets CB, Bryce J, Chan A, Epstein JB, Eaby-Sandy B, Lacouture ME. Clinical practice guidelines for the prevention and treatment of acute and late radiation reactions from the MASCC Skin Toxicity Study Group. Support Care Cancer. 2013;21(10):2933–48.
70. Théberge V, Harel F, Dagnault A. Use of axillary deodorant and effect on acute skin toxicity during radiotherapy for breast cancer: a prospective randomized noninferiority trial. Int J Rad Oncol Biol Phys. 2009;75(4):1048–52.

71. Watson LC, Gies D, Thompson E, Thomas B. Randomized control trial: evaluating aluminum-based antiperspirant use, axilla skin toxicity, and reported quality of life in women receiving external beam radiotherapy for treatment of stage 0, I, and II breast cancer. Int J Rad Oncol Biol Phys. 2012;83(1):e28–e34 25.

72. Baumann BC, Verginadis II, Zeng C, Bell B, Koduri S, Vachani C, MacArthur KM, Solberg TD, Koumenis C, Metz JM. Assessing the validity of clinician advice that patients avoid use of topical agents before daily radiotherapy treatments. JAMA Oncol. 2018;4(12):1742.

73. Shukla PN, Gairola M, Mohanti BK, Rath GK. Prophylactic beclomethasone spray to the skin during postoperative radiotherapy of carcinoma breast: a prospective randomized study. Indian J Cancer. 2006;43:180–4.

74. Miller RC, Schwartz DJ, Sloan JA, Griffin PC, Deming RL, et al. Mometasone furoate effect on acute skin toxicity in breast cancer patients receiving radiotherapy: a phase III double-blind, randomized trial from the North Central Cancer Treatment Group N06C4. Int J Radiat Oncol Biol Phys. 2011;79:1460–6.

75. Haruna F, Lipsett A, Marignol L. Topical management of acute radiation dermatitis in breast cancer patients: a systematic review and meta-analysis. Anticancer Res. 2017;37(10):5343.

76. Elliott EA, Wright JR, Swann RS, Nguyen-Tân F, Takita C, Bucci MK, Garden AS, Kim H, Hug EB, Ryu J, Greenberg M, Saxton JP, Ang K, Berk L, Radiation Therapy Oncology Group Trial 99-13. Phase III Trial of an emulsion containing trolamine for the prevention of radiation dermatitis in patients with advanced squamous cell carcinoma of the head and neck: results of Radiation Therapy Oncology Group Trial 99-13. J Clin Oncol. 2006;24(13):2092–7.

77. Wells M, Macmillan M, Raab G, MacBride S, Bell N, MacKinnon K, MacDougall H, Samuel L, Munro A. Does aqueous or sucralfate cream affect the severity of erythematous radiation skin reactions? A randomised controlled trial. Radiother Oncol. 2004;73(2):153–62.

78. Hemati S, Asnaashari O, Sarvizadeh M, Motlagh BN, Akbari M, Tajvidi M, Gookizadeh A. Topical silver sulfadiazine for the prevention of acute dermatitis during irradiation for breast cancer. Support Care Cancer. 2012;20(8):1613–8.

79. Shell JA, Stanutz F, Grimm J. Comparison of moisture vapor permeable (MVP) dressings to conventional dressings for management of radiation skin reactions. Oncol Nurs Forum. 1986;13:11–6.

80. Mak SS, Molassiotis A, Wan WM, Lee IY, Chan ES. The effects of hydrocolloid dressing and gentian violet on radiation-induced moist desquamation wound healing. Cancer Nurs. 2000;23:220–9.

81. Macmillan MS, Wells M, MacBride S, Raab GM, Munro A, MacDougall H. Randomized comparison of dry dressings versus hydrogel in management of radiation-induced moist desquamation. Int J Radiat Oncol Biol Phys. 2007;68:864–72.

82. Gollins S, Gaffney C, Slade S, Swindell R. RCT on gentian violet versus a hydrogel dressing for radiotherapyinduced moist skin desquamation. J Wound Care. 2008;17:268–270, 272, 274–275.

83. Bernier J, Bonner J, Vermorken JB, Bensadoun RJ, Dummer R, Giralt J, Kornek G, Hartley A, Mesia R, Robert C, Segaert S, Ang KK. Consensus guidelines for the management of radiation dermatitis and coexisting acne-like rash in patients receiving radiotherapy plus EGFR inhibitors for the treatment of squamous cell carcinoma of the head and neck. Ann Oncol. 2008;19(1):142–9.

84. Delanian S, Balla-Mekias S, Lefaix JL. Striking regression of chronic radiotherapy damage in a clinical trial of combined pentoxifylline and tocopherol. J Clin Oncol. 1999;17:3283–90.

85. Magnusson M, Höglund P, Johansson K, Jönsson C, Killander F, Malmström P, Weddig A, Kjellén E. Pentoxifylline and vitamin E treatment for prevention of radiation-induced side-effects in women with breast cancer: a phase two, double-blind, placebo-controlled randomize magnud clinical trial (Ptx-5). Eur J Cancer. 2009;45(14):2488.

86. Gothard L, Stanton A, MacLaren J, et al. Non-randomised phase II trial of hyperbaric oxygen therapy in patients with chronic arm lymphoedema and tissue fibrosis after radiotherapy for early breast cancer. Radiother Oncol. 2004;70:217.

87. Rossi AM, Nehal KS, Lee EH. Radiation-induced breast telangiectasias treated with the pulsed dye laser. J Clin Aesthet Dermatol. 2014;7:34.
88. Santos-Juanes J, Coto-Segura P, Galache Osuna C, et al. Treatment of hyperpigmentation component in chronic radiodermatitis with alexandrite epilation laser. Br J Dermatol. 2009;160:210.
89. Clarke B. Normal bone anatomy and physiology. Clin J Am Soc Nephrol. 2008;3(Suppl):S131–9.
90. Taichman RS. Blood and bone: two tissues whose fates are intertwined to create the hematopoietic stem cell niche. Blood. 2005;105:2631–9.
91. Gay HA, Barthold HJ, O'Meara E, Bosch WR, El Naqa I, Al-Lozi R, Rosenthal SA, et al. Pelvic normal tissue contouring guidelines for radiation therapy: a radiation therapy oncology group consensus panel atlas. Int J Radiat Oncol Biol Phys. 2012;83(3):e353–62.
92. Morrish R, Chan E, Silverman S, Myer J Jr, Fu K, Greenspan D. Osteoradionecrosis in patients irradiated for head and neck carcinoma. Cancer. 1980;47:1980–9.
93. Murray C, Henson J, Daley T, Zimmerman S. Radiation necrosis of the mandible: a 10-year study, Part I: factors influencing the onset of necrosis. Int J Radiat Oncol Biol Phys. 1980;6:543–8.
94. Hope R, Goffinet D, Bagshaw M. Carcinoma of the nasopharynx. Cancer. 1976;37: 2605–12.
95. Marks LB, Ten Haken RK, Martel MK. Guest editor's introduction to QUANTEC: a user's guide. Int J Radiat Oncol Biol Phys. 2010;76(3 Suppl):S1–2.
96. Cooper JS, Fu K, Marks J, Silverman S. Late effects of radiation therapy in the head and neck region. Int J Radiat Oncol Biol Phys. 1995;31(5):1141–64.
97. Dijkstra PU, Huisman PM, Roodenburg JL. Criteria for trismus in head and neck oncology. Int J Oral Maxillofac Surg. 2006;35(4):337–42.
98. Okoukoni C, Farris M, Hughes RT, McTyre ER, Helis CA, Munley MT, Willey JS. Radiation-induced bone toxicity. Curr Stem Cell Rep. 2017;3:333–41.
99. Dhakal S, Chen J, McCance S, Rosier R, O'Keefe R, Constine LS. Bone density changes after radiation for extremity sarcomas: exploring the etiology of pathologic fractures. Int J Radiat Oncol Biol Phys. 2011;80(4):1158–63.
100. Watsky MA, Carbone LD, An Q, Cheng C, Lovorn EA, Hudson MM, et al. Bone turnover in long-term survivors of childhood acute lymphoblastic leukemia. Pediatr Blood Cancer. 2014;61(8):1451–6.
101. Edwards BJ, Raisch DW, Shankaran V, McKoy JM, Gradishar W, Bunta AD, et al. Cancer therapy associated bone loss: implications for hip fractures in mid-life women with breast cancer. Clin Cancer Res. 2011;17(3):560–8.
102. Hopewell JW. Radiation-therapy effects on bone density. Med Pediatr Oncol. 2003;41(3):208–11.
103. Gierloff M, Reutemann M, Gülses A, Niehoff P, Wiltfang J, Açil Y. Effects of zoledronate on the radiation-induced collagen breakdown: a prospective randomized clinical trial. Clin Transl Oncol. 2015;17(6):454–61.
104. Okoukoni C, Randolph DM, McTyre ER, Kwok A, Weaver AA, Blackstock AW, et al. Early dose-dependent cortical thinning ofthe femoral neck in anal cancer patients treated with pelvic radiation therapy. Bone. 2017;94:84–9.
105. Okoukoni C, Lynch SK, McTyre ER, Randolph DM, Weaver AA, Blackstock AW, et al. A cortical thickness and radiation dose mapping approach identifies early thinning of ribs after stereotactic body radiation therapy. Radiother Oncol. 2016;119(3):449–53.
106. Green DE, Adler BJ, Chan ME, Rubin CT. Devastation of adult stem cell pools by irradiation precedes collapse of trabecular bone quality and quantity. J Bone Miner Res. 2012;27(4):749–59.
107. Cao X, Wu X, Frassica D, Yu B, Pang L, Xian L, et al. Irradiation induces bone injury by damaging bone marrow microenvironment for stem cells. Proc Natl Acad Sci U S A. 2011;108(4):1609–14.

108. Jacobson AS, Buchbinder D, Hu K, Urken ML. Paradigm shifts in the management of osteo-radionecrosis of the mandible. Oral Oncol. 2010;46:795–801.
109. Rana T, Schultz MA, Freeman ML, Biswas S. Loss of Nrf2 accelerates ionizing radiation-induced bone loss by upregulating RANKL. Free Radic Biol Med. 2012;53(12): 2298–307.
110. Wernle JD, Damron TA, Allen MJ, Mann KA. Local irradiation alters bone morphology and increases bone fragility in a mouse model. J Biomech. 2010;43(14):2738–46.
111. Oest ME, Damron TA. Focal therapeutic irradiation induces an early transient increase in bone glycation. Radiat Res. 2014;181(4):439–43.
112. Gong B, Oest ME, Mann KA, Damron TA, Morris MD. Raman spectroscopy demonstrates prolonged alteration of bone chemical composition following extremity localized irradiation. Bone. 2013;57(1):252–8.
113. Marx RE. Osteoradionecrosis: a new concept of its pathophysiology. J Oral Maxil Surg. 1983;41:283–8.
114. Bras J, de Jonge HK, van Merkesteyn JP. Osteoradionecrosis of the mandible: pathogenesis. Am J Otolaryngol. 1990;11:244–50.
115. Delanian S, Lefaix JL. The radiation-induced fibroatrophic process: therapeutic perspective via the antioxidant pathway. Radiother Oncol. 2004;73:119–31.
116. Rivero JA, Shamji O, Kolokythas A. Osteoradionecrosis: a review of pathophysiology, pre-vention and pharmacologic management using pentoxifylline, α-tocopherol, and clodronate. Oral Surg Oral Med Oral Pathol Oral Radiol. 2017;124(5):464–71.
117. Engleman MA, Woloschak G, Small W Jr. Radiation-induced skeletal injury. Cancer Treat Res. 2006;128:155–69.
118. Parker RG, Berry HC. Late effects of therapeutic irradiation on the skeleton and bone mar-row. Cancer. 1976;37:1162–71.
119. Alektiar KM, McKee AB, Jacobs JM, et al. Outcome of primary soft tissue sarcoma of the knee and elbow. Int J Radiat Oncol Biol Phys. 2002;54(1):163–9.
120. Yamamoto K, Nagao S, Suzuki K, et al. Pelvic fractures after definitive and postoperative radiotherapy for cervical cancer: a retrospective analysis of risk factors. Gynecol Oncol. 2017;147(3):585–8.
121. Small W Jr, Kachnic L. Postradiotherapy pelvic fractures: cause for concern or opportunity for future research? JAMA. 2005;294(20):2635–7.
122. Wood J, Bonjean K, Ruetz S, Bellahcène A, Devy L, Foidart JM, Castronovo V, Green JR. Novel antiangiogenic effects of the bisphosphonate compound zoledronic acid. J. Pharmacol. Exp. Ther. 2002;302(3):1055–61.
123. Pierce SM, Recht A, Lingos TI, Abner A, et al. Long-term radiation complications follow-ing conservative surgery (CS) and radiation therapy (RT) in patients with early stage breast cancer. Int J Radiat Oncol Biol Phys. 1992;23(5):915–23.
124. Meric F, Buchholz TA, Mirza NQ, et al. Long-term complications associated with breastcon-servation surgery and radiotherapy. Ann Surg Oncol. 2002;9(6):543–9.
125. Stephans KL, Djemil T, Tendulkar RD, Robinson CG, Reddy CA, Videtic GM. Prediction of chest wall toxicity from lung stereotactic body radiotherapy (SBRT). Int J Radiat Oncol Biol Phys. 2012;82(2):974–80.
126. Ross MD, Elliott RL. Thoracic spine compression fracture in a patient with back pain. J Orthop Sports Phys Ther. 2008;38(4):214.
127. Lindsay R, Silverman SL, Cooper C, Hanley DA, Barton I, Broy SB, et al. Risk of new ver-tebral fracture in the year following a fracture. JAMA. 2001;285(3):320–3.
128. Lindsay R, Burge RT, Strauss DM. One year outcomes and costs following a vertebral frac-ture. Osteoporos Int. 2005;16(1):78–85.
129. Vanderpuye V, Goldson A. Osteoradionecrosis of the mandible. J Natl Med Assoc. 2000;92:579.
130. Fan H, Kim SM, Cho YJ, et al. New approach for the treatment of osteoradionecrosis with pentoxifylline and tocopherol. Biomat Res. 2014;18:13.

131. Marx RE, Ehler WJ, Tayapongsak P, Pierce LW. Relationship of oxygen dose to angiogenesis induction in irradiated tissue. Am J Surg. 1990;160(5):51.

132. Marx RE, Johnson RP, Kline SN. Prevention of osteoradionecrosis: a randomized prospective clinical trial of hyperbaric oxygen versus penicillin. J Am Dent Assoc. 1985; 111(1):49.

133. Delanian S, Depondt J, Lefaix JL. Major healing of refractory mandible osteoradionecrosis after treatment combining pentoxifylline and tocopherol: a phase II trial. Head Neck. 2005;27:114–23.

134. Delanian S, Chatel C, Porcher R, Depondt J, Lefaix JL. Complete restoration of refractory mandibular osteoradionecrosis by prolonged treatment with a pentoxifylline-tocopherol-clodronate combination (PENTOCLO): a phase II trial. Int J Radiat Oncol Biol Phys. 2011;80(3):832.

135. Spadaro JA, Baesl MR, Conta AC, et al. Effects of irradiation on the appositional and longitudinal growth of the Tibia and Fibula of the rat with and without radioprotectant. J Pediatr Orthop. 2003;23:35–40.

136. Forrest CR, O'Donovan DA, Yeung I, et al. Efficacy of radioprotection in the prevention of radiation-induced craniofacial bone growth inhibition. Plast Reconstr Surg. 2002;109(4):1311–23.

137. Forro SD, Lowe JB. Anatomy, shoulder and upper limb, arm structure and function. SourceStatPearls [Internet]. Treasure Island (FL): StatPearls Publishing; 2019.

138. Hyland S, Varacallo M. Anatomy, bony pelvis and lower limb, popliteal region. SourceStatPearls [Internet]. Treasure Island (FL): StatPearls Publishing; 2019.

139. Rubin P, Andrews JR, Swarm JR, Gump H. Radiation-induced dysplasia of bone. AJR Am J Roentgenol. 1959;82:206–16.

140. Howland WJ, Loeffler RK, Starchman DE, Johnson RB. Postirradiation atrophic changes of bone and related complications. Radiology. 1975;117:677–85.

141. Ergun H, Howland WJ. Postradiation atrophy of mature bone. Crit Rev Diagn Imaging. 1980;12:225–43.

142. Dalinka MK, Mazzeo VP. Complications of radiation therapy. Crit Rev Diagn Imaging. 1985;23:235–67.

143. Jentzsch K, Binder H, Cramer H, et al. Leg function after radiotherapy for Ewing's sarcoma. Cancer. 1991;47:1267–78.

144. Stinson SF, DeLaney TF, Greenberg J, et al. Acute and long-term effects on limb function of combined modality limb sparing therapy for extremity soft tissue sarcoma. Int J Radiat Oncol Biol Phys. 1991;21:1492–9.

145. Welsh JS, Torre TG, DeWeese TL, O'Reilly S. Radiation myositis. Ann Oncol. 1999;10:1105–8.

146. Khan MY. Radiation-induced changes in skeletal muscle. An electron microscopy study. J Neuropathol Exp Neurol. 1974;33:42–57.

147. Schwenen MK, Altman KI, Schroder W. Radiation-induced increase in the release of amino acids by isolated perfused skeletal muscle. Int J Radiat Oncol Biol Phys. 1989;55: 257–69.

148. Phillips JL, Benak S, Ross G. Ultrastructural and cellular effects of ionizing radiation. Front Radiat Ther Oncol. 1972;6:21–43.

149. Willey JS, Long DL, Vanderman KS, Loeser RF. Ionizing radiation causes active degradation and reduces matrix synthesis in articular cartilage. Int J Radiat Biol. 2013;89(4): 268–77.

150. Damron TA, Horton JA, Pritchard MR, Stringer MT, Margulies BS, Strauss JA, Spadaro JA, Farnum CE. Histomorphometric evidence of growth plate recovery potential after fractionated radiotherapy: an in vivo model. Radiat Res. 2008;170(3):284–91.

151. Kwon JW, Huh SJ, Yoon YC, Choi SH, Jung JY, Oh D, Choe BK. Pelvic bone complications after radiation therapy of uterine cervical cancer: evaluation with MRI. Am J Roentgenol. 2008;191(4):987–94.

152. Long DL, Loeser RF. p38gamma mitogen-activated protein kinase suppresses chondrocyte production of MMP-13 in response to catabolic stimulation. Osteoarthr Cartil. 2010;18(9):1203–10.

153. Lindburg AB, Bielby SA, Willey JS, DesJardins DJ, Dean D. Society for Biomaterials 2011 Annual Meeting and Exposition. Effect of X-ray irradiation on porcine and murine cartilage modulus; 2011. p. 84.

154. Rubin D, Schomberg P, Shepard R, et al. Arteritis and brachial plexus neuropathy as delayed complications of radiation therapy. Mayo Clin Proc. 2001;76(8):849–52.

155. Hashmonai M, Elami A, Kuten A, Lichtig C, Torem S. Subclavian artery occlusion after radiotherapy for carcinoma of the breast. Cancer. 1988;61:2015–8.

156. Budin JA, Casarella WJ, Harisiadis L. Subclavian artery occlusion following radiotherapy for carcinoma of the breast. Radiology. 1976;118:169–73.

157. Delanian S, Lefaix JL, Pradat PF. Radiation-induced neuropathy in cancer survivors. Radiother Oncol. 2012;105(3):273–82.

158. Dong Y, Ridge JA, Ebersole B, Li T, Lango MN, Churilla TM, Donocoff K, Bauman JR, Galloway TJ. Incidence and outcomes of radiation-induced late cranial neuropathy in 10-year survivors of head and neck cancer. Oral Oncol. 2019;95:59–6.

159. Salner AL, Botnick LE, Herzog AG, Goldstein MA, Harris JR, Levene MB, Hellman S. Reversible brachial plexopathy following primary radiation therapy for breast cancer. Cancer Treat Rep. 1981;65(9–10):797.

160. Ram Doo A, Shin YS, Yoo S, Park JK. Radiation-induced neuropathic pain successfully treated with systemic lidocaine administration. J Pain Res. 2018;11:545–8.

161. Janovski NA, Paramanandhan TL. Ovarian tumors. Tumors and tumor-like conditions of the ovaries, fallopian tubes and ligaments of the uterus. Major Probl Obstet Gynecol. 1973;4:1–245.

162. Chemaitilly W, Mertens AC, Mitby P, et al. Acute ovarian failure in the childhood cancer survivor study. J Clin Endocrinol Metab. 2006;91:1723–8.

163. Orio F, Muscogiuri G, Palomba S, et al. Endocrinopathies after allogeneic and autologous transplantation of hematopoietic stem cells. ScientificWorldJournal. 2014;2014:282147.

164. Stillman RJ, Schinfeld JS, Schiff I, et al. Ovarian failure in long-term survivors of childhood malignancy. Am J Obstet Gynecol. 1981;139:62–6.

165. Wallace WH, Thomson AB, Kelsey TW. The radiosensitivity of the human oocyte. Hum Reprod. 2003;18:117–21.

166. Chambers SK, Chambers JT, Kier R, Peschel RE. Sequelae of lateral ovarian transposition in irradiated cervical cancer patients. Int J Radiat Oncol Biol Phys. 1991;20:1305–8.

167. Larsen EC, Muller J, Rechnitzer C, et al. Diminished ovarian reserve in female childhood cancer survivors with regular menstrual cycles and basal FSH <10 IU/l. Hum Reprod. 2003;18:417–22.

168. Ash P. The influence of radiation on fertility in man. Br J Radiol. 1980;53:271–8.

169. Chambers SK, Chambers JT, Holm C, et al. Sequelae of lateral ovarian transposition in unirradiated cervical cancer patients. Gynecol Oncol. 1990;39:155–9.

170. Wallace WH, Thomson AB, Saran F, Kelsey TW. Predicting age of ovarian failure after radiation to a field that includes the ovaries. Int J Radiat Oncol Biol Phys. 2005;62:738–44.

171. Lambertini M, Del Mastro L, Pescio MC, et al. Cancer and fertility preservation: international recommendations from an expert meeting. BMC Med. 2016;14:1.

172. Du Z, Qu H. The relationship between ovarian function and ovarian limited dose in radiotherapy postoperation of ovarian transposition in young patients with cervical cancer. Cancer Med. 2017;6:508–15.

173. Yin L, Lu S, Zhu J, et al. Ovarian transposition before radiotherapy in cervical cancer patients: functional outcome and the adequate dose constraint. Radiat Oncol. 2019;14:100.

174. Gao W, Liang JX, Yan Q. Exposure to radiation therapy is associated with female reproductive health among childhood cancer survivors: a meta-analysis study. J Assist Reprod Genet. 2015;32:1179–86.

175. De Vos M, Devroey P, Fauser BC. Primary ovarian insufficiency. Lancet. 2010;376:911–21.

176. Lushbaugh CC, Casarett GW. The effects of gonadal irradiation in clinical radiation therapy: a review. Cancer. 1976;37:1111–25.
177. Hamre MR, Robison LL, Nesbit ME, et al. Effects of radiation on ovarian function in long-term survivors of childhood acute lymphoblastic leukemia: a report from the Childrens Cancer Study Group. J Clin Oncol. 1987;5:1759–65.
178. Bisharah M, Tulandi T. Laparoscopic preservation of ovarian function: an underused procedure. Am J Obstet Gynecol. 2003;188:367–70.
179. Morice P, Castaigne D, Haie-Meder C, et al. Laparoscopic ovarian transposition for pelvic malignancies: indications and functional outcomes. Fertil Steril. 1998;70:956–60.
180. Donnez J, Godin PA, Qu J, Nisolle M. Gonadal cryopreservation in the young patient with gynaecological malignancy. Curr Opin Obstet Gynecol. 2000;12:1–9.
181. Newton H. The cryopreservation of ovarian tissue as a strategy for preserving the fertility of cancer patients. Hum Reprod Update. 1998;4:237–47.
182. Rodriguez-Wallberg KA, Oktay K. Fertility preservation during cancer treatment: clinical guidelines. Cancer Manag Res. 2014;6:105–17.
183. Sklar CA, Antal Z, Chemaitilly W, et al. Hypothalamic-pituitary and growth disorders in survivors of childhood cancer: an endocrine society clinical practice guideline. J Clin Endocrinol Metab. 2018;103:2761–84.
184. Izard MA. Leydig cell function and radiation: a review of the literature. Radiother Oncol. 1995;34:1–8.
185. Thomson AB, Critchley HO, Kelnar CJ, Wallace WH. Late reproductive sequelae following treatment of childhood cancer and options for fertility preservation. Best Pract Res Clin Endocrinol Metab. 2002;16:311–34.
186. Biedka M, Kuzba-Kryszak T, Nowikiewicz T, Zyromska A. Fertility impairment in radiotherapy. Contemp Oncol (Pozn). 2016;20:199–204.
187. Shalet SM. Effect of irradiation treatment on gonadal function in men treated for germ cell cancer. Eur Urol. 1993;23:148–51; discussion 152.
188. Rowley MJ, Leach DR, Warner GA, Heller CG. Effect of graded doses of ionizing radiation on the human testis. Radiat Res. 1974;59:665–78.
189. Mitchell RT, Saunders PTK, Sharpe RM, et al. Male fertility and strategies for fertility preservation following childhood cancer treatment. Endocr Dev. 2009;15:101–34.
190. Heller GC. Effects on the germinal epithelium. In: Langham WH, editor. Radiobiological factors in manned space flight. eNPW, DC: National Academy of Sciences, National Research Council; 1967. p. 124–33.
191. Sklar CA, Robison LL, Nesbit ME, et al. Effects of radiation on testicular function in long-term survivors of childhood acute lymphoblastic leukemia: a report from the Children Cancer Study Group. J Clin Oncol. 1990;8:1981–7.
192. Brauner R, Czernichow P, Rappaport R. Greater susceptibility to hypothalamopituitary irradiation in younger children with acute lymphoblastic leukemia. J Pediatr. 1986;108:332.
193. Sukhu T, Ross S, Coward RM. Urological survivorship issues among adolescent boys and young men who are cancer survivors. Sex Med Rev. 2018;6:396–409.
194. Skinner R, Mulder RL, Kremer LC, et al. Recommendations for gonadotoxicity surveillance in male childhood, adolescent, and young adult cancer survivors: a report from the International Late Effects of Childhood Cancer Guideline Harmonization Group in collaboration with the PanCareSurFup Consortium. Lancet Oncol. 2017;18:e75–90.
195. Shalet SM, Horner A, Ahmed SR, Morris-Jones PH. Leydig cell damage after testicular irradiation for lymphoblastic leukaemia. Med Pediatr Oncol. 1985;13:65–8.
196. Skaznik-Wikiel ME, Gilbert SB, Meacham RB, Kondapalli LA. Fertility preservation options for men and women with cancer. Rev Urol. 2015;17:211–9.
197. Wei C, Crowne EC. Recent advances in the understanding and management of delayed puberty. Arch Dis Child. 2016;101:481–8.
198. Agarwal A. Semen banking in patients with cancer: 20-year experience. Int J Androl. 2000;23(Suppl 2):16–9.

199. Bath LE, Wallace WH, Critchley HO. Late effects of the treatment of childhood cancer on the female reproductive system and the potential for fertility preservation. BJOG. 2002;109:107–14.
200. Damani MN, Master V, Meng MV, et al. Postchemotherapy ejaculatory azoospermia: fatherhood with sperm from testis tissue with intracytoplasmic sperm injection. J Clin Oncol. 2002;20:930–6.
201. Wei C, Crowne E. The impact of childhood cancer and its treatment on puberty and subsequent hypothalamic pituitary and gonadal function, in both boys and girls. Best Pract Res Clin Endocrinol Metab. 2019;33:101291.